The Life and Death of ACT UP/LA

The Life and Death of ACT UP/LA explores the history of the AIDS Coalition to Unleash Power, Los Angeles, part of the militant anti-AIDS movement of the 1980s and 1990s. ACT UP/LA battled government, medical, and institutional neglect of the AIDS epidemic, engaging in multitargeted protest in Los Angeles and nationally. The book shows how appealing direct action anti-AIDS activism was for people across the United States, as well as arguing for the need to understand how the politics of place affect organizing and how the particular features of the Los Angeles cityscape shaped possibilities for activists. A feminist lens is used, seeing social inequalities as mutually reinforcing and interdependent when examining the interaction of activists and the outcomes of their actions. This group's struggle against AIDS and homophobia and to have a voice in their healthcare, presaged the progressive, multi-issue, anti-corporate, confrontational organizing of the late twentieth century and deserves to be part of that history.

Benita Roth is Professor of Sociology, History, and Women's Studies at Binghamton University. Her research focuses on the intersections of gender, social protest, race/ethnicity, and sexuality. Her first book *Separate Roads to Feminism: Black, Chicana, and White Feminist Movements in America's Second Wave* (Cambridge University Press, 2003) won the Distinguished Book Award from the Sex and Gender Section of the American Sociological Association.

The Life and Death of ACT UP/LA

Anti-AIDS Activism in Los Angeles
from the 1980s to the 2000s

BENITA ROTH
Binghamton University

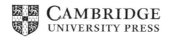

CAMBRIDGE
UNIVERSITY PRESS

CAMBRIDGE
UNIVERSITY PRESS

One Liberty Plaza, 20th Floor, New York, NY 10006, USA

Cambridge University Press is part of the University of Cambridge.

It furthers the University's mission by disseminating knowledge in the pursuit of education, learning, and research at the highest international levels of excellence.

www.cambridge.org
Information on this title: www.cambridge.org/9781107514171
10.1017/9781316226940

© Benita Roth 2017

First published 2017

Printed in the United Kingdom by Clays Ltd.

A catalogue record for this publication is available from the British Library.

ISBN 978-1-107-10631-4 Hardback
ISBN 978-1-107-51417-1 Paperback

Dedicated to the life and memory of Gerald Roth, alav hashalom, *with thanks for the lessons about survival he taught me;*

To the lives and memories of the many members of ACT UP/LA without whom there would be less justice in the world;

And to the lives and futures of my students, who give me hope.

Contents

Preface and Acknowledgments

In 1990, I was a graduate student in a sociology program at the University of California – Los Angeles (UCLA) and enrolled in a two-quarter course on ethnography in order to fulfill my methods requirement. I was interested in social change and social protest. We got to choose our research sites for the class. I lived in West Hollywood – having grown up there, I always joked that I was personally gentrifying my old neighborhood – and I had noticed flyers posted in various spots around the neighborhood announcing the formation of a women's caucus within the local incarnation of the AIDS Coalition to Unleash Power, or ACT UP. I had been following the rise of the anti-AIDS movement mostly through reading about it in the alternative press and free gay and lesbian papers that I could pick up around the neighborhood. I was intrigued by ACT UP – by the militance of its members, by their analysis of the injustices of the healthcare system, by their critique of heterosexism, and by the theatricality of their actions. I had also recently had a childhood friend disclose his HIV-positive status to me, and, in some ways, I was still reeling from that. With warnings from one professor against "going native" and losing my objectivity about the group's actions, but with the blessings of another professor, I made ACT UP/LA my research site and stayed active in the group for a little less than two years. I never thought I would write a book about the group; at the time, I was hoping for a good grade in the class and maybe a journal article. These happened, and now, many years later, after taking a job at the State University of New York, Binghamton, publishing a book on a racial/ethnic feminisms in post-World War II America, receiving tenure, and entering mid-career, I've written this book.

As the reader may ascertain from that last sentence, the path from my participant observation with ACT UP/LA in the early 1990s to writing this book in the second decade of the twenty-first century was not a direct one. But my path to writing *The Life and Death of ACT UP/LA*, if not direct, was not arbitrary. In short, I never forgot about my experiences in ACT UP/LA, and

I wanted to somehow follow-up on the group, which was "dead" by the time I left Los Angeles in 1998. I wondered about where some of the activists had chosen to take their considerable skills, knowledge, and energy because my readings in social movement studies had led me to expect that such intense commitment to a cause would not simply evaporate into thin air. My readings in feminist studies (which sometimes overlapped with social movement studies) had sensitized me to the pervasiveness of gendered politics, and the gendered divides which permeate movement struggles. And so, with the small amounts of research funding I had, I kept returning to Los Angeles again and again to interview former activists and to comb through archives. I started presenting bits and pieces of what I had found as conference papers and came to realize that I had the makings of a book.

Readers can determine for themselves how successfully I have traced the rise and fall of ACT UP/LA, whether it is a story worth reading about, and what kinds of theoretical contributions the case can make to movement/feminist studies. I, of course, must thank those who helped this book come into being without holding any of them responsible for its shortcomings. First, a variety of entities helped fund my research activity over more than a decade. I thank the sociology department of Binghamton University and the dean of BU's Harpur College of Arts and Sciences who supported travel to Los Angeles and to places where I presented research. In particular, a 2010–2011 "Harpur Dean's Research Award" aided me, as did my participation as a fellow in the 2010–2011 inaugural sessions of Harpur College's 2010–2011 Institute for Advanced Study in the Humanities, which supported my work with a course "buy-out" and travel funding. An earlier stint as the William S. Vaughn Visiting Fellow, Robert Penn Warren Center for the Humanities, Vanderbilt University in 2004–2005 helped inform this project; the Warren Center's interdisciplinary atmosphere was a crucial incubator for some of the ideas in the book, and I give special thanks to Mona Frederick, the center's director, for running such a special place. I received research funding in the form of the Heller-Bernard Fellowship from the Center for Lesbian and Gay Studies (CLAGS) at the Graduate Center of the City University of New York in 2007. A number of Individual Development Awards from my union, United University Professions, helped support my archival research and my conducting interviews.

I gave a number conference presentations and talks about ACT UP/LA at which I received valuable feedback, including at American Sociological Association meetings, at the Social Science History Association meetings, and at the Society for the Study of Social Problems meetings. I thank Deborah Gould, Jennifer Brier, and Nancy Whittier for discussants' comments at these talks.

As the book took shape over a number of years, people gave generously of their time and read bits and pieces of it at (very) early and late points in its existence. I would like to thank Bob Emerson and Joshua Gamson for their helpful comments very early in this process, Gianluca Miscione for his insights mid-stream, and Karen O'Neill and Dolores Trevizo for their help in the last stretch. Two Cambridge University Press reviewers read the manuscript and were generous in their comments; I'd like to thank Silke Roth – and despite our interests and our last names, we are not related – for "outing" herself as a reader and giving me the most thorough-going and helpful comments I have ever received on any piece of writing I have ever done.

I owe a huge debt to the archivists and staff at the One National Gay and Lesbian Archives, especially Bud Thomas, Michael Oliveira, Kyle Morgan, Loni Shibuyama, Ashlie Mildfelt, and director Joseph Hawkins. They were unfailingly helpful and made the experience of rummaging through boxes as pleasurable as it could be. I also owe more than I can say to the former ACT UP/LA activists who allowed me to interview them (and who are listed in the order they were interviewed): Jan Speller, J. T. Anderson, Stephanie Boggs, Peter Cashman, Jeri Deitrick, Phill Wilson, Mary Lucey, Nancy MacNeil, Ferd Eggan, Judy Sisneros, Gunther Freehill, Walter "Cat" Walker, Genevieve Clavreul, Richard "Doe" Racklin, Jeff Scheurholz, Pete Jimenez, Doug Sadownick, Helene Schpak, Ty Geltmaker, Wendell Jones, James Rosen, Terri Ford, and Brian Pomerantz. I thank John Fall, Larry Holmes, and Jake Epstine for their responses to the "email interview." I think that they will have many things to say about my inevitably partial distillation of ACT UP/LA's whirlwind of activity, but I hope to have captured some of their collective spirit in writing this book.

This book is dedicated to the life and memory of my father, Gerald Roth (*zikhrono livrakha*) who died in 2007 of brain cancer. My father was immensely proud of me and my work, and his death was a serious blow. Friends and family who helped me through difficult years coping with my father's illness while I researched this book know who they are, but I single out my sister Bella Roth Rizzo, my friends Sharon Fagen and Peter and Susan Sheridan for their special level of support.

Last, I wish to thank my students at Binghamton University for keeping me on my toes in terms of how I think about social protest and social change. They constantly push me to reconsider received wisdom about the world and what is possible in it, and they provide me more and more with examples of how to live in it.

I

Anti-AIDS Activism in the 1980s and 1990s

[M]isfortune is not the same thing as injustice. Death and illness are misfortunes. We are deeply upset over the prospect of a young man dying of incurable cancer, but we do not conceive it as a deep injustice which provokes a sense of outrage against a system productive of such misfortunes.

   – Ralph H. Turner, "The Theme of Contemporary Social Movements," 1972[1]

Oh, yeah?

   – Benita Roth, writing in the margins of the article above, 1990

INTRODUCTION: ANTI-AIDS ACTIVISM AND INJUSTICE REDEFINED

The preceding epigraphs are drawn from the work of one of the most respected and influential sociologists of the twentieth century – that would be the late Ralph Turner – and a snarky UCLA graduate student – that would be me. Juxtaposed, they show how much activism around questions of health and disease has shifted over the past several decades. Writing in 1972, Dr. Turner captured the general view that illnesses like cancer were equal-opportunity diseases. Very few of those suffering from cancer would have attributed the cause of that cancer to negligence by others, and therefore the means of generating the moral outrage that would turn misfortune to injustice was lacking.[2] But moral outrage around health issues was just around the corner. By the end of the 1970s, the feminist women's health movement was in full

---

[1] Turner, Ralph. 1972. "The Theme of Contemporary Social Movements," pp. 586–599 in *Sociology, Students, and Society*, edited by Jerome Rabow. Pacific Palisades, CA: Goodyear Publishing Company.

[2] I'm indebted to Dolores Trevizo for making the point that an injustice frame requires the alleged malfeasance of others. Cancer, especially, was seen as the product of a repressed personality and therefore self-inflicted: see Sontag (1988).

swing, challenging sexist health practices, doctors' paternalistic authority over women, inequalities in healthcare delivery, and prevailing standards in resource allocation for research. Views on what caused disease and who was responsible for health changed, and the feminist health movement spilled over (Meyer and Whittier 1994), spawning other movements that worked to pave the way for a large-scale democratization of the culture of medical treatment and research.[3]

One of the movements that spilled over, buoyed by the questioning spirit of feminist women's health activism, was the direct action anti-AIDS movement of the 1980s and 1990s. This book is about the life and death of an organization that was part of that movement, the AIDS Coalition to Unleash Power, Los Angeles, or ACT UP/LA.[4] ACT UP/LA was founded on December 4, 1987, when activists in Los Angeles called a "town meeting" for people who wanted to take direct action to fight AIDS.[5] The organization lasted for about ten years, ending sometime in 1997, when its three remaining members voted it out of existence.[6] ACT UP/LA's peak period of activism lasted from early 1989 to mid-1992, when it held weekly meetings attended regularly by eighty to one hundred people and sometimes twice that number. The group kept an office open until the mid-1990s, a bank account open beyond its final days, and maintained a network of contacts through an online listserve after it dissolved.

When I wrote my "Oh yeah?" comment in the margins of Turner's article, I myself was participating in ACT UP/LA, so I knew that the deaths of young men prompted outrage. Generating that outrage against the AIDS epidemic took effort and time. The first reactions of the lesbian and gay communities of Los Angeles, New York, San Francisco, and other American cities to the appearance of what came to be called AIDS was the widespread organizing of community-based social services for the sick.[7] In 1981, Gay Men's Health Crisis (GMHC) formed in New York City; in 1982, the organization that began as the

---

[3] On the women's health movement, see Sandra Morgen (2002); on the democratization of health research in the United States, see Steven Epstein (2009); on the spillover effects of the feminist health movement *and* AIDS activism on the anti-breast cancer movement see Klawiter (2008).

[4] I use "ACT UP/LA" throughout this book when writing about the Los Angeles group, as opposed to the generic "ACT UP" which has come to mean ACT UP/NY (see Brier 2009, note 1, p. 242). In using "ACT UP/LA," I follow the group's most common spelling of its name because there are variations in how the acronym is spelled in the group's documents; I preserve those variations when citing from documents.

[5] ACT UP/LA, "A Very Brief History of ACT UP/Los Angeles." Author's collection.

[6] As I discuss in Chapter 5, accounts of the end of ACT UP/LA differ. J. T. Anderson, Stephanie Boggs, and Peter Cashman, Interview with author, 1999; Jeff Scheurholz and Peter Jimenez, Interview with author, 2011.

[7] I use the terms "lesbian and gay" or "gay and lesbian" to denote what would now commonly be referred to as the "lesbian, gay, bisexual, and transgendered" (LGBT) community. I use the former terms because they were how the community referred to itself during the 1980s and 1990s. I consider this an imperfect solution to characterizing what was and is a diverse set of communities.

San Francisco Kaposi's Sarcoma Foundation and would eventually become the San Francisco AIDS Foundation had formed.[8] In October 1982, the information hotline that would become AIDS Project Los Angeles was set up by four "founders" who, along with a representative from the San Francisco Kaposi's Sarcoma Foundation, attended a meeting about what was then called Gay-Related Immunodeficiency Disease (GRID) at the Los Angeles Gay and Lesbian Community Services Center.[9]

These early community-based, service-oriented organizations were highly politicized responses by lesbians and gays to the sense "that public health entities were unlikely to address something considered a gay disease" (Brier 2009: 20). Organizing militant direct action against institutions seen as responsible for the AIDS crisis took a few years to coalesce as the pride of the community taking care of its own became rage at the continued unwillingness of the government to fight AIDS and at the homophobic backlash that ensued as the public became aware of the disease (Gould 2009; see Chapter 2). In March 1987, lesbian and gay activists in New York City formed the AIDS Coalition to Unleash Power/New York (ACT UP/NY). Although accounts of ACT UP/NY's founding vary, two things stand out. First, ACT UP/NY was not the first direct-action style protest group around AIDS that formed; second, the 300 or more "lesbians, gay men, and other sexual and gender outlaws" who attended the founding meeting of ACT UP/NY had the numbers and the desire to commit themselves to "the use of civil disobedience and direct action to fight the AIDS crisis" (Gould 2009: 131). ACT UP/NY became the largest, best known, and most widely emulated model for direct action anti-AIDS organizing. In particular, ACT UP/NY's appearance at the October 1987 March on Washington for Lesbian and Gay Rights left a strong impression on lesbians and gays from all over the United States who were fighting local battles for the resources to fight the epidemic.

One of the places where ACT UP/NY's model of militancy was catalytic was Los Angeles. ACT UP/LA arose in late 1987 because members of LA's lesbian and gay community were enraged by authorities who alternately ignored them and reviled them. The members of ACT UP/LA were extraordinarily ambitious. They addressed a wide variety of HIV/AIDS issues, matters of healthcare generally, and other political issues involving queer rights and human rights. Members worked on local matters – the establishment of the dedicated AIDS ward at the publicly run County/USC hospital, subsequent monitoring of the ward and of county-funded outpatient clinics – and they coordinated with other ACT UPs to mount national campaigns. A very partial list of issues that ACT UP/LA addressed include:

---

[8] See http://www.gmhc.org/about-us); http://www.sfaf.org/about-us/; and Gould (2009).
[9] See http://www.apla.org/about/history.html and Kenney (2001).

- Challenging the Immigration and Naturalization Service's policy regarding the immigration of HIV-positive people to the United States
- Protesting the reluctance of the Catholic Church and then Archbishop of Los Angeles Roger Cardinal Mahony to endorse safe-sex practices and education
- Speaking out against the Federal Drug Administration's slowness in approving life-saving AIDS drugs
- Asking for more visibility and more recognition for women's AIDS issues, including the fact that women were affected by different opportunistic infections than were men and subsequently demanding that the Centers for Disease Control in Atlanta change definitions of AIDS to be more inclusive of female "people with AIDS" (PWAs)
- Raising awareness about consent issues for clinical trials
- Protesting prison conditions and the lack of care for prisoners with AIDS
- Arguing for universal healthcare and health insurance
- Promoting needle exchange programs and services for intravenous drug users
- Challenging discriminatory policies and individual acts of discrimination against HIV-positive people

ACT UP/LA members were also involved with other progressive causes, such as Central American solidarity politics, abortion clinic defense, and, by the early 1990s, queer politics through the organization Queer Nation. In the words of the late Stephanie Boggs, one of ACT UP/LA's last members, "there were too many AIDS issues."[10]

ACT UP/LA members used a wide variety of tactics to address these issues: they "employ(ed) multiple mechanism of influence (including disruption, persuasion, and bargaining" as they contended with power (Andrews 2001: 75). Members lobbied elected officials and they wrote letters to those in power, but they also participated in disruptive "phone zaps" and "fax zaps," where members would deluge an official's office with endless calls or faxes. They protested by sitting in officials' offices; they held vigils, marches, and demonstrations at relevant sites. They distributed leaflets, but they also put up stickers and wheat-pasted posters on the walls of public spaces, defying laws about those activities. ACT UP/LA members appeared at gay and lesbian pride parades, staging die-ins at those events and in other spaces. They attended government meetings and participated on internal review boards at hospitals but were willing to disrupt those same meetings. As one might surmise by the variety of tactics used, some members of ACT UP/LA championed disruption and feared any form of cooperation with authority. Others were willing to "play ball" with authority. Still others were ready to be nice or nasty as the situation required.

What these lists of issues and tactics show is how wide a net ACT UP/LA cast in trying to capture energy to direct against the many-faceted AIDS crisis. ACT

---

[10] Interview with author, 1999.

UP/LA participants were for the most part lesbians and gay men whose politics were left-of-center or had been pushed left by the crisis. People came to the group out of concern and outrage over inaction regarding the crisis and over societal prejudice against those infected with HIV. This concern and outrage was often very personal because many members were themselves HIV-positive and had friends who had died of AIDS. Some ACT UP/LA members died in the course of their activism. The ambitious list of goals was accompanied by a set of great expectations about what the group could accomplish. While not all of their expectations were met, the ACT UP/LA members accomplished enough to change the landscape of AIDS funding, service provision, and awareness in Los Angeles. In the late 1980s and early 1990s, AIDS was a pandemic barely addressed by government, the medical establishment, and the social service sector, and every victory seemed hard-won and insufficient. At the same time, an "AIDS industry" was beginning to be built in both private and public settings as doctors, drug companies, not-for-profit groups, magazines, and media emerged in support of the AIDS community. As such, ACT UP/LA's effectiveness really depended on negotiating two related stances: (1) criticizing the shortcomings of institutions in fighting the AIDS crisis – the insufficient resources devoted to stopping AIDS, the lack of basic information about the virus, and the dearth of services for PWAs – and (2) insisting that these same institutions build new agencies and incorporate new spaces for dealing with the pandemic.

WHY STUDY ACT UP/LA?

I wish to make several interventions into the field of movement studies through examining ACT UP/LA's life and death. First, I wish to remedy the conflation of the ACT UPs, a broad and decentralized social movement, with ACT UP/NY, a conflation that misrepresents the widespread appeal and coalitional nature of direct action anti-AIDS activism in the 1980s and 1990s. Second, I make the case for greater attention to the politics of place in movement studies. Scholars have acknowledged the importance of studying the local movement field (Ray 1999) in order to understand activists' choices and organizational trajectories. I argue that the LA metropolitan area's structure of "segregated diversity" (Pulido 2006: 52), the County of Los Angeles' role in healthcare provision, and the local history of LGBT politics in Los Angeles affected ACT UP/LA's trajectory as a movement organization. Third, I argue that ACT UP/LA, like other ACT UPs, was an example and, in fact, an exemplar of progressive, multi-issue, anti-corporate, confrontational movements of the late twentieth century. Last, I argue that a feminist intersectional theoretical lens is essential for understanding the dynamics and trajectory of this social movement organization as members grappled with challenges to their intent to engage in democratic and coalitional politics. ACT UP/LA as an organization struggled with maintaining the coalitional solidarity that its members sought due to intractable social inequalities and increasing heterogeneity within the group. A feminist intersectional lens, which examines the mutually reinforcing hierarchies of oppression that impact interaction, makes it possible to see those social cleavages as they emerged.

CONFLATION AND HIDING THE COALITION NATURE
OF DIRECT-ACTION ANTI-AIDS PROTEST

Although ACT UP/NY was the first and the largest ACT UP, it was not the only ACT UP of consequence. The conflation of ACT UP with ACT UP/NY minimizes the scope and appeal of militant anti-AIDS activism in the mid-1980s to early 1990s. Some scholars have written about ACT UP/NY without conflating it with the rest of the movement (Carroll 2015); others have moved beyond the conflation (see Gould 2009; Stockdill 2003) to look at other ACT UPs. But popular media still sees ACT UP/NY as constituting all of ACT UP. Mainstream media in the United States remains centered in New York City: a recent story in *New York* magazine, "Pictures from a Battlefield," depicted ACT UP/NY founders "then and now," without any sense that ACT UPs existed outside New York City.[11] ACT UP/NY is also the most "researchable" ACT UP.[12]

In terms of social movement theory, the conflation of ACT UP with ACT UP/NY leads away from important explorations of the coalitional nature of social movements. What does a more accurate picture of the anti-AIDS direct action movement tell us about the kinds of coalitions needed to do direct action protest? Conflating ACT UP with ACT UP/NY portrays the anti-AIDS direct action movement as the project of a singular, vanguard organization rather than an example of real *social movement*. The ACT UPs were a loosely bound coalition of activists who used direct action along with other forms of disruption – and other forms of more routine political action – to make claims on authorities at the local, national, and, at times, international levels. The network of ACT UPs was internally fractured and at times fragile, but members were nevertheless able to coordinate actions *and* retain a measure of control over their participation. My study of ACT UP/LA contributes to the literature about coalitions in social movements and makes three larger points. First, the very way we speak about movements – the civil rights movement, the labor movement, the feminist movement, the anti-AIDS movement – minimizes differences among coalition members and minimizes the different kinds of challenges that coalition members face. As Van Dyke and McCammon (2010: vii) note

---

[11] David France, March 25, 2012, accessed April 2, 2012 http://nymag.com/news/features/act-up-2012–4/.

[12] ACT UP/NY's files have been made accessible at the New York Public Library (see http://www .nypl.org/archives/894); the excellent ACT UP Oral History Project focuses chiefly on activists who were in ACT UP/NY (see http://www.actuporalhistory.org/). Two recent documentaries – David France's Academy Award-nominated "How to Survive a Plague" (http://surviveaplague .com/) and Jim Hubbard's "United in Anger" (http://www.unitedinanger.com/) also focus on ACT UP/NY, although both filmmakers show ACT UP/NY members acting in concert with participants from other ACT UPs to pull off demonstrations outside the city.

many, if not most, movements are amalgamations of movement organizations. Many researchers assume that movements are simply homogenous social entities ... conceptualizing social movements as ... coalitional networks allows us to grasp more fully the varied constituencies, ideological perspectives, identities and tactical preferences different groups bring to movement activism.

The ACT UPs as a movement were such a coalitional network. As I discuss at a number of points in this book, ACT UP/LA had a tenuous relationship with the variously named national networks of ACT UPs that coordinated national actions, and it fought with the national network over questions of democratic decision-making and the distribution of resources. Conflating the whole of the ACT UPs with one social movement organization hides exactly what Van Dyke and McCammon advise us to uncover – the complex coalitional dynamics of ACT UP as a social movement made up of a variety of constituencies.

In fact, a number of social movement scholars agree that speaking of the existence of a social movement in the singular is no more than a "grammatical convenience ... in reality, movements are much sloppier affairs" (Meyer and Corrigall-Brown 2005: 329). Some scholars have put forward understandings of movements as networks; for them, social movements are unique political formations because they rest on the creation of a new network out of

formally independent actors who are embedded in specific local contexts (where "local" is meant in either a territorial or a social sense), bear specific identities, values, and orientations, and pursue specific goals and objectives, but who are at the same time linked through various forms of concrete cooperation and/or mutual recognition in a bond which extends beyond any specific protest action, campaign, etc. (Diani 2003: 301)

There is further recognition by scholars that the edges and borders of movements are often unclear. New networks of activists and new organizations are formed as individuals with multiple alliances shift their relationships with others, with issues, and with particular groups (Meyer and Whittier 1994; Roth 2008; Saunders 2007).

Second, much of the work that social movement scholars have written on coalitions has to do with how "grammatically convenient" movements affiliate (or don't) with other movements. In other words, scholars tend to focus on when and how individuals in organizations in different movements – defined as "different" on the basis of issues – come together in coalition across difference (see, among others, Agustin and Roth 2011; Beamish and Luebbers 2009; Dixon and Martin 2012; Ferree and Roth 1998; Krinsky and Reese 2006; Mayer et al. 2010; Meyer and Corrigall-Brown 2005; Mix and Cable 2006; Rose 1999; Roth 2010; Saunders 2013; Simmons and Harding 2009; Van Dyke 2003).[13] According to Meyer and Corrigall-Brown (2005: 327)

---

[13] For a look at intramovement coalition formation – again with the movement defined by an issue as such – see Staggenborg (1986).

(t)he decision of social movement organizations to join a coalition is akin to the process whereby individuals join social movements, involving an assessment of costs, benefits, and identity. As the political context changes, the costs and benefits are assessed differently and, for this reason, actively engaged coalitions are difficult to sustain over a long period as circumstances change.

Thus, scholars generally agree then that heterogeneity among social movements – of issues, of constituency, of ideology – is a challenge for joint political action.

Third, I wish to broach the question of how heterogeneity or diversity within a social movement organization is also a challenge for actors. Unlike social movements, social movement organizations generally have perceivable outlines and boundaries – in fact boundary-making by members of an organization between themselves and the outside is a key way of mobilizing and establishing collective identity (Taylor and Whittier 1992). Within a social movement organization, members often struggle with negotiating common interests while battling structural inequalities among members that lead to division. To give just one example, Ostrander (1999: 640) has written about how, even in progressive organizations, members engage in active practices to try to prevent structural inequalities from impeding action, such that "gendered and racialized patterns may both be very much in evidence and, at the same time, be regularly and actively challenged" (Ostrander 1999: 640). Silke Roth, in her work on the Congress of Labor Union Women (CLUW), a "bridging organization" (Roth 2003) that sought alliances with other related movements, argued that CLUW needed to use conscious strategies to maintain a collective identity that was "sufficiently broad as well as meaningful to a diverse constituency" (Roth 2008: 215). In particular, Roth emphasized that CLUW's organizational structure provided a means of integrating diverse elements because the group followed the formal, federated, and representation structure of the American labor movement in mobilizing members.

Using a very different template but also relying on structure to manage heterogenous interests, ACT UP/LA and other ACT UPs declared themselves to be coalitions of individuals. The name "ACT UP" itself – "AIDS *Coalition* to Unleash Power – showed that participants intended the group to be diverse in its make-up. ACT UP/NY established a participatory democratic structure of having a general assembly – or "General Body" – make decisions while having committees devoted to members' diverse interests and, less easily, their diverse identities. ACT UP/LA emulated ACT UP/NY's structure of "General Body plus committees" and made participation the sole criterion of membership. ACT UP/LA's founding was, as I discuss in Chapter 2, based on a coming together of a variety of groups working against AIDS and for lesbian and gay rights, and its founders wanted to maintain the new group as a coalition of individuals united by the desire to actively fight AIDS. In practice, the ACT UP/LA's coalition of individuals was maintained by channeling members into committees but also by allowing for participation "only" in the General Body or "only" at actions The structure that ACT UP/LA used came at a moment of heterogeneity within the larger lesbian and gay community, which had come to tolerate a great deal of diversity in organizing. By the late 1980s, the lesbian and gay movement, organized as it was around constituencies seeking changes in policy, seeking to celebrate identity, and looking for pleasure, had what Armstrong calls a "high tolerance for ambiguity," which helped foster cooperation among its constituencies (Armstrong 2002: 198). In this book, I show how ACT UP/LA's members negotiated the pressures of maintaining unity in the face of real structural differences among members.

THE POLITICS OF PLACE: THE SIGNIFICANCE OF LOCAL FIELDS FOR ACTION

A second contribution I wish to make with this examination of ACT UP/LA, one that dovetails with the coalitional perspective on social movements advocated earlier, is to suggest that scholars pay attention to the politics of place in exploring the actions of social movement participants and the trajectory of organizations. Local histories and relationships among political actors condition social movement activism and mean that actors working in coalition but situated in different physical spaces face different challenges. In social movement studies, scholars have usefully referred to local contexts as social movement *fields*, following Raka Ray's (1999) term. In her work comparing the two different settings for Indian feminist organizing of Bombay and Calcutta, Ray defined "field" as "a structural, unequal, and socially constructed environment *within* which organizations are embedded and *to* which organizations and activists constantly respond" (1999: 6, emphasis in the original). In Ray's view, a field encompasses the other political players – movement organizations, political parties, and state structures – that social movement actors confront. Significantly, a field also has a prevailing political culture, that is, a way that actors make and respond to claims. Political culture can be understood as being both the routine ways that politics is done in a given context and the embodied understandings of politics based on the experience of the founders and joiners of organizations (Roth 2003; Whittier 1997). Ray's conception of activists confronting the local as well as the national helped to bring questions of regional variation to the front of analyses of movements, and the term "field" has been used in social movement studies in a variety of ways to signify the environment that social movement participants act in beyond the organization. Although Ray meant the field to include social movement actors and the political institutions to which they made claims, others, for example, Armstrong (2002), have used "field" to mean the social movement sector itself, specifically that of LGBT organizing in the city of San Francisco. In another comparative work on feminist organizing within a national framework,

Guenther (2010) examines how feminist organizations in different parts of "reunified" Germany constructed different agendas linked to local contexts and political cultures. She makes a particularly strong case for how local histories and local political opportunities shape the character of local feminist organizations.

Following Ray's original definition of a social movement field as an environment for social activism that includes institutions, social movement organizations, and a history of political culture, in this book, I examine how ACT UP/LA operated in a social movement field characterized by features specific to Los Angeles as a metropolitan area: (1) the city as a sprawling urban metroscape of "segregated diversity" (Pulido 2006: 52) and the way that public health institutions were distributed within that urban space and (2) the specific history of lesbian and gay activism, some of it militant, in the Los Angeles metro area. First, as any visitor would know, LA is a huge, sprawling metropolitan area. That sprawl is a relatively recent phenomenon, and the hollowing out of the urban core due to the growth of suburbs is a post-World War II phenomena. Suburbanization in Los Angeles further divided the metro area by race and class. Political geographer Laura Pulido (2006: 34) has noted that while LA's postwar development was triggered by "a tremendous population explosion" and by "massive economic development, particularly in the military and aerospace industries," it proceeded along lines of race and class. As defense companies turned Los Angeles into a "martial metropolis" (Loyd 2014: 7), the new jobs provided opportunities both for people of color – with interned Japanese Americans returning from camps with nothing and no choice but to find new places to live – and for internal white working-class migrants, but segregation deposited them in different neighborhoods,

The "incorporation movement" in LA County further ensured racial and class segregation:

Between 1940 and 1960, almost sixty cities incorporated in the metropolitan area. . . . . [Incorporation] established a geographic base for unequal opportunity, as incorporated cities were able to exert far more control over who lives, entered, and shopped in their communities . . . the reproduction of white privilege was predicated on distancing oneself from the poor and people of color. (Pulido 2006: 34)

These "minimal cities" (Davis 1990: 166) were able to keep the Other – however the Other was defined – out, and they foisted responsibility for municipal functions onto Los Angeles County. At roughly the same historical moment, the federal government passed the 1946 Hill-Burton Act, which allowed for the construction of new public hospitals, with specific provisions that allowed the hospitals to be placed in "underserved" areas. The Act allowed counties and municipalities to justify racial discrimination on the basis of creating geographical "service areas" with racially separate medical facilities. According to Loyd (2014: 38),

[i]n Los Angeles, rapidly suburbanized, new hospitals constructed with Hill-Burton funding would effectively be segregated by virtue of where they were built. Between 1950 and 1959 ninety general hospitals were built in metropolitan Los Angeles, a stunning increase of almost 8,500 beds, 64 percent of which were in new hospitals.[14]

As public hospitals were being built, LA County saw the development of free clinics tied to the "community control" movement of the 1960s and 1970s (Loyd 2014: ch. 7). But these clinics were not able to wrest control from the new corporate health empires being established because hospitals, along with pharmaceutical companies and insurance companies, usurped power from the medical professionals and community activists who had sought free clinics in the first place (Loyd 2014: 204).

Thus, in the 1980s, direct action anti-AIDS activists in Los Angeles organized within a diverse but segregated metroscape and faced one major opponent in their quest for better resources for people with AIDS: the County of Los Angeles, the entity responsible for the provision of public health. The quest for resources was also shaped by the state of California's shifting of the burden for rising public healthcare costs onto smaller municipalities and counties as a means of politically insulating the state from criticism for the failures to control costs and provide care (Loyd 2014: 220). By the late 1970s, the thirty or so public hospitals operating in California provided almost 50 percent of "uncompensated care" (Loyd 2014: 223): that is, they were serving the poor and the uninsured. Confronting the County of LA's public health department and the County Board of Supervisors was a constant, central activity for ACT UP/LA's members, given that institution's central role in the (non-)provision of healthcare for people with AIDS.

The presence of prior LGBT activism in Los Angeles was also important in shaping the way that ACT UP/LA organized. Although standard narratives of LGBT activism in the United States present what Moira Kenney (2001: 1) calls "a tale of two cities, centering on New York and San Francisco," the way that lesbians and gays lived in LA – less visibly in more spread-out neighborhoods – was more like the way that most lesbians and gays lived in other cities:

The size and sprawl of the city necessitates a mobility of daily life that scatters ethnic, racial, religious, and other culturally defined communities, reducing the possibilities of the kind of geographic concentrations of community landmarks that characterize enclaves like Greenwich Village or the Castro. (Kenney 2001: 5)

For much of the twentieth century, the LA metro area did not have visible LGBT enclaves; that changed with the incorporation of West Hollywood, a story that I will turn to in a moment. But Los Angeles was nonetheless the site of important LGBT activism. As historians Lillian Faderman and Stuart

---

[14] The racializing provisions of Hill-Burton were deemed unconstitutional by the US Supreme Court in 1964 (Loyd 2014: 48–49).

Timmons (2006: 3) note "more lesbian and gay institutions started in Los Angeles than anywhere else on the planet." There were certain neighborhoods that attracted gays and lesbians, like the Silverlake district, where gay leftist men founded the first "homophile" organization, the Mattachine Society, in 1950 (Kenney 2001: 7). The ONE Institute and *ONE* magazine were also founded in Los Angeles in the 1950s; both were forums for gay scholarship, with the ONE Institute eventually comprising the largest archive of LGBT materials in the world (Kenney 2001: 7). The likely first US lesbian publication was circulated out of Los Angeles by "Lisa Ben" who "stole time from her secretarial job in Hollywood to write and publish *Vice-Versa*, the first lesbian publication circulated in the United States" in the late 1940s (Kenney 2001: 7). And the Metropolitan Community Church was founded in Los Angeles by the Reverend Troy Perry in 1968 (Faderman and Timmons 2009: 162–165), giving lesbians and gays a place to express their (Christian) faith.

All of the activism just described predated the June 1969 Stonewall Rebellion in Greenwich Village, the event most often used to mark the founding of militant lesbian and gay politics in the United States. LA also saw public and disruptive LGBT protest in the 1960s prior to Stonewall. The intolerable degree of harassment by Los Angeles police of gay bars led to demonstrations in the wake of egregious police brutality on New Year's Eve in 1967 at a bar called the Black Cat (Armstrong and Crage 2006: 733–735). Although the Black Cat Raid did not trigger the "commemorative" response that the raid on the Stonewall Inn did two years later, it was nonetheless a key moment for the LGBT activists in LA as homophiles went from routine forms of political interaction toward the consideration of more open display (Faderman and Timmons 2006: 153). One group that helped to organize the demonstrations against the Black Cat raid, Personal Rights in Defense and Education (PRIDE), eventually ended up starting *The Advocate*, still the premiere national LGBT magazine/media conglomerate.[15]

WEST HOLLYWOOD'S ROLE IN LESBIAN AND GAY POLITICS

By the 1970s, West Hollywood, a slice of unincorporated county in the relative middle of the LA metro area, had become an LGBT enclave, in part because it was "overlooked and relatively ungoverned" (Kenney 2001; 36–37) by the County. Since the 1920s, West Hollywood had been known for its night life, much of which was tied to the film industry studios next door in Hollywood. The county sheriffs who policed the area were less brutal than the LA Police Department (LAPD; Kenney 2001: 23). Attracted by West Hollywood's location, wedged between the studios of Hollywood and the riches of Beverly Hills, after World War II, hipsters, hippies, Jewish refugees from Europe, and,

---

[15] See Faderman and Timmons (2006: 159) and http://www.advocate.com/; http://web.archive.org /web/20080129125434/http://www.planetout.com/pno/news/history/archive/advocate.html).

later, Russians and Ukrainians moved in, rented cheap apartments, and shopped Santa Monica Boulevard, the soon to be city's main artery. West Hollywood incorporated in 1984, making it a relative latecomer to the incorporation movement, but it was a very different kind of political entity than had been seen in the metro area. Along with the so-called "People's Republic of Santa Monica," West Hollywood's founders styled themselves as progressive, and many were unabashedly lesbian or gay. The city's first city council election featured forty candidates, nineteen of whom were openly gay or lesbian (Kenney 2001: 49).

The incorporation and ongoing success of West Hollywood as a city nonetheless contributed to LA County's landscape of segregated diversity. While West Hollywood was internally diverse in terms of its inhabitants, with people of different ages, religions, and sexualities sharing its densely packed streets, it was still largely white and distant from the neighborhoods where people of color lived. Some gays and lesbians of color saw going to "WeHo" as "an excursion into whiteness" (Faderman and Timmons 2009 281). In contrast, another neighborhood within Los Angeles City's boundaries, Silverlake, was a place where lesbians and gays worked in coalition with that area's working-class Latino families (Faderman and Timmons 2009: 298–299). Because Silverlake was part of the larger city of Los Angeles, gays and lesbians could not take the kind of control they did in West Hollywood; for this and other reasons, Silverlake was West Hollywood's not quite as glamorous, not quite an enclave, counterpart. West Hollywood remained the center of LGBT life in LA County, a city where lesbian and gay citizens had real power to shape social agendas, and, when the AIDS epidemic struck, it was in West Hollywood where social services were most easily set up for PWAs (Kenney 2001: 9).

ACT UP/LA came to embody the bipolar LGBT world in how and where it chose to organize. Its Monday night "General Body" meetings took place in West Hollywood's Plummer Park, and its office space was located in a downmarket (then, anyway) stretch of Sunset Boulevard in Silverlake. The politics of place – the social movement field – that ACT UP/LA occupied was thus characterized by LA County's geography of segregated diversity and the County's centrality in providing healthcare to poorer PWAs from different racial/ethnic neighborhoods and by a political culture of activism by lesbians and gays that culminated in the establishment of the LGBT power enclave of West Hollywood, a progressive city that was still far, symbolically and actually, from many of those affected by AIDS.

The failure to consider the politics of place also renders invisible the way that all the ACT UPs, including ACT UP/NY, *oscillated between local and national actions* during the 1980s and 1990s. ACT UP/NY also made use of local targets to make its voice heard about the AIDS crisis. Actions at spaces like the New York Stock Exchange, Shea Stadium, Grand Central Station, and St. Patrick's Cathedral received national attention, but they were *local* targets.[16] This oscillation between the local and the national in terms of actions was mirrored by other ACT UPs; it was certainly what ACT UP/LA did.

In order to understand how a decentralized, networked coalition of social movement organizations actually proceeds, we have to understand this oscillation between the local and the national because the ACT UPs were *never* solely about taking nationally coordinated action against national targets. The many ACT UPs that existed engaged in local and nationally coordinated actions and similarly made use of local landmarks in their actions; activists made claims on political authorities for resources, and some of these authorities were cities, counties, and states. Both local and national struggles could be invigorating or enervating; certainly, on the whole, locally based anti-AIDS activists benefited from the national networks that they chose to be a part of, but national coordination among the ACT UPs was always fraught. I think it is significant that not a single activist I interviewed saw his or her participation in the national actions as the only reason to be in ACT UP/LA; instead, almost all recounted stories of oscillation between local and national actions, as I will show in the chapters to come.

ACT UPS AS EXEMPLARS OF LATE TWENTIETH-CENTURY ACTIVISM

A third way that my study of ACT UP/LA contributes to movement studies is by showing how the ACT UPs collectively embodied the decentralized structure of many late twentieth-century and early twenty-first-century social movements, as well as the set of interlocking concerns about inequality, democracy, and justice that went beyond healthcare. The ACT UPs were decidedly left-wing organizations, and recentering direct action anti-AIDS organizing within the narrative of progressive protest in the late twentieth and early twenty-first centuries helps to address the traditional left's neglect of issues of "sex, sexuality, desire, and gender" (Highleyman 2002: 116) as well as redress a history of protest politics that does the same (Pulido 2006; Valocchi 2001).

The direct action anti-AIDS movement was decentralized and networked in an era largely before the communications revolution that the Internet ushered in (Juris 2008a). ACT UP/LA and the other ACT UPs made copious and sophisticated use of what was, in the 1980s and 1990s, a barely emerging new set of communication technologies. Activists coordinated actions by teleconferencing, used cell phones, and, toward the end, sent messages via email, listserves, and bulletin boards. At its height, the ACT UP network included over one hundred ACT UPs in the United

---

[16] Tamar Carroll (2015: 5) has helpfully pointed out in her work on anti-AIDS mobilization in New York City that the city's local landmarks have iconic status for the rest of the United States (think the Statue of Liberty). That, as well as the importance of the city for finance, culture, immigration, and media, have led to New York City being "perceived as simultaneously distinctive and representative of America."

States (Halcli 1999), and the name "ACT UP" was used by anti-AIDS groups in Sydney, Paris, London, and even Moscow.[17]

In the United States, the individual ACT UPs retained their autonomy while they coordinated national actions involving hundreds and sometimes thousands of participants. The ACT UPs were dedicated to participatory democracy and organizational informality. They operated without membership lists for the most part (although fundraisers compiled mailing lists for direct mail campaigns), and yet they were able to mount repeated local and national challenges to institutional authority. Informality was part of identity; ACT UP/LA members, like those in other ACT UPs, engaged in activism that was simultaneously instrumental in its goals and explicitly expressive of members' identities. Many, if not most, who participated in ACT UPs were dismissive of assimilative, integrationist "rights" politics that were becoming more prominent in the lesbian and gay community (Armstrong 2002; Seidman 2005). But, at least in ACT UP/LA, those same activists were equally dismissive of mere expressivity in political action, and most were uninterested in single-issue politics. AIDS was at the center of a politics that linked the crisis to homophobia; racial, class, and gender inequality; and the lack of real democracy in people's everyday lives.

Some scholars have noted the way that the ACT UPs simultaneously embodied militancy against AIDS *and* other kinds of injustice, and they have noted how the ACT UPs exemplified the decentralized, late-twentieth-century social movement. Shepard and Hayduk, in their 2002 collection, *From ACT UP to the WTO: Urban Protest and Community Building in the Era of Globalization*, assert a link between anti-AIDS activism, particularly the ACT UPs, and anti-corporate globalization struggles. In their contribution to that volume, Lesley J. Wood and Kelly Moore (2002: 28) argue that

ACT UP pioneered a new political stream by drawing upon the affinity group model used by American anti-nuclear activists, using the anarchist, pacifist, and civil rights tradition of localized decision-making; the direct action techniques of pacifists who physically confronted systems of power through "misuse" of spaces; and the feminist emphasis on process.

The affinity group model of "small, face-to-face groups that form the basic units for a protest" had existed in protest movements for decades and, more immediately, was used in US left and anti-Vietnam War protest in the 1960s and 1970s (Kauffman 2002: 36). Affinity groups were an important safety valve for ACT UP/LA, a way for participants to engage in disruptive protest and, at the same time, protect the "General Body" of ACT UP/LA as an organization.

---

[17] Stride and Lee (2007) have argued that institutionalized nonprofits and charities using branding in order to promote the values of the organization to the public; in the 1980s and 1990s, the ACT UP brand, much like the Occupy brand of 2011–2012, denoted a modular style of direct-action protest that could be adapted to local circumstances. On the international appeal of the ACT UP brand, see Nguyen (2010), who has noted that an anti-AIDS group in Abidjan, Ivory Coast, renamed itself "ACT UP Abidjan" to link itself to the ACT UP style of activism.

They were also an explicit and structural acknowledgment that individuals had the right to protest as they saw fit, without necessarily asking for the majority's approval.

ACT UP/LA members targeted a number of institutions and power centers, including the state; they used a variety of tactics that ranged from disruptive to routine; and they built an agenda based on the interests of members of their community. The multiple targets of LGBT activists – the way that activists focus on centers of power beyond the state – have led some in movement studies to see gay and lesbian organizing as "a subcultural movement that embraces tactics that are expressive and internally oriented, rather than instrumental and externally oriented" (Taylor et al. 2013: 220). Because ACT UP/LA was built on a foundation of members' interests, questions arose concerning who the ACT UP/LA community was and how united the participants could be under the ACT UP/LA banner. ACT UP/LA members had to grapple with difference – different interests, different positions within the lesbian and gay community, different positions within the larger matrices of power relations – in the making of solidarity, ACT UP/LA, like many movement organizations before it, had to struggle with creating links among heterogenous individuals situated in structurally unequal space. Because ACT UP/LA's members were diverse, I argue that a feminist intersectional theoretical approach works well for understanding the group's trajectory, and I next turn to an explanation of what feminist intersectional theory can bring to the understanding of ACT UP/LA and social movement organizations generally.

THE FEMINIST INTERSECTIONAL LENS ON ACT UP/LA

A last theoretical intervention I wish to make is to argue for using a feminist intersectional perspective to unpack the ways in which activists in ACT UP/LA and other social movement organizations like it dealt with complex inequalities (Stein 2013) in interaction. I argue that a feminist intersectional perspective on movement studies is useful because the very concept of intersectionality is rooted in the idea of (oppositional) communities being composed of coalitions of actors whose social locations exist at the intersection of mutually co-constructed inequalities.

The concept of "intersectionality" is usually attributed to critical race law scholar Kimberlé Crenshaw (1989, 1991) who is given credit for coining the term because her work both encapsulated and extended the ideas present in the emerging interdisciplinary field of women's studies.[18] Crenshaw argued that in

---

[18] Crenshaw's work remains a touchstone for scholars across a number of disciplines working in intersectionality studies in the US and internationally. See Brah and Phoenix (2004); Carastathis (2013); Carbado (2013); Cho, Crenshaw, and McCall (2013); Choo and Ferree (2010); Chun, Lipsitz, and Shin (2013); Davis (2008); Jordan-Zachery (2007); Lewis (2013); MacKinnon (2013); Ferree (2009); McCall (2005); Mohanty (2013); Patil (2013); Valentine 2007; Verloo

looking at the situation of marginalized groups – women, Blacks, people living in class-segregated communities – scholars needed to account for the "multiple grounds of identity when considering how the social world is constructed" (1995: 358). Following her conceptualization of individual identities shaped by mutually co-constructed inequalities, Crenshaw theorized that oppositional communities were actually coalitions rather than homogenous groups in which all members had identical interests. Some members were relatively privileged in terms of how they were treated by dominant institutions; others decidedly less so.

Definitions of intersectionality have proliferated over time, and the term's "ambiguity and open-endedness" helped ensure its widespread adoption (Davis 2008: 67). Thus, any scholar using the concept of intersectionality needs to specify what she means by it (Choo and Ferree 2010). Recently, in a special issue of the journal *Signs* devoted to intersectionality studies, Crenshaw and co-authors Sumi Cho and Leslie McCall (2013: 795) characterized intersectionality as

... best framed as an analytic sensibility ... What makes an analysis intersectional – whatever terms it deploys, whatever its iteration, whatever its field or discipline – is its adoption of an intersectional way of thinking about the problem of sameness and difference and its relation to power. This framing – conceiving of categories not as distinct but as always permeated by other categories, fluid and changing, always in the process of creating and being created by dynamics of power – emphasizes what intersectionality does rather what intersectionality is.

The view that Cho, Crenshaw, and McCall take of intersectionality as sensibility has several advantages for thinking about power, sameness, and difference, and I found their view of intersectionality as sensibility important in researching ACT UP/LA. Thinking about intersectionality as sensibility severs the substantive link between the researcher's methodology and the progressive ideology of the group being studied. Even a group like ACT UP/LA that emerged from a marginalized community and sought to organize itself in an intersectional manner – conscious of difference and the pervasiveness of relations of power – should be studied as if it can be affected by the very same power relations it rejects.

As a sociologist, I do take some issue with Cho, Crenshaw, and McCall on the question of fluidity; here, I follow Mignon Moore's (2011: 7) approach of seeking not to "dismantle categories ... [but] to understand how people whose lives have historically been structured by categories make sense of them and use them in different ways." As my research will show, activists chose subject positions and, indeed, inhabiting a relatively stable subject position was a necessity for action. ACT UP/LA's members, like any other social movement

(2013); and Yuval-Davis (2006). For earlier, "pre-coinage" expressions of intersectional perspectives, see the Combahee River Collective (1979, 1981); Thornton Dill (1983); King (1988); Sacks (1989); and Spelman (1982).

participants, needed to construct a collective identity in order to act together. In social movement studies, scholars have focused on the processes by which participants establish collective identities strong enough to enable mobilization across difference (Jasper and Polletta 2001; Kosbie 2013). Scholars have rightly conceptualized the accomplishment of collective identity as an achievement, not a given, and thus have led us away from assuming that marginalized group members automatically share common interests. But marginalized groups do find common cause even as they contend with internal heterogeneity. The ongoing achievement of collective identity oriented toward action should be seen as a resource in itself, although an ultimately unstable one, and intersectional analysis can uncover "politicized identity categories to be held together variously by tacit, unspoken, deliberate, and explicit acts of alignment, solidarity, and exclusion" (Carastathis 2013: 942). It is also useful, I think, to consider heterogeneity as socially constructed and to consider what it means to establish a collective identity based on the idea of embracing difference. As Ghaziani (2008: 2) has argued in his work on the organizing of large-scale marches for LGBT rights in the 1970s through the 1990s, even conflict can have positive effects for coalitional work because "conflict is one of the major ways activists make decisions about goals and strategies" (Ghaziani 2008: 2). However, conflict across organizations is likely experienced quite differently than conflict within organizations; an intersectional approach should also pay attention to the ramifications of social difference experienced in specific interactional settings.

Another advantage of having an intersectional sensibility is that it mandates thinking *structurally* about people's interactions; that is, thinking about the way the "macro" influences choices made on a more "micro" scale. As Chun, Lipsitz, and Shin (2013: 922) have argued, "(t)he idea of intersectionality helped shift the focus of academic feminist and anti-racist contestations away from preoccupations with intentional prejudice and toward perspectives grounded in analyses of systemic dynamics and institutional power." In sociological terms, the view of intersectionality as structural and interactional dovetails well with Choo and Ferree's (2010: 134) characterization of "process-centered" intersectional analysis, in which the researcher uses an intersectional view to reveal "structural processes organizing power." Process-oriented intersectionality is necessarily constructionist and, as such, "examine(s) how individuals are 'recruited to' categories and yet have choices in the 'subject positions' they adopt in these complex locations." Process-oriented intersectional analysis does more than generate lists of groups who are "given voice" in analysis – what Choo and Ferree refer to as the "inclusion" model of intersectionality; instead, process-oriented intersectionality proposes that intersecting inequalities are "characteristic of the social world in general" (2010: 133), and this always important for analysis.

Process-oriented intersectional analysis is what drives my analysis of ACT UP/LA in this book. I argue that specific inequalities – being gay or lesbian, being female or male or transsexual, being a specific race, even having a specific set of AIDS issues – are incarnated in specific settings. For example, gay men in ACT UP/LA were marked by their non-mainstream sexuality, but, at the same time, they were men, members of a socially privileged group in society at large. Their gayness may have hampered easy access to that privilege, but questions of male dominance were part of ACT UP/LA's internal discussions almost from its beginning. A process-oriented intersectional perspective posits that *everyone* has an inherently intersectional social location, an inherently interactional set of resources to employ. This insight about everyone's intersectional location/ resources/burdens holds whether or not members with disparaged statuses actually make claims *on behalf* of redressing the injuries caused by disparaged statuses because it matters that claims are being made *by* those with disparaged statuses. At the same time, process-oriented intersectionality allows the researcher to consider the question of which social cleavages caused by inequalities are salient in given social situations, allowing that "in specific historical situations and in relation to specific people there are some social divisions that are more important than others in constructing specific positioning" (Yuval-Davis 2006: 203).

I noted earlier that Crenshaw's work inspired scholars to think of oppositional communities as coalitions, and this is a particularly important aspect of the feminist intersectional perspective for movement studies. Social movement theorists of late have drawn more pronounced and sustained attention to the question of coalitions in movement politics (see the essays in Van Dyke and McCammon 2010). Intersectionality scholars have long maintained that, not only are collective action groups coalitions, but also that, because of intersecting inequalities, these "strategic group positions ... are always partial, perspectival, and performative" (Chun et al. 2013: 923). If chosen "strategic group positions," including collective identities, are always partial, an intersectional perspective can help to uncover the way that "politicized identity categories [are] held together variously by tacit, unspoken, deliberate, and explicit acts of alignment, solidarity, and exclusion" (Carastathis 2013: 942).

In this work then, I am interested in the way that ACT UP/LA's members worked as a coalition intentionally, and I am interested in how and when social inequalities shaped the results of their intentions. There is still a lot to be said about what kinds of inequality mattered for direct action anti-AIDS activists, and there is more to be said for how a feminist intersectional perspective can help us understand inequalities in action in any social movement organization. Others, for example, Stockdill (2003), have argued for taking an intersectional approach to understanding the shaping of oppositional consciousness in movements, but, in this book, I am less concerned with the making of individual oppositional consciousness than I am with the shaping of organizational and movement dynamics.

In taking an intersectional look at ACT UP/LA, I hope to complicate the overly simple "gender story" that has been told about the demise of the ACT UPs by the mid-1990s. Gendered divisions are cited as playing a large role in splitting ACT UP activists into two camps: one, purportedly composed of white men, argued for actions that would lead to more "drugs into bodies"; a second, purportedly composed of white women *and* men and women of color, argued for the need to go beyond the "drugs into bodies" approach and fight for universal healthcare as a social right (Altman 1994; Corea 1992; Epstein 1996; Gould 2009; Halcli 1999; Leonard 1990). However, in this reading of gender splits as central to the demise of the ACT UPs, the paradigmatic rupture is the one that affected ACT UP/NY. In June 1992, ACT UP/NY's Treatment and Data Committee – devoted to putting drugs into bodies – became a separate organization, the Treatment Action Group (TAG; Halcli 1999, http://www .treatmentactiongroup.org/history). TAG's actions supposedly broke ACT UP/NY beyond repair – and they may have done so, but the reality of gender politics in the other ACT UPs was more complicated than the drugs into bodies/ universal healthcare dichotomous picture provides.[19] It is true that, nationally, a growing network of activist ACT UP women chose to focus on issues involving women and AIDS. While they worked on questions of universal healthcare, their activism was also focused on the health and welfare of a particular constituency of PWAs: women. This makes the implicitly stark division between the genders – one of self-interest on the part of white men and selflessness on the part of all others – open to question.

Once again, it is useful to think of particular and local coalitions rather than network-wide cleavages. What is one to make, for example, of the fact that in ACT UP/LA, many men, including HIV-positive ACT UP/LA co-founder and leader Mark Kostopoulos, were strong and consistent advocates for universal healthcare? What is one to think of the fact that, although ACT UP/LA had an active Women's Caucus (WC) supported by almost all ACT UP/LA men, not all women in ACT UP/LA worked on women's issues or wanted to? Last, why didn't ACT UP/LA's Treatment and Data Committee spin off from the larger group, and why did another committee focused on needle exchange cause much more disruption to the group's solidarity? As I argue through my examination of the case of ACT UP/LA, the gender dynamics that led to the deaths of individual ACT UPs by the mid- to late 1990s were local stories about gender, but were also about other lines of social cleavage, like race and sexuality. Gender is certainly a part of the story of the fall (and, for that matter, the rise) of ACT UP/LA, but gender's role in the organization's trajectory needs to be considered in a situated and intersectional manner.

---

[19] As Carroll (2015: ch. five) notes, an earlier schism in ACT UP/NY – its housing committee becoming the social service organization "Housing Works" – did not doom ACT UP/NY. Carroll also gives an alternative reading of the relationship between anti-AIDS direct action and women's health activism in New York City as being one of synergy and not schism. She in fact sees ACT UP/NY and the other ACT UPs as continuations of feminist health activism from the previous decades, a reading that supports the idea of anti-AIDS protest as a spillover movement relative to the women's health movement.

To summarize, a feminist intersectional perspective emphasizes the coalitional quality of oppositional communities due to existing inequalities; an intersectional perspective focuses on the meaning and (re)iteration of inequalities in the lived experiences of activists; and looking at the internal dynamics of a social movement organization from an intersectional perspective puts front and center the question of how inequalities are (or may be) implicated in internal conflicts. An intersectional feminist perspective alerts us to look for consequential social interactions predicated on co-constructed inequalities. If gender and other significant markers of social inequality are always elements of interaction – that is, are always being localized – then those same markers of social inequality always matter for inquiry as to what activists do. I take activists' words about their intentions in their activism very seriously in this work, as the reader will see, activists disagree: if there are disagreements, it is reasonable to ask if these are patterned by social inequalities and if the disagreements themselves reference tensions about divisions caused by social inequality. It is therefore important to ask how, when, and why inequalities mattered.

This last point – about how an intersectional feminist perspective orients the research toward finding out about the effects of inequalities – segues into the area of methodology. I find affinities among feminist intersectional theory, grounded theory, and extended case views of how to look at social protest, which I discuss in more depth in the appendix. The appendix also covers the kind of data used for this study – participant observation, archival, and interview data – with further discussion of how I acquired each kind of data and how they illuminate the case when used in tandem. A reader interested in these questions of method and data may wish to read the appendix first: for others, I turn next to the plan of the book.

PLAN OF THE BOOK

The book provides an overall view of ACT UP/LA's rise and fall and an analysis of the internal struggles and external relationships that led to its demobilization. I end the book with a substantive chapter about the relationship between the inside and the outside in ACT UP/LA and its role in the lives of several former activists, followed by a conclusion and a methodological appendix for those inclined to think about qualitative methods and approaches.

In Chapter 2, "Beginning, Building, and Being ACT UP/LA," I look at the founding of ACT UP/LA, its structure, and the actions members took during the group's mobilization and peak years of activity. I focus especially on (1) how activists oscillated between local and nationally coordinated ACT UP actions; (2) how local activists sometimes captured a national stage through audacious, theatrical actions; (3) how the greater prominence of women's AIDS issues in ACT UPs nationally manifested in Los Angeles with actions that involved both women and men; (4) how ACT UP/LA was challenged by coalitional anti-Gulf War work and the emergence of Queer Nation; and (5) how ACT UP/LA members during the group's heyday addressed difficult and unpopular causes, working on behalf of the rights of prisoners with AIDS and taking on the local Catholic Church over safe sex issues.

In Chapter 3, "Battling for Women's Issues and Women's Visibility in ACT UP/LA," I explore how feminists within ACT UP/LA formed a women's caucus as they worked toward making women's AIDS issues a more visible place within the larger group. I also examine the broader impact of feminist politics on ACT UP/LA – the way that feminism had "spillover" (Meyer and Whittier 1994) effects onto ACT UP/LA – by looking at the phenomenon of feminist men in the group who came to the aid of the WC explore how ACT UP/LA feminists kept a focus on women's AIDS issues through interactional strategies such as counting men in attendance at meetings and actions and by reminding others of the presence of women in the group. ACT UP/LA Women's Caucus members became the group's "official women," inhabiting paradoxical roles in which they received male deference on women's AIDS issues but were also made solely responsible for a women's AIDS agenda. I conclude that WC members' actions made a feminist AIDS agenda an integral part of ACT UP/LA's trajectory in part by underscoring the inherently coalitional basis of the oppositional organization and, by extension, the larger anti-AIDS community.

In Chapter 4, "Intersectional Crises in ACT UP/LA," I consider how gender, racial, and sexuality politics were embedded, but underexamined, in moments of conflict within ACT UP/LA. I briefly consider the meaning of conflict in the lesbian and gay community and then go on to examine three moments of intersectional crises for the group: (1) the influx of new members after California governor Pete Wilson's veto of a gay and lesbian rights bill in 1991, (2) ongoing controversy within ACT UP/LA over a needle exchange program and the implications of expanding ACT UP/LA's purpose and community through the provision of a social service, and (3) arguments about "competing actions" at the 1993 March on Washington for Lesbian, Gay, and Bisexual Rights and Liberation. I argue that intersectional crises fractured the hard-won solidarity of group members and that ACT UP/LA's trajectory as a movement organization is inexplicable without understanding the way that gendered, raced, and, at times, sexual divisions affected the group.

In Chapter 5, "Demobilization: ACT UP/LA in the Years 1992–1997," I explore ACT UP/LA's extended period of demobilization. While the timing of ACT UP/LA's demobilization roughly corresponds with that of other ACT UPs (see Halcli 1999), in keeping with my focus on the politics of place, I argue that a combination of more localized factors led to the demobilization of ACT UP/LA. ACT UP/LA was enervated by its struggle with the County of Los Angeles over making sure that adequate provisions were made for PWAs reliant on public healthcare, a lack of success and the deaths of key leaders demoralized activists, and the numbers of participants fell. National coalitional work with other ACT UPs were more fraught and failed to infuse ACT UP/LA with energy in the same way that earlier oscillations between national and local actions had. I chronicle internal efforts to heal rifts within the group and show how, over a period of five years, low numbers of participants led to ACT UP/ LA's death as a viable direct action anti-AIDS organization.

In Chapter 6, "From Streets to Suits: The Inside(r)s and Outside(r)s of ACT UP/LA," I look at how the case of ACT UP/LA undercuts received wisdom about the supposedly clear dichotomy between insider and outsider activism. Scholarship by feminists and others have challenged the idea that institutions are eager to co-opt activists, and insights about the possibility of institutional activism have also led to a reassessment of the varied relationships between insider and outsider politics. I chronicle extensive debates in ACT UP/LA about how to relate to political insiders, as well as the group's actual accommodation of different tactics, which derived from the premium members put on participation. I look at a subset of activists who used insider and outsider spaces at various times to fight against AIDS. I conclude that ACT UP/LA's former activists carry "ACT UP" attitudes while doing their insider work and that, while institutions directly shape the possibilities for these activists, the time they spent with ACT UP/LA was crucial to their understandings of the institutional activism they do now.

In Chapter 7, "Looking Back on the Life and Death of ACT UP/LA," I discuss the importance of recapturing the direct action anti-AIDS movement's history for our understanding of how social change was made. I summarize the main arguments in the chapters outlined earlier and then consider the implications that the case has for the study of social movement organizations; namely, that a feminist intersectional lens can reveal how inescapable complex inequalities are in social movement praxis; that the politics of place and the shape of the local social movement field matter for activists; and that, contrary to our common sense understandings, outsider and insider spaces are interwined in activists' lives and practice. Last, I consider the ACT UPs' legacy for the ongoing AIDS crisis; that is, how this kind of loosely bound, networked, and self-consciously coalitional organizing is still needed in the struggle to end AIDS.

In the appendix, I discuss my use of archival, participant observation, and interview-based sources, as well as the limitations of each way of gathering data and the usefulness of using multiple data sources in conducting historical sociological work. In the second part of the appendix, I argue for why the methodological perspectives of grounded theory and extended case method are appealing for the feminist intersectional researcher, and I describe how they informed the way that I did research for this book.

Beginning, Building, and Being ACT UP/LA

After eight years and nearly 25,000 official deaths, AIDS still rages out of control as a result of our local and national government's inadequate and harmful actions. . . . Across the nation people are coming together to demand a change. Now is the time for more than politics as usual.

Act to build a militant grassroots organization to end AIDS.

– ACT UP/LA (Flyer advertising first meeting, December 1987)[1]

If you were to poll the man on the street, the vast majority of people would not have any interest in AIDS funding.

– Los Angeles County Supervisor Pete Schabarum on the prospect of opening a dedicated AIDS ward at Los Angeles County's main public hospital (1989)[2]

INTRODUCTION

This chapter chronicles the emergence of AIDS Coalition to Unleash Power, Los Angeles (ACT UP/LA). In it, I explore the ramifications of its structure as an organization, examine the question of how leadership functioned in a group that saw itself as leaderless, and highlight the pattern of oscillating actions between the local and the national during the group's peak period of mobilization from late 1987 through 1991. Activists in Los Angeles emulated ACT UP/NY's left-wing participatory structure when they formed a schedule of "General Body" meetings – meetings of all participants – coupled with committees who formed based on members' interests for more specialized work. This structure enabled them to manage a member-driven, ambitious agenda that appeared to energize participants as they worked to get concrete

---

[1] ACT UP/LA. "Bring the Spirit of Washington Home!" Flyer, December 1987; ONE Collection.
[2] Schabarum's statement, first reported by the *Los Angeles Times* in May of 1989 (Merina 1989), became infamous within the AIDS activist community and beyond (Geltmaker 1992; Martinez 1989).

gains for those with HIV/AIDS and to make sure the public did not forget about the AIDS crisis.

The reader should keep several warnings in mind while reading this chapter. First, I am making a somewhat artificial demarcation between ACT UP/LA's peak period and its demobilization, which I discuss in Chapter 5. The line between mobilization and demobilization is not an easy one to draw in retrospect. My second caveat follows from the first in that I see inherent limitations to presenting a group's actions in the form of a retrospective narrative. I have tried to give the reader a coherent picture of ACT UP/LA's actions, but, in order to do that, I have had to eliminate from the narrative much of what the group discussed and did. I cannot convey through narration the reality of the simultaneity of actions – the whirlwind of activity – that members undertook. I "curated" the group's activities in order to avoid making an unreadable laundry list, which means that, in this chapter, as well as in the rest of the book, some issues and actions have been left out or given less attention than they deserve. My last warning to readers is that, despite this book's title, in this chapter, I present what can only be a partial picture of anti-AIDS organizing in Los Angeles in the 1980s and 1990s. Since my focus is in on ACT UP/LA, I discuss other groups or institutions only when they intersect with ACT UP/LA's actions. I begin by briefly recounting the circumstances of ACT UP/LA's actual founding; then I turn to an examination of the group's structure and stances on leadership. I then narrate the oscillating pattern of ACT UP/LA's local and national actions, the group's move toward activism on behalf of marginalized constituencies in the AIDS community (e.g., women and prisoners), and its responses to changes in the social movement field of LA anti-AIDS activism. By 1991, four years into its life, ACT UP/LA was a force in that field of activism, and members were looking back at its accomplishments and planning future battles against AIDS.

THE CALL TO ACTION: DECEMBER 4, 1987

The first ACT UP/LA meeting was held at Plummer Park in West Hollywood on December 4, 1987. West Hollywood had just incorporated as a city after having existed as unincorporated LA County for decades. It was home to disparate communities of artists, musicians, film industry folk, newly arrived immigrants from the soon to be former-USSR, aging Jews who had moved there after World War II and stayed put while their children moved to the suburbs, and gays and lesbians. West Hollywood was the most visible gay and lesbian enclave in the Los Angeles metro area and therefore a logical place for the first meeting of ACT UP/LA.

The founders of ACT UP/LA intended for the group to be visibly lesbian and gay, visibly a coalition of anti-AIDS activists, most of whom lived beyond the city limits of "WeHo," and visibly progressive. The flyer that advertised the first "town meeting to beat AIDS" urged people to "bring the spirit of Washington home," referencing the Second National March for Lesbian and Gay Right that had taken place in Washington, DC, on October 11, 1987.[3] The Washington event had featured a large number of ACT UP/NY members who had formed their group in March 1987, and ACT UP/NY's militant stance against AIDS made a strong impression on others. As in other urban areas where the lesbian and gay community had been organizing itself to deal with the pandemic through the provision of community-based social services (Brier 2009; Gould 2009), groups providing services and self-help to people with AIDS (PWAs) had already formed in Los Angeles. Twenty-one groups and organizations endorsed the town meeting that led to ACT UP/LA, including the AIDS Positive Action League, Being Alive, Black and White Men Together, Lesbian Nurses, Mothers of AIDS Patients, The Women's AIDS Project, The Women's Building (a local feminist arts center), and several lesbian and gay college campus groups. Eight individuals endorsed the meeting, including the Reverend Carl Bean from Minority AIDS Project; Morris Kight, a longtime gay activist; Betty Brooks, a long-time activist in the feminist anti-violence movement; and Ron Rose, listed as a "member, Board of Directors, National Association of People with AIDS" ("Bring the Spirit of Washington Home!" Flyer, 1987).

The facilitators at the town meeting were Andy Corrigan, who was listed as being part of the LA March on Washington Committee, and Phill Wilson, who was working with the Minority AIDS Project and the Los Angeles Gay and Lesbian Services Center (see Chapter 6 for more on Wilson). The agenda for the meeting included speakers from social service agencies and self-help groups and a presentation by Mark Kostopoulos, who, until his death in June 1992, was a central figure and leader in ACT UP/LA. Kostopoulos, and other members of the Lavender Left, a gay and lesbian socialist group, were instrumental in organizing the town meeting, but they were not alone as founders, nor was their style of left-wing politics uncontested. John Fall was part of the organizing group, and he recalled that the actions of ACT UP/NY at the October 1987 March on Washington were crucial for those attending from LA, because the march in DC brought together people from LA whom had not previously known each other.[4] Fall wasn't affiliated with the Lavender Left, nor was Michael Weinstein, who attended the meeting and went on to found the AIDS Hospice Foundation (later the AIDS Healthcare Foundation). Fall saw some Lavender Left members as only interested in "talk and argument," but he felt that others, like Kostopoulos, were more committed to action. Fall retrospectively saw tensions inherent at the very forming of ACT UP/LA between 1960s-style protest veterans – "products of the George Jackson era, say 1967 to 1972. Inspired by the Summer of Love, broken by the RFK and MLK assassinations, and resurrected by George Jackson's plight, the Black Panthers, and the Weather Underground" – whom he described as

[3] ACT UP/LA. "Bring the Spirit of Washington Home!" Flyer, December 1987; ONE Collection.
[4] Email interview with author, 2012.

"dogmatic," and a younger cohort of activists whom he saw as "pragmatic . . . willing to listen and to negotiate."[5]

Walter "Cat" Walker was also at the founding December 1987 meeting. Like Fall, Walker saw the example set by ACT UP/NY at the March on Washington as key to the formation of ACT UP/LA: "I think by that point there was a feeling in a lot of the gay community that we needed to do something because things were bad. . . . ACT UP[NY] [was] doing something and that we should do something too. . . . I had already had that feeling."[6] Walker recalled that about 120 people attended the town meeting, and he pointed to Kostopoulos as a particularly impressive participant: "he was sort of the leader of the meeting and I found him very charismatic and I was impressed by him." Walker remembered that the wisdom of forming an ACT UP/LA was not an easy sell in the gay and lesbian community. When I asked Walker about whether there were people in the lesbian and gay community who were scared of ACT UP/LA's promise of direct action against AIDS, Walker answered "Uh, yes" (and then we both laughed, presumably because we both knew what the answer was). He continued:

I don't think they should have been [scared] but they were. . . . I had a lot of friends in the gay community that weren't part of ACT UP . . . and some of them were appalled that I was in ACT UP and they would ask me questions and I would try to explain to them what we were doing . . . to them it seemed kind of frightening in a way both because they thought it would be really scary to do what we were doing as far as going out in the street and demonstrating and encountering the police and things like that . . . they thought that we were being kind of rude . . . like there was like nice ways to get our point across . . . [Imitates others talking to him] "Can't you just like write letters and things like that. . . ." We were actually doing a lot of different things – it's just that the attention went to like, the grittier parts of it and so, like, some people were turned off by that.

The town meeting attendees decided that ACT UP/LA's first demonstration would be an action against the Immigration and Naturalization Service's (INS) policy of testing immigrants and asylum seekers for HIV in order to bar the entrance of those who tested positive.[7] Seventy-five protestors demonstrated at the downtown location of the INS.[8] The reporter chronicling the event for the *Los Angeles Dispatch*, a short-lived local lesbian and gay periodical, quoted ACT UP/LA's John Fall as to the group's displeasure with the INS's failure to ensure, at the very least, confidentiality in the test-taking process. The reporter

---

[5] Email interview with author, 2012. Fall's recollection generally jibes with Kostopoulos's depiction of the group's founding four years later (Jim McDaniel, "Interview with Three Founding Members of ACT UP/LA," *ACT UP/LA News* 4:5 (December 1991/January 1992), pp. 6–7.

[6] Interview with author, 2011.

[7] McDaniels, 1991.

[8] *ACT UP Los Angeles* newsletter 1:1 (January 1988). The first newsletter contained information about the INS action in a reprint of article from the *Los Angeles Dispatch* 1:4 (January 6, 1988) by Chris Uszler entitled "Activists Demonstrate against INS AIDS Testing."

also noted that, although the demonstration received next to no mainstream press coverage, Fall saw the action as a success because "(t)he INS knew we were there."

ACT UP/LA'S STRUCTURE: EMBODYING COALITION

The first ACT UP/LA town meeting agenda included a discussion about how the group would structure itself. Participants introduced an internal structure composed of a General Body (GB) in which all members of the group would meet on Monday nights in Plummer Park, coupled with a committee structure in which interested members could get together to talk apart from the General Body. In putting forth the General Body plus committees structure, ACT UP/LA's founders directly mimicked the way that ACT UP/NY functioned. GB meetings were held for most of the group's life either weekly or biweekly; when they were held on a weekly basis, every other GB meeting was a "working meeting," wherein committees were given the time to meet; committees also had set times to meet outside of the GB in various community spaces (and sometimes in members' homes). At the group's height, anywhere from eighty to two hundred people would attend GB meetings. The agenda for the GB meeting was set the night before by a Coordinating Committee that was composed of co-facilitators from committees; the Coordinating Committee itself was "officially" proscribed from making policy decisions.[9] The Coordinating Committee usually met the night before the GB meeting in order to coordinate an agenda, but agendas were not set in stone, and items could come from the floor at GB meetings. James Rosen, who attended Coordinating Committee meetings at the time as a co-facilitator of the Treatment and Data committee, emphasized that "you could alter a [GB] meeting very very easily" no matter the set agenda.[10] The combined GB plus committees structure lasted for most of ACT UP/LA's life, until dwindling numbers made the committee structure untenable.[11]

The GB plus committee structure was an expression of ACT UP/LA's intentions to be a democratic, participatory coalition of anti-AIDS activists; it embodied the group's desire to accommodate individuals' interests and, at the same time, put decision-making in the hands of all participants. Through its committee structure, ACT UP/LA's members acknowledged from the very beginning the existence of political heterogeneity in the form of interests and, as I will explain, came to acknowledge heterogenous identities – that of people with AIDS, women, and people of color – as caucuses formed that acted very much like committees in terms of their relations to the GB. ACT UP/LA (and for that matter ACT UP/NY and other ACT UPs that were similarly structured)

---

[9] ACT UP/LA. "ACT UP/LA Structure." Two-page unsigned document, c. March 1990; ONE collection.
[10] Interview with author, 2012.
[11] ACT UP/LA. "ACT UP LA Agenda for 12/4/85 [sic]," ONE Collection.

thus embodied the coalitional networked logic common in other progressive, late twentieth-century movements, like the anti-globalization movement (Juris 2008b).

The GB plus committees structure fit with ACT UP/LA's ethos of participation and its member-derived agenda because committees worked both on permanent matters of interest (like Treatment and Data or Fundraising) and on an ad hoc basis on specific projects. During ACT UP/LA's height of activity, one could spend three weeks out of every month going to GB, caucus, and committee meetings, leaving only Friday and Saturday nights free, unless there were other ACT UP/LA events or fundraisers to attend. As Larry Holmes, who joined the group in 1988, put it, "I walked into Plummer Park, not knowing anyone, and pretty much didn't look up for 2½ years."[12]

The GB plus committee structure also channeled individuals into places where they could feel comfortable with a variety of tactics. Andrews (2001: 75) has argued that movement "infrastructures that allow the movement to employ multiple mechanisms of influence (including disruption, persuasion, and bargaining) will have the greatest impact on policy implementation." Recognizing that ACT UP/LA was only one organization, and without making claims about ACT UP/LA's effect on outcomes regarding AIDS policy in the Los Angeles metro area, the GB plus committee structure did allow for multiplicity; individuals were encouraged to find a comfortable point of entry into the group. Some, like Holmes, walked into the GB meeting on a Monday night and stuck around, and others – like me – came to a Women's Caucus meeting in a different place at a different time and then started going to GB meetings. It was difficult to limit one's participation in ACT UP/LA solely to committees, although some may have done so, and certainly there were members who strongly specialized in work on particular issues. However, the GB was impossible to ignore, not least because much committee work required attending at least the GB working meetings.

The GB made decisions for the group – about actions, about financial outlays, about endorsements and support of other groups – and anyone who came to the Monday night meetings was allowed to vote. As a serious joke, the FBI were routinely asked to leave the room at the beginning of GB meetings. The GB voted on proposals that came from committees and caucuses as well as those that came from the floor. During the time that I attended GB meetings, a simplified version of *Robert's Rules of Order* was in use, and two co-facilitators ran the meetings. A majority of votes was needed to pass a motion, but most votes were not particularly close and only a few required a count. John Fall recalled that, in the earliest days of ACT UP/LA, consensus was used to make decisions but that as the group grew in numbers, consensus became "more and more unwieldy and ultimately impossible" to use.[13] Fall recalled that consensus worked especially

---

[12] Email interview with author, 2012.
[13] Email interview with author, 2012.

badly in the Coordinating Committee meetings despite that group's small numbers because Kostopoulos would often play the holdout in terms of setting the agenda. Certainly, the tenor of GB meetings shifted over time as the group's numbers waxed and waned. Writing for the January 1990 ACT UP/LA *News*, Joe Bledsoe reflected on what attending GB meetings felt like in March 1988, a few months after the group's founding:

The ACT UP/LA meetings then were very different from the meetings we know today. They were very small and argumentative. My first impression was that I was surrounded by the political fringe, the mentally unbalanced and the irredeemably sociopathic. And yet, I felt immediately at home. ... Our meetings have become more cohesive and somewhat less contentious. But ACT UP/LA still provides a forum for ideas, some sound, some lunatic. I don't think there is a single member who hasn't left a meeting furious at some decision made or some opinion expressed.[14]

No membership lists were kept, although mailing lists were kept for the newsletter and for committees, caucuses, and attendance at some specific actions. Informality was an important part of being in ACT UP/LA; James Rosen recalled that at one point someone told him that they were "quitting" ACT UP/LA, to which he replied "what do you mean, how can you quit? Whoever said you joined?"[15] Since there were no members who officially joined, there were no membership dues; instead, a bucket was passed around the room for donations.[16] With the agenda set the night before, a typical GB meeting would consist chiefly of committee reports, but, depending on issues and upcoming events, some committees took much more GB meeting time than others. Announcements in the form of updates about what other groups with network connections to ACT UP/LA were doing were given at the end of meeting. At each GB meeting, a table with flyers, pamphlets, and other kinds of printed material was set up in the back of the room.

My experience of GB meetings was that the atmosphere was intense, but that things were run with a startling amount of efficiency; meetings began on time at 7:30 p.m. and were almost always over by 10. At the time, I felt ACT UP/LA's GB meetings were the best-run that I had ever attended, and having sat through many years of meetings as an academic and union activist, I haven't changed my mind. Efficiency was accompanied by something that felt like fun. There were moments of laughter, outbursts of applause, snapping one's fingers to indicate approval, booing and hissing to display dismay and disgust, and there were a lot of people standing in the back of the room by the literature tables gossiping or scanning the room to get a better view (of particular people).

Most members of ACT UP/LA saw the group's raison d'etre as direct action and wanted a structure and a process that facilitated actions. ACT UP/LA's

---

[14] Joe Bledsoe, "From the Inside Looking Out," ACT UP/LA *News* 2:6 (December 1989/January 1990), p. 8.
[15] Interview with author, 2012.
[16] ACT UP/LA, "ACT UP/LA Structure."

appeal was its instrumentality. For example, Helene Schpak was led to ACT UP/LA because it was an effective venue for action against AIDS:

I didn't feel the need to simply be expressive. I really felt like I needed concrete change. I felt like what I was doing in ACT UP was not for the fun of it, it was very purpose-driven . . . there were specific things that we wanted to see change, there were wrongs that we wanted to address . . . and really pushed the envelope to try and get there.[17]

When reflecting back on how the structure of ACT UP/LA came to be, Mark Kostopoulos and David Lee Perkins both emphasized that participation was the intended basis for membership in the group.[18] Kostopoulos noted that the group's organizers "wanted active members. You couldn't be a member unless you did something." Perkins further defined the quality of participation: "We don't only want you to come and lick envelopes. We want your mind, your voice, your thoughts and your abilities. We want you as a whole person there doing things."

LEADERSHIP IN A LEADERLESS GROUP

ACT UP/LA was officially leaderless and informally full of leaders, and this tension between a desire for leaderlessness and the reality of informal leadership was present from the group's start. While ACT UP/LA's members wanted a participatory and democratic structure that put all on a horizontal plain, activists were aware that there were places where power congealed. Probably the most important unofficial leader of ACT UP/LA was Mark Kostopoulos who, as noted earlier, was part of the network of socialist gay and lesbian activists who were instrumental in founding the group. Kostopoulos was a long-time activist; he was HIV-positive, physically attractive, and articulate. Kostopoulos had been intimately involved with several other ACT UP/LA members; at the time of his death, he was living with another informal leader, the late Gunther Freehill. While it would be a gross exaggeration to attribute all of ACT UP/LA's successes to Kostopoulos's efforts, it would also be wrong to discount his charismatic influence. Geneviève Clavreul typified how a number of activists with whom I spoke felt about Kostopoulos; while she acknowledged that no one led ACT UP/LA, she saw informal leadership as centered around Kostopoulos, and she did not think that was a good thing.[19] Helene Schpak felt very differently about Kostopoulos as a person, but echoed Clavreul's assertion that Kostopoulos was the leaderless ACT UP/LA's leader:

I think Mark Kostopolous was so amazingly adept at what he did. I don't think there would have been an ACT UP/LA without Mark Kostopolous. He was an unparalleled

---

[17] Interview with author, 2011.
[18] McDaniels, 1991.
[19] Interview with author, 2011.

leader, I feel. In his knowledge, in his grace, his openness. He was welcoming to every person, every concept every ability. I think to a person everyone who I have ever spoken to feels that their time in ACT UP/LA brought them to a place where they got to be their better person, they got to shine at doing something that they felt really good about doing. And Mark brought that out in people, he set the tone. I don't think I've ever met anyone with his abilities, before or since.[20]

Other interviewees described Kostopoulos as "incredible" (Peter Cashman), a "really important figure" (Doug Sadownick), "a unifying leader" (Brian Pomerantz), and "a strong leader" (Cat Walker).[21]

But Kostopoulos's leadership abilities also led to clashes with others; if ACT UP/LA's organizers were hoping, as David Lee Perkins put it, to have "a whole person there doing things," well, they got whole persons. James Rosen remembered Kostopoulos as being "a great guy on a million levels but he was . . . totally hard core . . . he believed that there had to be a leader." Rosen described Kostopoulos as having vanguardist socialist politics, as believing that ACT UP/LA formed the "troops" who could enlist the "masses" in fighting AIDS and fighting for universal healthcare. Rosen recalled having a conflict with Kostopoulos that became heated to the point of almost being a "fist fight" over the extent to which ACT UP/LA should be involved with Health Access, an organization for universal healthcare that Kostopoulos was heavily involved in. Rosen's complex take on Kostopoulos was echoed by other activists. Jan Speller, who lived with Kostopoulos and Freehill, loved Kostopoulos and described him as "incredibly pragmatic" and "diplomatic." She nonetheless described being taken aback by the ferocity of his sexual politics, which she described as "really far left," and she had trouble, which she recalled with good humor, understanding both his stance on public sex and his libertarian view of safe sex (i.e., provide information for people and don't police them).[22] And ACT UP/LA activist Wendell Jones's described Kostopoulos as "too much of a leader. Sometimes he would get into that traditional male, my way or the highway, mimicking the patriarchy . . . I don't want to just diss Mark . . . this is something any of us, including myself, were capable of, especially men."[23] Even Freehill acknowledged that Kostopoulos's personal style of leadership was both compelling and problematic:

There were these curious, curious contradictions. . . . Mark was . . . a lot of things. He was very controlling, you know, he wanted his way . . . and went to great lengths to make his arguments carefully and persuasively. But in ways that I thought were always respectful of other people. Not everyone agreed with that. He was seen as someone who really manipulated everybody, because he was energetic, he would talk to everybody . . . he

---

[20] Interview with author, 2011.
[21] Interviews with author, 2012.
[22] Interview with author, 2000.
[23] Interview with author, 2011.

would talk to people who were mean to him ... so people would be mean to him and he would go and talk to them ... because of that he was seen as manipulating everybody.[24]

The variegated portrait of Mark Kostopoulos can't settle the question of how much influence he or other highly involved, charismatic unofficial leaders had within (or over) ACT UP/LA. The variety of views about Kostopoulos crystallizes the contradictions found in ACT UP/LA – and other ACT UPs – where the official policy of leaderlessness contributed to the formation of internal, friendship-based elites, as predicted by Freeman (1972–1973) in her well-known article "The Tyranny of Structurelessness." But ACT UP/LA was not structureless; if anything, its GB plus committees structure encouraged a proliferation of informal leaders, not all of whom were friends with each other. This was probably to the group's benefit; as Andrews (2001: 76) argues, a "leadership structure with a diversity of skill and experiences will be better able to use mass-based tactics as well as routine negotiation with outside groups." Still, charisma cannot be turned off, even if it can be challenged. Part of what kept Kostopoulos at the center of a group he helped create was his ability to embody the passionate politics that characterized ACT UP/LA. Jake Epstine, a nurse and an active ACT UP/LA participant, remembered being at an LA County Board of Supervisors meeting where

Finally Mark Kostopoulos screamed out: "They want us to die." I thought he was crazy in that moment; the next moment, I saw my dead friends, my dead patients, my sick patients, I knew he was right. These men wanted me to die. I was a marked man. The second memory [of Mark] I have is being at a demonstration in Chicago [1990], my arms linked with other activists, we were walking down a major street, I felt someone pushing at my back, really prodding me to go forward. I turned around to see a horse's snout in my face, a menacing cop on the horse, his eyes letting me know that in a moment he could have his horse ... trample us. He wanted us to die.[25]

ACT UP/LA IN ACTION: OSCILLATIONS BETWEEN THE LOCAL AND THE NATIONAL

I remember early on we collected plastic bags for people getting chemo (for KS) to throw up in. That's how basic the need was. People with KS were getting chemo in a hallway at County Hospital and there wasn't even a bucket for them to be sick into.

– Larry Holmes[26]

Inspired by the strong local response to their forming a direct action anti-AIDS group, ACT UP/LA's GB met every other week throughout 1988. In order to disseminate information about their actions, the group began publishing a

---

[24] Interview with author, 2000.
[25] Email interview with author, 2012.
[26] Email interview with author, 2012.

newsletter in 1988, which continued to be published monthly or bimonthly until 1992, when publication became more sporadic. In the early 1990s, the newsletter was mailed out to more than 2,200 names and available free at coffeehouses, bars, and other gathering places in lesbian/gay neighborhoods in LA. Since the newsletter was chiefly published on a bimonthly basis, members used it to "recap" their experiences at actions and share their personal concerns about the AIDS crisis. Even in its bimonthly, not up-to-the-minute format – or perhaps because of that format – the newsletter was an important filter for understanding which actions and issues were important to the group.[27]

With members' interests driving the action agenda, ACT UP/LA took on a host of primarily locally based action items, interspersed with participation in national actions coordinated by other ACT UPs. Sometimes, the local and the national melded, as in the INS action, where members targeted the local office to protest federal policy. This oscillation between the local and the national continued throughout most of the organization's life. ACT UP/LA's focus on local concerns – in particular, its multiyear struggle to get the County of Los Angeles to respond the public health crisis of AIDS – was always accompanied by coordinated work with other ACT UPs on "national" AIDS issues, and its most active members worked at both local and national (and occasionally international) levels. The group's pattern of oscillating action always came back to the local; while ACT UP/LA chose a name, a structure, and a stance congruent with ACT UP/NY and other ACT UPs, its actions were conditioned by relationships at the local level. As Guenther (2010) has noted, local incarnations of seemingly national movements can be quite different; the politics of Los Angeles as a place influenced who joined ACT UP/LA, what kinds of issues members focused on, and especially who their targets were.

One constant local target was the LA County Board of Supervisors, insofar as the Supervisors controlled the funds used for the provision of public health. In 1988, ACT UP/LA involved itself in the controversy over the County's regulation and closure of gay bathhouses. The Supervisors ordered the closing of several baths in a sporadic campaign that targeted baths at least through 1990.[28] The Supervisors had initially voted to monitor sex in the bathhouses in December of 1985, prompting a coalition of left and lesbian and gay community groups, including the Lavender Left, to denounce the interference in the bathhouses as a smokescreen for the County's failure to lobby the federal government for more funding to fight AIDS, its failure to pass an anti-discrimination act to protect lesbians and gays from discrimination, and its

---

[27] The newsletter name and format shifted over the course of ACT UP/LA's life. At times, it was called "*ACT UP/LA*," and at other times it was called "*ACT UP/LA News*." The numbering of the issues was irregular. I refer to the newsletter by what it was called at the time that it was published.

[28] Ray Reece, "Déjà vu: Back to the Baths." *ACT UP/LA* 3:5 (October/November 1990) p. 14.

opposition to AIDS education in schools.[29] In 1987, the County began to more tightly regulate the baths, using the rationale that the baths were health hazards and neighborhood nuisances.

In early 1988, ACT UP/LA's Agitating Committee recommended that the group write an "open letter to the community" about the County plans to close gay bathhouses.[30] ACT UP/LA voted to go on record as opposing the closing of bathhouses, and the GB charged the "Educating" committee with writing a new position paper in lieu of a demonstration.[31] As directed, members of the Education Committee wrote a position paper on the bathhouse issue.[32] They argued that more than 4,000 people had been diagnosed with AIDS in LA County, rejecting the idea that closing the baths would affect the spread of the epidemic. They noted that rates of sexually transmitted disease – the best available proxy for understanding the rate of HIV infection – were actually declining in the gay community. The ACT UP/LA authors feared that the Supervisors would use the safety rationale of closing the baths as an excuse to shut down gay bars, and they asked the Supervisors to forget about the baths and instead address the AIDS crisis by providing funds for in-home and hospital care of PWAs, especially at the County-USC public hospital, putting more money into "explicit education efforts within the County's 'high risk' communities," and developing "a comprehensive, long-range master plan for confronting the AIDS epidemic."

Another home-grown and fairly frequent target of ACT UP/LA's displeasure was the County Sheriffs who policed West Hollywood. The group saw Los Angeles County Sheriff Sherman Block as a real enemy because Block had co-sponsored a state proposition on HIV/AIDS that appeared on the November 1988 ballot, Proposition 96, and was passed by voters.[33] Proposition 96 allowed judges to order defendants to undergo AIDS tests when police or other law enforcement officers had been exposed to their blood "or other bodily fluids." The "other bodily fluids" phrasing was significant because it allowed testing based on a claim by an officer that he or she had been spat on (say by an activist).[34] In March 1988, ten ACT UP/LA members infiltrated the

---

[29] ACT UP/LA. "Demonstration against AIDS Hysteria and for Lesbian and Gay Rights," Unsigned press release c. January 1988; ONE Collection.

[30] Minutes, General Body meeting, January 25, 1988; ONE Collection.

[31] Education Committee of ACT UP/LA (Larry Day, Jim Burke, Ed Williams, and Brad Confer), "ACT UP/LA Position Paper: Los Angeles County Bathouse Closure." February 29, 1988; ACT UP/LA, "Appendix Bathhouse Background in the Context of the AIDS Epidemic." Three-page unsigned document c. February 1988; Jim Burke, "An Open Letter to the Community," c. February 1988, written by Burke "at the request of the Agitating Committee." ONE Collection.

[32] ACT UP/LA Education Committee. "ACT UP/LA Position Paper: Los Angeles County Bathhouse Closure," dated February 29, 1988; ONE collection.

[33] Edwin Chen, "Judge Orders First AIDS Test Under Prop. 96 Provisions." *The Los Angeles Times*, November 11, 1988.

[34] Kevin Roderick, "Proposition 96–Mandatory Aids Testing: The Other AIDS Initiative on Tuesday's Ballot." *The Los Angeles Times*, November 5, 1988.

graduation ceremony for the Los Angeles County Sheriff's Academy, unfurling a banner that read "AIDS Education, Not Testing," leafleting, and shouting questions like "Why won't you give prisoners condoms to protect themselves?" in order to voice their opposition to Block's support of the proposition and to demand the distribution of condoms in Los Angeles' County Jail.[35]

Early 1988 also saw the beginning of ACT UP/LA's long struggle with LA County over the creation and adequate staffing of a dedicated AIDS ward at LA County/USC public hospital. Perhaps a third of the PWAs in Los Angeles County were wholly dependent on the public health system. As ACT UP/LA's Ty Geltmaker (1992: 620) wrote,

(a)ny discussion of AIDS in Los Angeles County must be prefaced with the reminder that, of the eighty-seven independent municipalities within the County's 4,000-square-mile-territory, only Long Beach and Pasadena operate a public health and hospitals department. ... Like the rest of the state, the other eight-five towns and cities of Los Angeles County – including the City of Los Angeles itself – depend on the County Department of Health Services for public health education and care, as mandated by the county charter and state-funding mechanisms.

Geltmaker noted that, despite LA County's high AIDS caseload, "not one cent of public money was specifically earmarked for AIDS education or care in a County budget until fiscal year 1989/90, nine years into the epidemic. ... The County's AIDS Program Office was not established until 1985–86 and the Commission on AIDS was not convened until 1987" (622–633). Geltmaker described the Supervisors as overseeing "sprawling districts as private fiefdoms, dispensing 'discretionary' funds to competing alliances of homeowners and 'developers' more concerned with their own backyards and police protection of their own domains than with overall County-run services such as public health care."[36]

Although officially a nonpartisan entity, the Board was dominated in the 1980s and early 1990s by conservative supervisors Pete Schabarum, Deane Dana, and Mike Antonovich. The two more liberal supervisors – Kenneth Hahn and Edmund Edelman, whose district included West Hollywood and part of Silverlake – were thus outnumbered three to two. While the conservatives on the Board were particularly detested by members of ACT UP/LA, all of the Supervisors and most County public health officials were seen to be proponents of systematic and ingrained heterosexism; Mark Kostopoulos asserted that the County public health system was as poor as it was because of "a large streak of homophobia which runs through the hospital administration all the way to the County Board of Supervisors."[37] In 1988,

[35] Paul Feldman, "AIDS Protesters Carted Out of Sheriff's Academy Rites," *The Los Angeles Times*, March 5, 1988.

[36] Geltmaker, p. 621.

[37] Mark Kostopoulos, "People with AIDS: Care and Uncaring," *ACT UP LA* 1:3 (April/May 1988), p. 4.

ACT UP/LA began a multiyear campaign to get the County to establish and adequately staff a dedicated AIDS unit at County-USC hospital, starting with a picket at the hospital on April 30, followed by an overnight vigil in the hospital lobby; some sixty people participated. Three ACT UP/LA members – Mark Kostopoulos, John Fall, and David Niblett – were cited and given a court date for their violation of an order to disperse.[38]

The April protest at County/USC Hospital was followed by another action at the hospital in July. On Saturday, July 9, eighty ACT UP/LA members brought sleeping bags for a sleep-in at the hospital, including Chris Brownlie, who was part of a County-convened "Dedicated AIDS Ward Task Force" and who spoke to the assembled group and to media about the need for an AIDS ward. The sleep-in, complete with cots the activists brought in and lit by candles, was meant to represent a mock AIDS ward. It was monitored but not broken up by law enforcement; the protestors themselves ended the encampment early the next morning. ACT UP/LA's Peter Cashman described the scene:

The men and women of ACT UP, having shared their experiences with each other earlier in the evening … finally settle in. Here and there through the night strangers arrive, curious about the strange gathering. They stop and perhaps learn, then go on; others stay to share and enjoy food and a place to sleep in safety, if not in comfort. The homeless and the AIDS activists have common ground tonight and both learn. Candles flicker among the cots; a pound doggie sleeps contently with his new found women friends. The Sheriffs, once numbering five, have dwindled to two who lounge uncomfortably on a bus bench. ACT UP's own night watchers amble around the now quiet gathering of cots and candles and people who care, formed in a safety circle. Picket signs, now stilled, adorn the railings from side to side of the hospital plaza.[39]

The next month, in August 1988, the LA County Commission on AIDS voted unanimously to recommend to the Board of Supervisors that County-USC Hospital open a dedicated AIDS ward for up to twenty patients. The Commission's recommendation as to the number of beds fell short of what activists – and the County itself – thought was needed, since on any given day, the hospital housed twenty-five to forty PWAs, and a hospital-based clinic was already handling 1,400 outpatient visits a month.[40] Several days after the Commission voted, the Board of Supervisors voted unanimously – although only three supervisors were present – to open a dedicated AIDS ward at County-USC hospital and gave the County Department of Health Services (DHS) thirty days to develop a plan for the ward. County officials expressed concern about

---

[38] Fall and Niblett were placed on a year's probation and fined $400 each; Kostopoulos' case was treated separately (Larry Day "What a Week It Was!" *ACT UP/LA* 1:4 (June 1988) p. 3; Peter Cashman "ACT UP Fights Lying Down," *ACT UP/LA* 1:6 (August 1988), p. 3.).

[39] Cashman, p. 4

[40] Janny Scott, "Panel Favors Specialized AIDS Ward at County-USC," *The Los Angeles Times*, August 20, 1988.

the ability to find room for the ward, to staff the ward, and estimated it would be at least six months until the ward could be opened.[41]

The Supervisors' vote – which prompted the headline "We've Won an AIDS Ward" in the September 1988 *ACT UP/LA* newsletter – was in reality only the beginning of a long struggle to get the Supervisors and County health officials to make good on their promises. The editor of the newsletter, Enric Morello, wrote

While we can all be happy at having won a so long and so hard-fought victory, all has not yet been won. There still remains at least two important issues to be settled satisfactorily. The first is the question of the number of beds the AIDS Ward will have. Currently, there are 45–50 PWA or AIDS related patients scattered throughout County Hospital. ... Whether or not the hospital administration will recommend that a sufficient number of beds be allocated remains to be seen. ... The second issue is WHO will administer the dedicated AIDS Unit. There have been reports that certain staff originally, and perhaps still, inimical to the idea of a dedicated AIDS unit are seriously being considered to provide top-line leadership and assume responsibility for running and staffing the Unit. Should these people be appointed we may once again have to take to the streets to ensure adequate quality care for the patients in the Unit.[42]

Morello was right that the County would not respond quickly to the needs of hospitalized PWAs. In a September 1988 memorandum addressed to the Supervisors, the County's Director of Health Services Robert C. Gates reported on efforts to establish the twenty-bed ward. Gates's proposed timeline for the ward's creation seemed calculated to at once mollify the Supervisors and infuriate activists. Rather than actually deliver the AIDS ward in six months, Gates and his staff developed a plan for "Phase I" and "Phase II" actions; Phase I was to consist of the gathering of special teams of HIV/AIDS specialists (doctors, nurses, social workers) to be created by January 1 of 1989 – months away – and only during Phase II would the County actually open the ward, more than six months later than what the Supervisors had asked for.[43] Gates's memo exemplified why ACT UP/LA would, throughout its life, battle with the County. Activists wanted the government to respond to the AIDS crisis as if it were a crisis, and both elected and appointed officials in LA County seemed unable (or unwilling) to do so.

In 1989, ACT UP/LA, in existence for a little over a year, continued to press LA County for swifter action on implementing a dedicated AIDS ward and for improvements to County-USC Hospital's outpatient clinic, known as "5P21" (its room number in the huge hospital); the 5P21 clinic was already seeing twice the number of patients than expected. The group made plans for a week-long, 24-hour vigil coordinated with other AIDS activist groups because ACT UP/LA had decided that the County was not "operating in good faith or in the best interest of

---

[41] Janny Scott and Victor Merina, "Supervisors OK County-USC AIDS Ward," *The Los Angeles Times*, August 24, 1988.

[42] Enric Morello, "We've Won an AIDS Ward," *ACT UP/LA* 1:7 (September 1988) pp. 1–2.

[43] Memorandum dated September 23, 1988, from Robert C. Gates, Director of Health Services, LA County to LA County Supervisors; ONE Collection.

PWAs."[44] Mark Kostopoulos described the vigil as "one of the biggest projects ACT UP/LA has ever undertaken" and, indeed, coordinating the vigil – getting cots, blankets, and sleeping bags for protestors, arranging security, feeding them, let alone making sure that the vigil itself was always staffed – was a huge project.[45]

The week-long vigil at County-USC Hospital took place January 21–27, 1989, with the support not only of ACT UP/LA, but of AIDS service organizations and dozens of other groups who put together a long list of demands for the County. Supporters of the vigil included AIDS Project LA, AIDS Hospice Foundation (later the AIDS Healthcare Foundation), the California Nurses Association, and at least forty more local organizations.[46] Demands were drawn up at a December 1988 community meeting and were both aspirational – giving every PWA at County-USC the right to be in the AIDS ward – and focused on specific problems at 5P21. Activists also demanded that the County involve "all affected communities" in drawing up a plan to deal with AIDS in LA County.[47] The vigil included speak-outs by PWAs unable to procure proper AIDS care and memorial ceremonies with protesters calling out the names of friends and love ones who had died of AIDS. Hundreds of people visited the vigil site. Performers in a political drag show – the "Fascist Fashion Show" – took a sardonic look at the politics of AIDS as they dressed as a variety of figures that played with anti-AIDS themes. In one example, a "safe sex bride" appeared covered head to toe in white "latex and lace," including a white hood and a face mask; another performer came out dressed in a "hospital gown" that included a skirt of black ostrich feathers and an IV drip.[48]

On the last night of the vigil, Supervisor Edmund D. Edelman visited the site, and although many protestors welcomed him, he was confronted by smaller group of very angry activists who heckled him even as he agreed with them that the County had failed PWAs.[49] Edelman called the recent disclosure that $8

---

[44] Unsigned. "Emergency Community Meeting," *ACT UP/LA* 1:9 (November/December 1988), pp. 5–6; ONE Collection. Note: both the October 1988 and the November/December 1988 newsletters are listed as 1:9.

[45] Mark Kostopoulos "ACT UP/LA's January Action," *ACT UP/LA* 1:9 (November/December 1988) p. 3.

[46] Unsigned. "Vigil Support." ACT UP/LA 2:1 (February/March 1989). p. 3.

[47] Unsigned. "Condensation of Demands to Be Presented to the County as Formulated by Being Alive," *ACT UP/LA* 1:9 (November/December 1988) pp. 3–4.

[48] The performers were photographed by Brad Fowler and the images became postcard sets of ten that were sold as a limited edition as a fundraiser. Each postcard had captions under the photos; for example, the dress for the "safe sex bride" was described as being for "the bride who wants to live to see what lies beyond the honeymoon. . . . Helen says 'I do, I do' again and again, knowing that she will be around next year for a repeat performance." (Set of ten postcards/color photos in art paper envelope entitled "Los Angeles County Health Care a Fashion Victim" credited to "1989 Stiffsheets/photo: Brad Fowler." ONE Collection.)

[49] ACT UP/LA Unsigned. "Dateline: 21–27 January 1989." Article from the AIDS Project LA Newsletter," reprinted January 20, 1992, as part of *From the Archives* "an occasional publication of the ACT UP/LA Archives." ONE Collection.

million of the County's AIDS budget had been left unspent "intolerable" and told the crowd "We need to do a better job. . . . We can't afford to keep the status quo." The hecklers caused Edelman to leave abruptly, saying within earshot of a reporter "(i)t's not just up to me." In response to another activist's thanks for coming, Edelman reportedly said "I appreciate it. Don't ask again."[50]

Despite the contretemps with Edelman, the vigil was seen as a success by ACT UP/LA. Enrico Morello wrote that the 168 hours of the vigil gave the group "cause for guarded optimism that some really positive movement regarding improved treatment will take place soon."[51] Morello was heartened by "the diversity of groups and organizations" in the lesbian and gay community who participated, and he felt that "a significant portion of our community wanted the vigil to succeed." Numerous local telecasts had covered the vigil, as had print media in the Spanish-speaking community, and workers at the hospital had expressed support. Morello even put a positive spin on the Edelman semi-debacle, noting that Edelman seemed to understand the AIDS community's needs on "a much deeper level" after the vigil and that "it was a far different Edelman at the meeting the Monday after the vigil, a man who seemed convinced of the rightness of our effort and who insisted that the County Department of Health Services be responsive to our demands."

Morello and others saw the vigil as a success, but it did not yield immediate results. ACT UP/LA reported to its members that despite the Board having directed the County's DHS to find space for the AIDS ward quickly, the DHS dragged its heels. Consequently, ACT UP/LA scheduled an April demonstration at the DHS headquarters at which protestors demanded the resignation of DHS director Robert Gates, the director of AIDS services Robert Frangenberg, and the chief administrator of County-USC, Peter Heseltine.[52] At the DHS demonstration, approximately eighty protestors presented Gates with beds for the ward and came "equipped with miles and miles of red tape and a huge clock bearing the word: 'The time has come.'"[53] At the end of April, someone began outlining bodies in red spray paint in front of the County Hall of Administration and at Robert Gates' parking space, along with graffiti demanding Gates' resignation and calling Supervisor Pete Schabarum "a murderer."[54] The graffiti incident prompted Schabarum to suggest that the money needed to clean up the graffiti come out of the County's AIDS funding. It also apparently prompted the County Sheriffs to engage in a campaign of harassment against ACT UP/LA members, which ended only when the ACLU demanded that the Sheriffs stop and made a

[50] Unsigned. "Edelman Back Bigger AIDS Ward in Speech at Vigil Site." *Los Angeles Times*, January 29 1989.

[51] Enrico Morello, "From the Editor," *ACT UP/LA* 2:1 (February/March 1989) p. 2.

[52] Unsigned. "Times Is Up!" *ACT UP/LA* 2:2 (April/May 1989).

[53] Chris Roy, "Health Services Action." *ACT UP/LA* 2:2 (April/May 1989).

[54] Doug Sadownick, "ACT UP and the Politics of AIDS," *LA Weekly* (October 6–12, pp. 20–25).

formal request to hand over any surveillance records.[55] Along with confrontational protests, members of ACT UP/LA attended meetings of the "LA County/USC Medical Center AIDS Community Advisory Council [CAC]," along with representatives from the AIDS Hospice Foundation.[56] Meetings with this CAC and with other County officials continued for years as ACT UP/LA members monitored the County's actions regarding provisions for PWAs. In late September, the AIDS ward at County-USC opened with only 12 out of the 60 beds that were promised.

THE BEGINNINGS OF A NATIONAL NETWORK: ACT UP/LA AND ACT NOW

ACT UP/LA's local actions against recalcitrant County officials oscillated with the group's participation in the national network of ACT UPs and other direct action anti-AIDS groups called "ACT NOW (AIDS Coalition to Network Organize and Win)." By March 1988, there were close to twenty groups calling themselves "ACT UP."[57] ACT NOW's purpose was to work to coordinate national actions, funded by money channeled to it from local direct action groups. ACT NOW coordinated demonstrations in October 1988 at the Federal Drug Administration (FDA) and the Department of Health and Human Services (DHHS).[58] ACT UP/LA voted to send volunteers to participate on the steering committee for the October 1988 actions and donated an extra $300 to defray other costs associated with a national meeting.[59] ACT NOW, which was later renamed and reshaped as the "ACT UP Network," was to have a tumultuous history, consisting as it did of loosely coordinated groups who were overwhelming opposed to institutionalizing their voices of protest. From the beginning, ACT UP/LA members had questions about their relationship with ACT NOW. ACT UP/LA members initially wanted a clearer

decision making structure for Act Now, which would allow Act Now to make decision [sic] of a national nature, but not be necessarily binding on local groups. The general body requested the Act Now representatives have a written agenda with demands and propositions for the October Act Now conference ready for the generals body [sic] perusal at the nest [sic] meeting.[60]

---

[55] Sadownick, ibid. p. 24.

[56] Larry Day, "ACT UP/LA Attends LAC/USC AIDS Community Advisory Council Meeting." ACT UP/LA 2:3 (July 1989)

[57] Minutes, General Body meeting, March 28, 1988; ONE Collection.

[58] John Fall, "A Brief Personal View of the Happenings in Washington October 8–11." *ACT UP/LA* 1:8 (October 1988), p. 4.

[59] Minutes, General Body meeting, June 13, 1988; Minutes, General Body meeting, July 11, 1988; ONE collection.

[60] Minutes, General Body meeting, September 12, 1988; ONE collection.

ACT UP/LA showed its mixed feelings about ACT NOW in flip-flops about funding the attendance of participants at an October 1988 ACT NOW conference; the group initially voted not to fund participation and reversed itself two weeks later.[61] John Fall, who attended the DC protests and the activist conference that went along with it, reported that while the actions were successes – particularly the large-scale protest against the FDA that involved blocking the building's entrance – the ACT NOW conference that accompanied the actions quickly descended from a "confrontational atmosphere" into something close to an actual physical "brawl."[62] Fall blamed incompatible expectations on the part of attendees for the discord because some expected decisions to be made at the conference and others had only attended with the express promise that ACT NOW *not* make any decisions that would affect local ACT UPs. Fall also cited the problem of ACT UP/NY's dominant position vis à vis other ACT UPs as causing friction, especially ACT UP/NY's practice of fundraising in areas that had their own ACT UPs.

Some ACT UP/LA members began to punctuate their local work with international activism. A number of activists attended the contentious Fifth International AIDS Conference in June 1989, in Montreal, Canada. Mark Kostopoulos represented both ACT UP/LA and ACT NOW at the meetings and reported on attempts by ACT NOW to coordinate national protests despite the fact that ACT UP/NY did not formally participate in ACT NOW.[63] ACT NOW laid out an agenda that included a nationally coordinated action in Chicago, in April 1990, built around the theme of access to healthcare, and ACT UP/San Francisco voiced desire for another activist conference to take place on questions of healthcare access when the Sixth International Conference on AIDS came to San Francisco in the summer of 1990. Kostopoulos highlighted one of the key events of the Montreal meetings – the dissemination of "Le Manifeste de Montreal [The Montreal Manifesto]: Declaration of the Universal Rights and Needs of People Living with HIV Disease."[64] The Manifesto, a joint production of ACT UP/NY and AIDS Action Now, a Toronto-based group, listed a "preamble" about the rights and needs of those struggling with HIV disease followed by ten demands addressed chiefly to governments and national health organizations on the treatment of PWAs. The Manifesto raised questions about gender and HIV, stating that "[t]he unequal social position of women affecting their access to information about HIV transmission must be recognized and also their rights

[61] Minutes, General Body meeting, September 26, 1988; ONE Collection.

[62] Fall, 1988.

[63] Mark Kostopoulos, "Montreal AIDS Conference." *ACT UP/LA* 2:3 newsletter (July 1989), p. 10.

[64] The "Montreal Manifesto" appeared on page 11 of *ACT UP/LA* 2:3 under the long heading "AIDS ACTION NOW! Toronto, Canada & ACT UP/NEW YORK, USA jointly issue: Le Manifeste de Montreal Declaration of Universal Rights and Needs of People Living with HIV Disease."

to programs redressing this inequality, including respect for women's right to control their own bodies." On October 6, 1989, the national and the local came together for ACT UP/LA as they demonstrated at the Los Angeles offices of the US Food and Drug Administration (FDA) at the "Federal Building" in Westwood. Approximately four hundred protestors shut the building down.[65] The Federal Building sits at the corner of Wilshire Boulevard and Veteran Avenue, which is one of the busiest intersections in the entire city. As it had in the County vigil action, ACT UP/LA once again led a coalition of groups, which by this time included other ACT UPs in Long Beach and San Diego. Activist and journalist Robin Podolsky participated in the FDA action:

While this action was initiated by ACT UP/LA, the coalition which has emerged to pull it off extends way beyond ACT UP/LA's usual base. There is a large group of pro-choice activists, mostly women, substantially heterosexual, whose friendship has [been] won in the course of abortion clinic defense. There is a Latino contingent, gay and heterosexual, brought in through the efforts of Arturo Olivas, Project Director of Cara a Cara, which outreaches to gay Latinos. There are anti-nuclear activists for whom non-violence is a passionate life commitment and West Hollywood gay men who have never been political before. Dave Johnson, LA's AIDS Coordinator and Torie Osborn, the Gay & Lesbian Community Services Center's Director, are among the arrestees. ACT UP/LA has propelled itself into a position of great responsibility, and from the looks of this action, they are handling it fine.[66]

Both *The Los Angeles Herald Examiner* and *The Los Angeles Times* covered the demonstration, noting that eighty protesters were arrested.[67] *The Herald Examiner* reported that ACT UP/LA had prevented about 1,500 employees from entering the building as they blocked entrances and "plastered the structure's plate-glass windows with stickers bearing the names of dead AIDS victims and the epitaph, 'Don't Forget Me.'" The arrests at the action were chiefly for trespassing, but a small number of demonstrators were charged with resisting arrest, and one, Pete Sigal, was charged with assault for allegedly spitting on an officer. Robin Podolsky reported that, according to witnesses, not only did Sigal *not* spit at anyone, he was singled out by law enforcement, arrested, forced to wear a germ mask, arraigned, and later ordered released by a federal magistrate, at which point he was not set free but taken to a holding cell and threatened with detention over the upcoming long holiday weekend.[68] Sigal was also taken to County-USC Hospital, where police tried to coerce him into taking an HIV test, which he refused. When the federal magistrate was informed by ACT UP/LA's legal

[65] ACT UP/LA "Proposal for Fall Action." August 7, 1989; ONE collection.

[66] Robin Podolsky, "Shutting Down the Feds." *ACT UP/LA* 2:6 (December 1989/January 1990).

[67] Darrell Dawsey, "80 Arrested as AIDS Protest Is Broken Up." *Los Angeles Times* (October 7, 1989); Emilia Askari, "Officers in Gloves Jail 80 at AIDS Protest: Activists Angry with Inaction by Federal Officials," *Herald Examiner* (October 7, 1989).

[68] Podolsky, 1989, p. 4–5.

representative that Sigal had not been released, the incensed magistrate ordered Sigal's re-release.[69]

ACTIONS IN 1990: A NATIONAL STAGE FOR LOS ANGELES ACTIVISTS

By the beginning of 1990, ACT UP/LA had made a name for itself – not always a positive one – within the lesbian and gay community, and it was well-known to its targets. ACT UP/LA's 1990 activities started off with an action that was technically not an ACT UP/LA action at all. An affinity group called S.A.N.O.E (Stop AIDS Now Or Else, and pronounced "Say No") attempted to stop the Pasadena Tournament of Roses Parade. S.A.N.O.E. began its life in San Francisco; local members, almost all of whom were in ACT UP/LA, tried to stop the parade in order to unfurl a banner that read "Emergency – Stop the Parade – 70,000 Dead from AIDS" (Faderman and Timmons 2009: 315). The attempt to stop the Rose Parade – an event attended in person by hundreds of thousands and watched by millions more on television – was audacious, dramatic, and, to hear participants tell it, extremely scary. The plan to stop the parade was a symbolic disruption of business as usual: "(b)acked by more than 50 behind-the-scene supporters, the nonviolent demonstrators intend to bring the … parade to a halt, sounding an alarm in America's conscience."[70] The S.A.N.O.E. protestors weren't targeting an agency and expecting a particular policy outcome; they were taking advantage of the Rose Parade as a local event that drew national coverage. They wanted everyone watching to wake up and respond to the AIDS crisis.[71]

The late Gunther Freehill was among the fourteen or so activists, some chained together, who were arrested for trying to stop the parade. He described the action as being "a real high," but also described feeling like he was in danger during it. Half-jokingly, he told me "there was no doubt in my mind that I was going to die."[72] When I asked him why he had felt this way, Freehill said that the action exposed the group to a great deal of anger from both the crowd and the police. Describing a photograph taken of the action at the point where the demonstrators were apprehended, Freehill recounted that

the photograph was actually taken at the moment of my greatest fear because there was … you can't see my face because there's a cop sort of kneeling down … he's on one knee … and the knee that is up … my face is right behind it. … And this is in the middle of the street

---

[69] Sigal was charged with one count of misdemeanor assault and one count of disorderly conduct; a prosecutorial warrant for a blood test was not pursued. Podolsky ibid. p. 5.

[70] S.A.N.O.E.'s "AIDS Activists to Stop Rose Parade," Press Release, January 1 1990; ONE collection.

[71] Kevin Farrell, "Why Stop the Rose Parade?" *ACT UP/LA* 3:1 (February/March 1990), p. 3.

[72] Interview with author, 2000.

and the cop is telling me to face the wall and I thought I was gonna die, because I can't face the wall and he is going to beat me to death right here, for not facing the wall . . .

BR: Did you get beat up?

FREEHILL: Yeah. But I said things like "You keep telling me to face the wall! There's no wall! [laughs]."[73]

Helene Schpak was part of S.A.N.O.E. and echoed Freehill's sentiment that the Parade action had been frightening: "It's scary because the whole idea of chaining yourself to one another . . . we knew we were going to go down . . . but we didn't know it was going to be that harsh . . ..I certainly heard the crowd go hugely negative."[74] Jan Speller, who was part of the group chained together during the action stated in her interview that

[w]e thought we were gonna be shot at the Rose Parade . . ..And it was really really scary. So I pull that file out [of clippings, etc.] sometimes to say well if you could do that, if you could chain yourself to seven other people and run out in front of the Rose Parade, not really knowing what you were doing but doing it then you can do this other thing . . .[75]

According to the *Los Angeles Times*, S.A.N.O.E. was able to stop the parade and unfurl their banner in front of a float sponsored by the Ronald Reagan presidential library for about a minute before they were arrested.[76] At the 1991 Rose Parade, eleven members of ACT UP/LA proper went back to Pasadena to take the much less confrontational action of passing out leaflets about the growing numbers of AIDS deaths. Accordingly to ACT UP/LA's David Lacaillade, most parade-goers accepted the leaflets, but apparently older attendees were not pleased once they realized what they had been handed, and activists got into trouble with the county sheriffs after they had started to place their leaflets on parked cars. The sheriffs themselves were apparently conflicted about the legality of ACT UP/LA's actions, stopping the activists once to say that they could put the leaflets on cars and a second time to say that they couldn't. The second stop piqued a passer-by's curiosity; she asked for a leaflet, which "was passed to her in full view of all ten sheriffs. The sheriffs were silent. No riot ensued."[77]

---

[73] Hector Tobar, "Protest by AIDS Activists Halts Procession for a Short Time." *The Los Angeles Times*, January 2, 1990.

[74] Interview with author, 2011.

[75] Interview with author, 2000.

[76] Tobar, 1990. Tobar put the arrests of the S.A.N.O.E. activists in context, reporting that there were 192 arrests at the parade that day for "alcohol-related violations," 9 for assault, and 30 more for theft.

[77] David Lacaillade, "Back to the Rose Parade: American are Still Dying for Health Care." ACT UP/LA *News*, 4:1 (January/February 1991), p. 6. Terri Ford, who at the time of her interview with me was the director of global advocacy for AIDS Healthcare Foundation, mentioned that AHF sponsored a float dedicated to Elizabeth Taylor for the 2011 Rose Parade; it was the first float ever to focus on AIDS/HIV. See http://www.towleroad.com/2011/12/roseparade.html.

ACT UP/LA members oscillated back to the national in April 1990, participating in large-scale, nationally coordinated actions in Chicago that were focused on two main issues: getting Cook County to open up its dedicated AIDS ward to women and challenging the major insurance companies to stop discriminatory practices against HIV-positive people and PWAs.[78] Protestors gathered at the intersection of Michigan and Randolph in downtown Chicago to rally against Prudential Insurance Company and the Cook County Board of Supervisors.[79] Prudential was singled out because of its purported refusal to pay for pentamidine, a drug used to treat pneumocystis pneumonia. ACT UP/LA members had already confronted Prudential at their local offices in Los Angeles' Hancock Park six months prior to the Chicago protests in November 1989.[80] ACT UP/LA's "Not Ready for Cancellation Players" staged a mock funeral procession across Wilshire Boulevard and avoided run-ins with the police, although Prudential threatened to bring charges for vandalism for plastering their front doors with "SILENCE = DEATH" stickers. Richard Beecher wrote about ACT UP/LA's charges against Prudential; the group accused the company and other insurers of discriminatory practices, including refusing to reimburse policy holders for the costs of experimental drugs, redlining zip code areas considered "high risk," and large rate increases for PWAs who had to convert from group policies to individual ones after their COBRA coverage ran out.

The 1990 Chicago actions drew ACT UP activists from around the country. The actions resulted in many arrests, but it led to Cook County's agreement to allow women into dedicated AIDS wards. A number of the former ACT UP/LA members interviewed described the events at Chicago as alternately frightening and exhilarating. Wendell Jones, who was arrested in Chicago, remembered that fellow activist Doug Sadownick had been cut off from a group of marchers at one point and that Sadownick had "actually jumped under a police horse to get [back] to where we were."[81] Sadownick briefly described the same moment in his interview; he recalled being in the middle of an "awful demonstration, the police went crazy on us, I dove under a horse, there's a picture of me doing it . . . and it was really scary."[82] Geneviève Clavreul, an ACT UP/LA participant whose resumé as a research nurse and membership in the "mainstream" gay and lesbian civil rights group Municipal Elections Committee of Los Angeles (MECLA) did not prepare her for violence at demonstrations, remembered being kicked by a horse and having broken ribs as a result.[83] Clavreul characterized the Chicago demonstrations as having some logistical problems,

---

[78] Unsigned. Three page report for General Body meeting, March 5, 1990; ONE collection.

[79] Unsigned. "National AIDS Actions for Healthcare." Flyer/schedule regarding Chicago events April 20–23, 1990; ONE collection.

[80] Richard Beecher, "ACT UP Throws a Piece of the Rock!" ACT UP/LA 2:6 (December 1989/ January 1990), pp. 1–2, 12

[81] Interview with author, 2011.

[82] Interview with author, 2011.

[83] Interview with author, 2011.

but nonetheless felt that the Chicago actions were effective in getting large insurance companies to change their ways and in getting Cook County to open up a women's AIDS ward.

Ty Geltmaker went to Chicago with his partner, James Rosen. Geltmaker recalled that many LA activists did not intend to get arrested; some had intended "to play cat and mouse" with the police. Geltmaker and Rosen helped to block a door to an insurance company that was designated as having denied insurance to HIV-positive people. They were arrested and thrown into a police wagon. Geltmaker described being in the wagon:

I've never felt so claustrophobic in my life. Because we were in this wagon for about an hour before they took us to ….[the] precinct but they put us in an auditorium. That was the easiest arrest I ever had because we just sat there in like this school auditorium but in this police precinct for the day … and they finally processed us and we were out.

Geltmaker recalled that he and Rosen were charged with "mob action" and given a court date. Eventually, they pled guilty and an openly sympathetic judge sentenced them to community service in Los Angeles.[84]

The Chicago actions were accompanied by a two-day ACT NOW conference attended by representatives from more than twenty ACT UPs, including ACT UP/LA.[85] ACT UP/LA's Mark Kostopoulos gave a presentation to attendees about universal healthcare, outlining different systems of nationalized care in other countries. A unanimous vote of attendees urged ACT NOW to address the role of "isms" – like racism and sexism – while simultaneously cautioning activists against turning "isms" into "special interest groups within the AIDS activist movement." Doug Sadownick covered the conference as a journalist for the alternative paper *LA Weekly*, depicting ACT NOW as full of tensions among activists who disagreed about the kinds of demands that ACT UPs could make of the federal government. Some felt that asking the government to fast-track experimental AIDS drugs was one thing and demanding the overhaul of the entire healthcare system was quite another.[86] Sadownick reported as well on the growing distance between ACT UP/NY, which was not "officially" a part of ACT NOW, and the rest of the ACT UPs. He characterized members of ACT UP/NY as dismissive of the focus of the Chicago demonstrations and quoted Ferd Eggan, a founder of ACT UP Chicago who later moved to Los Angeles and became LA City's third AIDS policy coordinator, as saying that ACT UP/NY had felt that the Chicago actions were poorly conceived and organized.

ACT UP/LA activists came back from Chicago and joined their compatriots in their continuing battle with the LA County Board of Supervisors and County

[84] Interview with author, 2011.
[85] Unsigned. "Minutes – ACT-Now General Membership Meeting in Chicago – April 22, 1990." ONE Collection.
[86] Doug Sadownick. 1990. "ACTing UP Against the Health-Care System: National AIDS Activists' Conference Debates Tactics." *LA Weekly* May 4–10, p. 12.

public health officials. On May 22, 1990, ACT UP/LA protestors forced the Board to suspend their meeting.[87] There were twenty-seven arrests, with perhaps as many as three dozen law enforcement officers and security staff involved in quelling the demonstrators (and wearing rubber gloves while doing so). According to the *Los Angeles Times* reporter, ACT UP/LA demonstrators began chanting "and justice for all" immediately following the recitation of the Pledge of Allegiance that opened every Board meeting. Banners were unfurled reading "AIDS Is Ignored by the County Board." ACT UP/LA demanded that the supervisors increase the $60 million budgeted for AIDS care (out of a proposed County budget of $10 billion). ACT UP/LA protestors also demanded that supervisors act on the two-month wait for an appointment at the 5P21 outpatient clinic at County-USC Medical Center. The protest underscored what were already clear fault lines between the City and the County of Los Angeles over AIDS policy; the *Times* reporter recounted an exchange at the meeting between Dave Johnson, the AIDS policy coordinator for the City of Los Angeles, and Pete Schabarum, the conservative supervisor much hated by the AIDS activist community. Johnson, referring to an anti-AIDS message scrawled in lipstick by demonstrators on a glass screen in the meeting room, told supervisors

"It's very easy to sit here and talk about whether or not we should condone demonstrations. It's very easy to take a squeegee and wipe the red paint off the glass." "You're not condoning that conduct, are you?" Supervisor Pete Schabarum interrupted. "If you are, you lose me right now." Johnson continued, "People who depend on the county for health care are dying with AIDS faster because we finally have drugs that can help them, and we are not getting those drugs to people. . . ."

The LA County budget that passed during the summer of 1990 contained cuts in healthcare generally, with only a small increase in the AIDS budget mostly targeted for home healthcare.[88] ACT UP/LA's Connie Norman contended that home healthcare providers with whom the County contracted had refused to go to minority-dominated areas of Los Angeles after dark and that some of the home care companies did not accept Medicare or MediCal (the healthcare insurance program for poor Californians). Norman further stated that the 5P21 outpatient clinic was still understaffed to the point that it was not uncommon to wait four (not two) months for a first appointment. Norman, who had engaged and would engage extensively in lobbying efforts with government entities, simply did not believe in the good faith of the Board of Supervisors:

While I have been consistent in my belief that we must work with the system as well as applying pressure from without, I cannot stress enough that I have come to a point where

---

[87] Richard Simon, "27 Arrested in Protest to County Over AIDS Budget." *The Los Angeles Times*, May 23, 1990.

[88] Connie Norman, "LA County Board of Stupes." *ACT UP/LA* 3:5 (October/November 1990), p. 5.

I question the validity of trying to work with this Board of Stupes [Supervisors]. We spent a full year in the Planning Council [for the budget]. . . . While I am proud of the document we came out of the planning process with, I am outraged that it seems to have been a waste of time.

In response to what they saw as shortcomings in the County Budget, ACT UP/LA members participated in the "The Alternative Budget Coalition [ABC]," which consisted of about fifteen organizations, including homeless shelters and two locals of the Service Employees International Union.[89] The Coalition staged "Alternative Budget Hearings"; they rented the Board's meeting room and held a mock hearing regarding the spending priorities of the LA County's $10 billion-plus budget; ACT UP/LA argued that the County budget was deficient in terms of overall provision for public health.[90] The County's provisions for public health always lagged behind need; when a new AIDS outpatient clinic was opened in 1991, it was only staffed to about 60 percent capacity, with wait times of weeks for a first appointment (Geltmaker 1992: 631).[91]

A NEW FOCUS ON WOMEN AND AIDS IN LATE 1990: "THE WEEK OF OUTRAGE"

The oscillating local and national actions that ACT UP/LA members undertook culminated in a series of protests in late 1990 on women's AIDS issues. Women's AIDS issues had started to become a visible subject for anti-AIDS direct action activists. For example, in June 1990, activists took the opportunity of the International Conference on AIDS in San Francisco to stage many actions, a number of which focused on emerging concerns about women's AIDS issues.[92] One demonstration, a sidewalk picket/march, was coordinated by a team of ACT UP women from Chicago, New York, Seattle, DC, San Francisco, and Los Angeles, as well as other cities.[93] The women's sidewalk picket, which men were encouraged to attend, turned into a march to the Moscone Center, where a "mock AIDS conference was held," as "(w)omen chained themselves to police barricades in red (tape) chains." The group then went to busy Market Street to hold a die-in, and arrests of several waves of activists began. ACT UP/LA's Jan Speller concluded that "[in] San Francisco, women gathered and I think for the first time began to expose the multiple layers

---

[89] Alternative Budget Coalition, "The 'ABC's' of the LA County Budget." Two-page position paper, c. June 1990, ONE Collection; Edmund Newton, "'Supervisors' Rip Priorities of Real Board," *Los Angeles Times*, June 10, 1990. http://articles.latimes.com/1990-06-10/local/me-415_1_board-meeting, (accessed June 18, 2012).

[90] Larry Day, "Campaign Continues." *ACT UP/LA* 3:4 (August/September 1990) p. 2

[91] Geltmaker also gave the General Body a report on the ongoing discussions with County over 5P21 ("Hospital Update," June 10, 1991, author's collection).

[92] jan speller, "Women Demand Action." *ACT UP/LA* 3:4 (August/September 1990), p. 8. Speller used lower-case for her name in the original article.

[93] speller, p. 8.

of issues surrounding women and AIDS in this country, and left with the sense that there is a great deal of work to be done."[94]

Women's issues were the main focus of a series of nationally coordinated actions that took place in late 1990 at the Centers for Disease Control (CDC) in Atlanta. The "Week of Outrage" demonstrations were aimed at changing the CDC surveillance definition of AIDS, which activists claimed did not take into account the opportunistic infections from which female PWAs suffered.[95] The CDC actions were planned by a network of feminists in ACT UP who called themselves the "ACT UP Women's Caucus" and by ACT NOW, which had morphed into the "ACT UP/Network" after a meeting with representatives from twenty-five ACT UPs and other AIDS activists groups over Labor Day weekend in San Francisco.[96] The new ACT UP/Network intended to be more task-oriented, with any national actions the result of a "loose, consensual confederation of corresponding organizations." The Network also decided that the Week of Outrage should take place on or around World AIDS Day, December 1.

The Week of Outrage events in at Atlanta featured a large and boisterous demonstration on December 3 at the CDC itself, with more than thirty ACT UP/LA members participating.[97] Mauri Tausner, who was part of the recently formed ACT UP/LA Women's Caucus, reported back to ACT UP/LA about the Atlanta events stating that, despite activists' best efforts to practice civil disobedience, police arrested *only* ninety-three demonstrators (with sixteen of the arrestees being from Los Angeles).[98] The *Los Angeles Times* actually covered the Atlanta action, with reporter Marlene Cimons quoting at some length from an ACT UP position paper about changing the definition, as well noting that there was a class-action suit pending against Surgeon General Louis Sullivan regarding the restrictions on access to Supplemental Security Income (SSI) benefits placed on women by the restrictive definition.[99] Cimons quoted a Social Security Administration spokesperson to the effect that the agency had stopped using the CDC's definition because it was "apparent that HIV infection (is) manifested by additional severe impairments not encompassed in the CDC definition."[100]

---

94 speller p. 16.
95 See Brier (2009: chapter five) for a discussion of the national ACT UPs' Women's Caucus's role in spearheading the effort to change the CDC definition.
96 Ferd Eggan, "ACT NOW to Network." *ACT UP/LA* 3:5 (October/November 1990), p. 9
97 Mauri Tausner, "93 Arrested in National CDC Action," *ACT UP/LA News*, 4:1 (January/February 1991). p. 3; Author's field notes, General Body meeting, December 10, 1990.
98 *The Atlanta Journal and Constitution* reported that there had been approximately 300 protestors present. (Elizabeth Coady, "300 Protest Definition of AIDS: ACT UP Group Claims CDC Is 'Killing Women,'" December 4, 1990, p. D-2.)
99 Marlene Cimons, "Activists Call for Expanded Definition of AIDS in Women." *Los Angeles Times*, December 27, 1990, p. A5.
100 Lawrence K. Altman, "Widened Definition of AIDS Leads to More Reports of It," *The New York Times*, April 30, 1993 (accessed online 3/16/2013).

With timing suggested by the ACT UP Women's Caucus and ACT UP/ Network, the recently formed ACT UP/LA's Women's Caucus, in concert with the GB, planned a series of local actions that took place from mid-November to early December 1990.[101] The Week of Outrage started with a "Teach-in" on issues involving women and AIDS.[102] Other events followed: a night of "Safe Sex Vending" where ACT UP/LA women and men visited bars and handed out kits that included bleach for cleaning syringes, condoms, and dental dams;[103] a guerilla theater "Dance of Death" aimed at weekend crowds gathered at the Venice Boardwalk and Santa Monica's Third Street Promenade, popular pedestrian-only spaces on in Los Angeles beach communities; and the largest action, a demonstration at Frontera Women's Prison about the conditions that HIV-positive women prisoners faced.[104]

ACT UP/LA demonstrated at California's Frontera Women's Prison in Chino, located approximately an hour east of Los Angeles, on World AIDS day, December 1, 1990. The demonstration, which I and approximately one hundred others attended, was in protest of egregious conditions suffered by HIV-positive prisoners. By going to Frontera – one of the largest women's prisons in the United States – ACT UP/LA chose to highlight discrimination against HIV-positive women as well as prisoners' AIDS issues. By scheduling the Frontera action on World AIDS Day and as part of the Week of Outrage, ACT UP/LA activists meshed their concerns with the priorities of the ACT UP/Network and the national ACT UP/Women's Caucus. The idea to demonstrate outside the prison was nevertheless a home-grown one.[105]

The conditions that HIV-positive prisoners faced at Frontera in the segregated part of the facility for HIV-positive prisoners named "Walker A" eventually became a very public scandal, covered mainly by the *Orange County Register*; at the same time, the problems of women prisoners with AIDS was a very personal issue for ACT UP/LA members.[106] One of the ACT UP/LA Women's Caucus's founders (see Chapter 3), Mary Lucey, a former resident of Walker A. Lucey, sent to Frontera for parole violations, was put in

---

[101] ACT UP/LA. "Week of Outrage /November 26 to December 3, 1990." Flyer. Collection of author.

[102] See Chapter 3 for a more extensive discussion of the gendered dynamics of the Teach-in.

[103] Dental dams are small sheets of latex used by dentists for endodontic procedures. They were adapted by safer sex activists for use as a barrier to prevent the transmission of bodily fluids during cunnilingus and anilingus. They were not easily obtained, and safer sex activists often improvised by cutting nonlubricated condoms into squares.

[104] Minutes, Women's Caucus meeting October 28, 1990; author's field notes November 11, 1990.

[105] Minutes, Women's Caucus October 28, 1990; David Lee Perkins, "Press Release for Frontera," November 30, 1990. Author's collection.

[106] *The Orange County Register* had conducted an exposé of unqualified state officials and shoddy practices involved in the care of HIV-positive prisoners at Frontera; see Donna Wares and James V. Grimaldi "Secret Frontera Pact Confirmed: State Officials to Sign Deal with Suspended Medical Chief," November 15, 1990, pp. 1, 26, and Donna Wares and James V. Grimaldi, "Inspectors Assail Frontera Infirmary," November 16, 1990, pp. 1, 4.

The Women's Caucus of ACT UP/LA calls upon you to unite in action as we demonstrate at Frontera Women's Prison friday, november 30–1p.m.

As a part of **ACT UP**'s nation-wide **"Week of Outrage"** focusing on concerns of women with AIDS, we will protest Frontera's treatment of women with AIDS. Frontera has an AIDS ward where all incarcerted women in California with AIDS are sent. The medical treatment these women receive is completely inadequate: there is money alloted for an infectious disease doctor, yet there is no such doctor; women have no acces to AZT until they become very ill; the infirmary has no state license resulting in no facilities for I.V.s or oxygen tubes; women in this ward are not allowed to receive visits from their children; the food these women receive is of sub-human quality. We demand that these women be treated properly and receive appropriate health care!

WE DEMAND:

* CONDITIONS: ACCESS TO PROPER MEDICATIONS FOR HIV POSITIVE INMATES ACCORDING TO ACCEPTED PROTOCOLS ALONG WITH SPECIAL DIETS TO MEET THE NEED OF SAME.

* TREATMENT: PROVISION OF A MEDICAL AIDS SPECIALIST/I.D. DOCTOR AND THE UPGRADING OF THE PRISON INFIRMARY FOR STATE LISCENSING TO PROVIDE ACUTE CARE SERVICES.

* EDUCATION: DISTRIBUTION OF AND ACCESS TO DENTAL DAMS, CLEAN "WORKS", SAFE SEX EDUCATION AND SAFE "WORKS" EDUCATION FOR ALL INMATES AND STAFF.

* IMMEDIATE IMPLEMENTATION OF THE FOLLOWING: DAILY SICK CALLS, WEEKLY MONITORING OF PWAs, MONTHLY PHYSICALS (INCLUDING PAP SMEARS) FOR HIV POSITIVE INMATES AND BI-ANNUAL GYN EXAMS FOR ALL.

THE DEMONSTRATION BEGINS AT 1:00 p.m.
**We will meet to carpool out to Chino at PLUMMER PARK in West Hollywood–
SOUTH PARKING LOT–11:15 a.m.**

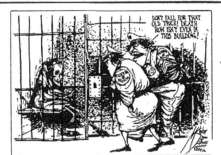

DIRECTIONS TO FRONTERA
WOMEN'S PRISON:

from L.A. take the 60 Freeway East
to Euclid Avenue. Take Euclid Avenue
south (right) for 5.3 miles to Pine Street.
Make a left on Pine Street and get into
the right turning lane—make your first
right onto Chino-Carona Street. The
prison is within one block.

ACT UP/LA WOMEN'S CAUCUS IS UNITED IN ANGER AND COMMITTED TO DIRECT ACTION TO END THE AIDS PANDEMIC. WE DEMAND PROPER TREATMENT OF HIV POSITIVE WOMEN AND QUALITY HEALTHCARE FOR ALL. WE EDUCATE THE PUBLIC ON ALL ISSUES RELATED TO WOMEN AND AIDS. WE ARE NOT SILENT.

for more info. call the ACT UP office at (213) 669-7301

FIGURE 2.1: Flyer, Demonstration at Frontera Women's Prison, November 1990.

Walker A because she was HIV-positive. She testified to the ill-treatment that she and other HIV-positive incarcerated women faced, telling of "the cops who work the unit [who] did not even want to touch you. We had one officer who instead of giving you leftover food said, 'I'd rather throw it away than give it to the women in Walker A.'"[107] Lucey was using AZT to control HIV before her incarceration; once inside, her AZT was confiscated.[108] She and other inmates of Walker A were fed "cold oatmeal for breakfast, cold ham for lunch and cold green franks for dinner – the kind of food women with HIV shouldn't eat." She was kept from mingling with other prisoners; she and other HIV-positive women were not allowed to work or take classes; they were verbally abused by prison staffers and deprived of visits with spouses and children.

The Frontera demonstration was marked by a complicated dance that ACT UP/LA often played with law enforcement, authorities, other sympathetic organizations, and the media. Originally, ACT UP/LA had wanted to do civil disobedience at the prison but changed plans after being told by the American Civil Liberties Union (ACLU) that breaking the law on prison grounds was a felony. In any case, the legal demonstration was the first ever at Frontera's gates, which, as activist Ellen Yellowbird reported, threw prison administrators "into a state of alarm."[109] I attended the demonstration, riding from West Hollywood on a bus that brought approximately half the demonstrators to the prison. As we gathered in the Plummer Park parking lot, I noticed men who seemed to be plainclothes police videotaping us. One ACT UP/LA member confronted the videotapers about what they were doing; they reportedly told him that they were waiting for their wives, to which he responded, "you're waiting for your wives and videotaping 60 homosexuals?"[110] There were more "undercover" videotapers on the scene when we arrived at Frontera.

The *Los Angeles Times* covered the Frontera demonstration,[111] and the *Orange County Register* continued its investigative coverage, noting that the head doctor at Frontera was being looked at for "irregularities" in his dealings with prisoners.[112] ACT UP/LA would continue to focus on prisoners' AIDS issues. Shortly after Frontera, a committee called "Prisoners with AIDS Advocacy Committee United" (or PWAACU, pronounced "Pwack-you" to rhyme with a common epithet) formed. As discussed later, in May 1991, ACT UP/LA members went to the state capitol of Sacramento as part of a statewide

---

[107] Mark Satterlees, "InterViews/You," *ACT UP/LA News* 4:2 (April/May 1991), p. 3.

[108] Doug Sadownick, "AIDS Treatment, Steerage Class: AIDS Programs for Women in (and out of) Prison, Say Critics, Are Nonexistent or Worse," *LA Weekly*, November 30–December 6, 1990.

[109] Ellen Yellowbird, "Frontera: The Struggle for Humane Conditions Continues," *ACT UP/LA News* 4:1 (January/February 1991), pp. 1, 8.

[110] Author's field notes, December 1, 1990.

[111] Jennifer Warren, "Protestors Decry Segregation of HIV Inmates," *Los Angeles Times*, December 1, 1990, p. A30.

[112] James V. Grimaldi and Donna Wares, "Frontera Wants Doctor Charged," *Orange County Register*, December 6, 1990, p. 1, 26.

coalition to testify before the state legislature and protest outside the Capitol Building about ongoing mistreatment of HIV-positive prisoners.[113]

CHALLENGES TO UNITY IN 1991: WAR AND QUEER NATION

ACT UP/LA had participated in a dizzying array of local and national actions against AIDS in 1990. A "Women's Caucus" formed (see Chapter 3), representing a potential challenge to unity, but working on women's AIDS issues locally and nationally seemed to energize the group. However, the year 1991 did not start out well for progressive Americans. On January 17, 1991, the Persian Gulf War – Operation Desert Storm – commenced after Operation Desert Shield, a month-long build-up of American-led coalition troops in the area. ACT UP/LA participants voiced strong opposition to the war, with most resenting the money devoted to war efforts that, in their calculation, should have gone to fighting AIDS. An excerpt from my field notes from a GB meeting in early January, right before the war began, illustrates the internal politics involved in ACT UP/LA's anti-war stance:

The next item on the agenda is "Stop the War Vigil/Apartheid March." A large, youngish, Asian man stands up. ... I miss his name. He is the liaison to the LA Coalition Against Intervention in the Middle East ... and he has been sent to get ACT UP's endorsement on a flyer advertising one of the Coalition's events. ... He says words to the effect that something has to be done to show that "self-righteous moral hypocrite in the White House" that we mean to protest the war. He sits down. A man speaks, and says "what's this got to do with AIDS?" He goes on to say that he feels that these issues should be kept separate, and that we should focus on one thing at a time. He doesn't think we should endorse the vigil. Hands shoot up all around the room. Patrick calls on a man in a yellow shirt, who speaks in a very impassioned voice about how war means no money for AIDS and how the two issues are therefore very much connected. Patrick then calls on Gypsy. She says that even though "the war machine will be doing whatever it wants to anyway no matter what we do," that the issue is one of endorsement vs. sponsorship. She doesn't have any problem with endorsing the vigil – sponsorship would generally require more effort and/or money. In contrast to the others, she is very matter of fact in her manner. Barry is the next person to speak. He also is very passionate in his presentation and states that the "ACT UP philosophy" is opposed to war, any war period. Louise then asks the original Coalition liaison if ACT UP can table at the event. He says "absolutely" and says that ACT UP can also send speakers. Patrick calls for a vote on the endorsement and it passes. The original objector votes no.[114]

[113] In April 1992, ACT UP/LA, Being Alive, and others helped win a compassionate release from prison for Judy Cagle, a Frontera inmate with AIDS whose doctors gave her less than a year to live. (Scott Harris, "Freed AIDS Patient Seeks Prison Reform," *Los Angeles Times*, April 2, 1992, p. B2). Mary Lucey represented ACT UP/LA at a news conference that Cagle gave and told the press that Cagle was the first PWA granted compassionate release, which the California Department of Corrections officials would not confirm or deny.

[114] Author's field notes, January 7, 1991.

The first Gulf War put ACT UP/LA into coalition with local anti-war progressives and others fighting social inequality, and, as illustrated from the extract from my notes, most members were happy to be in such a coalition because their vision of fighting AIDS aligned with other social justice concerns. Many of ACT UP/LA's participants had always been active in "non-AIDS" groups, with clinic defense – countering Operation Rescue's attempts to block access to abortion clinics – a particularly popular choice.[115]

While participation in anti-war efforts or clinic defense didn't seem to challenge ACT UP/LA as an organization, a new group that formed within the lesbian and gay community seemed to be more of a potential threat. An LA "chapter" of Queer Nation (QN) was formed during the summer of 1990. QN arose first in New York City, coming out of discussions among some members of ACT UP/NY in April 1990, but, by the next month, the group had its own identity and began meeting separately from ACT UP/NY (Fraser 1996). QN members wanted to attack homophobia through direct action in a variety of arenas and to shift the focus of the fight from one of fighting AIDS to one of fighting for alternative sexualities. In Los Angeles, as in other cities, QN activists were also at least initially drawn from ACT UP, and QN was especially important to those who were concerned that ACT UPs were losing their specifically lesbian and gay identity as they embraced other constituencies affected by the epidemic.[116]

Several ACT UP/LA members I spoke with recalled being very active in QN Los Angeles. Ty Geltmaker and James Rosen hosted one of the "private before public" QN meetings in the summer of 1990. Geltmaker recalled QN as being a response to "this moment where there was an effort to sort of 'dehomosexualize' ACT UP."[117] Geltmaker believed that this moment of seeking to change ACT UP/LA's image so that "it wasn't so out-there gay white guy" came as the group sought greater linkages with "other" communities affected by HIV-disease, especially women and people of color. Geltmaker and Rosen hosted a meeting of QN LA in the backyard of their Silverlake home. "We put a cardboard pink triangle – I still have it somewhere – on our front gate," Geltmaker said to show people where the meeting was. He recalled about fifteen members at the first meeting, and, he said, "all of these people rose to the occasion and it took on a life of its own."

In their interviews, ACT UP/LA activists Cat Walker, Richard "Doe" Racklin, Pete Jimenez, Jeff Scheurholz, Judy Sisneros, James Rosen, and Ty Geltmaker all recalled being somewhat or very involved in QN. Sisneros, Rosen, and Geltmaker recalled that QN's first big protest was at a star-studded event at AIDS Project Los Angeles (APLA): the fourth annual "Commitment to Life" fundraiser, which featured, among others, Madonna, David Hockney, Rod

---

[115] Author's field notes, January 7, 1991.
[116] Ty Geltmaker, email to author July 9, 2012.
[117] Interview with author, 2011.

Stewart, Ian McKellan (who had just recently come out), Melissa Etheridge, and celebrity "ushers" drawn from the entertainment industry's A-list.[118] Approximately ten QN protested targeted three Hollywood moguls for being in the closet, calling their donations to APLA and to the American Foundation for AIDS Research (AmFar) "blood money," and asking them to end their hypocrisy by being public about their sexuality.[119] The next QN action was a better attended "kiss-in" with about fifty protestors at the Beverly Center, an upscale shopping mall just outside the boundaries of West Hollywood. The "kiss-in" was greeted by the LAPD, who apparently said words to the effect of "you're out of here people."[120] Rosen recalled that the police came in riot gear and that there were more than two hundred of them, which struck him as ridiculous since QN had sent out a fax to the news media announcing the kiss-in, which specifically stated that no one intended to get arrested.[121] According to Geltmaker, the QN demonstrators were told that they were unlawfully assembled. He recalled thinking that "we don't have nurses at County [i.e. in the AIDS ward and clinic] so where do these cops come from, that they're on call ... ?"[122]

Geltmaker, Rosen, and others from inside and outside ACT UP/LA were attracted by QN's politics of public queer identity. QN was even more loosely organized than ACT UP/LA, which caused some frustration for ACT UP/LA members who were used to a kind of disciplined informality. For example, Rosen was the treasurer of QN for several months, but the other group members would not let him open a bank account:

That was too corporate, it was too patriarchal ... so I had a box, which we kept under a bed in our house, which had all the money, and it had everything from pennies to nickels and quarters and dimes to hundreds of dollars in singles ... and the group would agree to do something and I'd just dole it out and finally one day I said, "you know what? I just cannot do this anymore."[123]

While QN was an important activist venue for a number of ACT UP/LA members, others, like Jan Speller and Ferd Eggan, believed in retrospect that

[118] Interviews with the author, and David J. Fox, "Star Studded AIDS Fundraiser" *Los Angeles Times*, September 7, 1990, http://articles.latimes.com/1990-09-07/entertainment/ca-778_1_aids-research (accessed July 10, 2012); Jeanine Stein, "Stars Turn Out to Support AIDS Benefit," *Los Angeles Times*, September 10, 1990, http://articles.latimes.com/1990-09-10/news/vw-76_1_aids-benefit, (accessed July 10, 2012).

[119] Email from James Rosen, July 9, 2012. Rosen recalled that Ian McKellan, one of the fundraiser's honorees, gave the group a ticket so that one member got into the benefit itself.

[120] Ty Geltmaker, interview with author, 2011.

[121] Interview with author, 2012.

[122] Geltmaker and Rosen also recalled that the QN protestors planned to have dinner at the Beverly Center's Hard Rock Café after the action, and they therefore made a reservation under the name "Queer Nation." The reservation was not honored; the group was apparently given the choice to be seated under another name.

[123] Interview with author, 2012

QN represented a challenge to ACT UP/LA since, in practice, QN attracted many of the same activists as ACT UP/LA. QN continued to conduct actions in the LA area for the next several years and played a role in leading largely spontaneous demonstrations against Governor Wilson's veto of AB 101 in the fall of 1991 (see later discussion and Chapter 4).

ANOTHER NATIONAL STAGE FOR ACT UP/LA: THE OSCARS ACTION

ACT UP/LA members began planning an action directed at the Academy Awards – otherwise known as "the Oscars" – in late January/early February of 1991. In an unsigned four-page proposal to the GB, the protest proponents argued that Hollywood had neglected the AIDS epidemic; that Hollywood movies sent out "racist, homophobic and anti-women" messages; and that the Oscars themselves "epitomize Hollywood at its most superficial and irresponsible level."[124] The members proposing an Oscars action made three basic demands: (1) that Hollywood become "more responsible" about portraying the AIDS crisis; (2) that changes be made in national healthcare and that Los Angeles be a laboratory for that change; and (3) that the media stop hiding "behind the glamour of the Oscars."[125] ACT UP/LA actually mailed "Silence=Death" buttons adorned with rhinestones to Academy members two weeks before the ceremony, asking them to wear the button at the awards.

Los Angeles, as no one needs reminding, is one of the centers of global entertainment production. Angelenos and transplants alike refer to the entertainment industry simply as "The Industry," as if there wasn't any other in the area. The Oscars, the signature self-congratulatory awards show hosted by the Academy of Motion Picture Arts and Sciences (AMPAS), has been held in Los Angeles since 1929.[126] While the oft-repeated estimates that one billion people watch the awards broadcast is a serious exaggeration, the Oscars ceremony is still one of the most watched events broadcast on American television, and the festivities receive a great deal of local press.[127] AMPAS held its sixty-third annual Oscars ceremony on March 25, 1991, at the Shrine Auditorium in downtown Los Angeles. According to the *Los Angeles Times*, "(i)n the wake of the Persian Gulf War, security was tight at the Shrine Auditorium. ... The Shrine had been checked by teams of bomb-sniffing dogs, and the 6,000 formally dressed guests were guided through metal detectors before entering."[128] The *Times* did

---

[124] ACT UP/LA, "Proposal for National Action." c. February 1991 – Unsigned four page proposal laying out the rationale for the Oscars action. Quote is from page 1. Author's collection.

[125] Ibid., p. 2.

[126] http://oscar.go.com/oscar-history/year/1929

[127] On the "one billion viewers" myth, see Daniel Radosh, "One Billion" *The New Yorker*, February 28, 2005, at http://www.newyorker.com/archive/2005/02/28/050228ta_talk_radosh.

[128] Nina J. Easton, "Dances with Wolves, Irons, Bates Win Oscars," *The Los Angeles Times*, March 26, 1991, http://articles.latimes.com/print/1991-03-26/news/mn-916_1_supporting-role (accessed July 10, 2012).

not report that security had been breached – by two ACT UP/LA protestors who infiltrated the auditorium. One of them loudly, if briefly, interrupted the telecast. Nor did the *Times* say much about the fifty ACT UP/LA protestors who swarmed the red carpet area outside the Shrine, where they held up posters of the Oscar statuette half covered by a condom, "with the caption AIDS-PHOBIA – PROTECT YOURSELF FROM HOLLYWOOD."[129] ACT UP/LA protestors also handed out "Silence=Death" buttons to actors and actresses going into the ceremony. Only actress Susan Sarandon was photographed wearing hers into the awards, although actor Bruce Davison reportedly wore his button throughout the ceremony.[130]

While the Oscars action received little coverage in the local mainstream media, the event was written about in the lesbian and gay press and in the entertainment newspapers *The Daily Variety* and *The Hollywood Reporter*. *Daily Variety* writers appeared to have actually spoken to the ACT UP/LA protestors, quoting ACT UP/LA spokesperson Dwayne Turner extensively about the rationale for the protest. Referring to the independent film "Longtime Companion" and the Oscar-winning documentary "Common Threads" (about the Names Project AIDS memorial quilt), *Daily Variety* reported that protestors unfurled a banner outside the Shrine that read "102,000 Plus Dead From AIDS – Two Films Not Enough." Turner was quoted as saying that "lots of stars coming here tonight live in LA County. We need their voices and their help to speak out to County officials about helping increase the budget for fighting AIDS."[131]

David Lacaillade was the protestor who actually got in, and he was able to shout out "102,000 dead!" before he was grabbed by security. Lacaillade's disruption was heard by others in the auditorium, but it came at a break during the television coverage and was not heard by those watching the ceremony live on television. Lacaillade wrote about his experience for the April/May 1991 *ACT UP News*:

I was seized by security guards, half-carried, half-dragged out of the orchestra through the lobby to the north end of the building, pushed face forward against the wall, and handcuffed. I was asked whether I was intoxicated. I was asked what grudge I had against Chevy Chase, [the] show presentation I interrupted. I was asked how I had gotten into the Shrine. I was frisked several times for knives until an officer of the Los Angeles

---

[129] Bruce Mirken, "Best ACT UP Award at the Oscars Show" *LA Reader*, March 29, 1991. Mirken's article and others were collated and distributed as an "Oscars Media Coverage Packet" to the General Body; ONE collection and author's collection.

[130] In the "Oscars Media Coverage Packet," Sarandon's photo appeared in clipped form, taken from the *Daily News* (the San Fernando Valley paper) on March 26, 1991. Davison had appeared in one of the first films to address the AIDS crisis, "Longtime Companion." Terri Ford and Judy Sisneros participated in the action and wrote about it for the ACT UP/LA *News* as "Lights! Camera! AIDS Action Now! ACT UP Hits the Oscars," (4:2, April/May 1991, p. 1).

[131] Amy Dawes and Claudia Eller, "Security Tight, Skies Clear, Traffic Smooth at Shrine," *Daily Variety* March 3, 1991. In "Oscars Media Coverage Packet." Author's collection.

Police Department pointed out to excited Shrine security guards that I had already passed through a metal detector upon admittance and therefore could not have smuggled in a weapon.[132]

Lacaillade was held by security for a short time until the producer of the Oscars telecast, Gil Cates, came forward to make a citizen's arrest.[133] The charge against him, "disturbing an assembly without authority of law, a misdemeanor," was later rejected by the LA City Attorney.[134] At least three of the activists I interviewed, Judy Sisneros, Terri Ford, and Cat Walker, participated in the action, Walker from the inside of the auditorium as support for Lacaillade; once Lacaillade was arrested, Walker recalled wondering what he was supposed to do at that point, and, worried about security finding him, he left.

Walker may not have been able to enjoy the show, but the Oscars action was regarded as a success by ACT UP/LA members despite the fact that it was not directed at a particular authority; it was more like the Rose Parade action than one at the Board of Supervisors. But ACT UP/LA members intended for the Oscars action to make the group visible to a local elite; in that sense, the Oscars was a local action, with the potential for having a national audience hear an anti-AIDS message merely a bonus. The Oscars action actually drew participants from other ACT UPs, and having the Oscars as a target seemed to foster creativity in tactics; one allied affinity group involved several protestors who turned up at the post-Oscars Governors' Ball disguised as waiters, putting "Action=Life" stickers on programs as well as sneaking fact sheets about AIDS statistics in LA County into programs as they were handed to ball-goers.

Through the Oscars action, ACT UP/LA turned the staging grounds inside and outside the ceremony into a temporary space for communicating their messages about what the entertainment industry should be doing for PWAs and for lesbian and gay people. Writing in the ACT UP/LA *News*, Terri Ford and Judy Sisneros noted that huge amounts of money were spent on films, amounts that dwarfed the annual County budget for AIDS programs of just under $14 million. Ford and Sisneros promised ACT UP/LA sympathizers that "Hollywood's silence on AIDS is no longer acceptable . . . and Hollywood will be reminded of it until something is done."[135]

PRISONERS' RIGHTS: ACT UP/LA IN THE ACT UP/CALIFORNIA COALITION

Working as part of a statewide coalition "ACT UP California," ACT UP/LA followed up on the local action against the Frontera Women's Prison in May

---

[132] David Lacaillade, "Shrine Tours Interrupts Oscars, ACT UP/LA Member Arrested," ACT UP *News* 4:2 (April/May 1991), p. 6.
[133] Lacaillade, p. 6.
[134] Ford and Sisneros, p. 8; Lacaillade, p. 6.
[135] Ford and Sisneros, p. 8.

1991, when members went up to the state capital of Sacramento to protest on behalf of prisoners with AIDS in California institutions. Protestors picketed and lobbied at the State Capitol building and held a sit-in at the offices of the James Gomez, Director of the Department of Corrections, and Dr. Nadim Khoury, Assistant Deputy Director of Health Care Services.[136] The protestors demanded a long list of changes to better the conditions of all HIV-positive prisoners in the state, but special attention was paid to the situation of women prisoners housed at Frontera. ACT UP/LA distributed a four-page informational handout, which included a page listing the sources for the statistics cited and drew from a 1989 US Department of Justice report on "AIDS in Correctional Facilities," as well as the series on prison abuses that had recently appeared in the _Orange County Register_.

Conditions for HIV-positive prisoners in California's huge system were generally abysmal. Prisoners known to be HIV-positive were sent to one of four prisons. At the Vacaville prison's California Medical Facility (CMF), segregated prisoners lacked general prison privileges, and inmates formally complained about lack of adequate care, insensitivity by staff who had no education about AIDS issues, and inconsistencies in their treatment. At the women's segregated ward at Frontera Walker A, the situation was considerably worse; the infirmary was still not licensed, which meant that no outside monitoring of the care given there was done. Segregated women prisoners lacked access to work furlough and education programs, and they were not allowed to use the _library_ at the prison. They were also denied visiting rights. Worse still, from a civil liberties perspective, female HIV-positive prisoners were segregated in Walker A whether or not they were actually ill.[137] In response to these conditions, ACT UP/California made twenty-eight different far-ranging demands that were circulated prior to and at a legal picket on May 6, 1991, outside the Capitol Building.[138] The legal picket was accompanied by civil disobedience, a teach-in, a rally, a fundraiser art auction, and parties in San Francisco on the nights leading up to the picket. Organizers had wanted the legal picket to be very large; about one hundred people showed up, with perhaps fifty, including me, coming from ACT UP/LA. ACT UP/California announced that the legal picket would be "aggressive and boisterous," and it was, despite the small turnout.[139]

The Sacramento actions on prisoners' rights were propelled forward by the local struggle by ACT UP/LA over Frontera. After the November 1990 Frontera demonstration, ACT UP/LA had presented officials with specific demands aimed at improving the conditions in Walker A.[140] The statewide coordination of the

[136] ACT UP California. "Prisoners & AIDS: Some Facts," handout c. May 1991. Author's collection.

[137] "Prisoners & AIDS: Some Facts," ibid.

[138] ACT UP California, "ACT UP Demands." Flyer c. May 1991. Author's collection.

[139] ACT UP/LA. Flyer announcing May 6th Sacramento protest. Author's collection.

[140] Bruce Merkin, "'AIDS Is a Disaster! Prisoners Die Faster!'" ACT UP/LA _News_ 4:3 (June–July 1991), p. 1

Sacramento actions was planned to put more pressure on the state and the Department of Corrections to remedy problems being caused by policies of neglect, or conversely, hypercaution through segregation. But the legal picket was not where the real action occurred; at the same time, ACT UP/LA conducted some "unannounced" civil disobedience by occupying the offices of the Director of the Department of Corrections and the Assistant Deputy Director of Health Care Services for the department. Nineteen activist were charged with disturbing the peace and vandalism.[141] Later in the day, Khoury actually met with a small group of the released demonstrators, all the while denying that the suddenly scheduled meeting had anything to do with the sit-in. Khoury apparently promised ACT UP a response to its demands within a month.

There was also an "unexpected surprise" that occurred about one hour into the legal picket, one that was not seen by the legal picketers who remained outside:

A group of nine ACT UP members had gone into the capitol rotunda, intending to do some attention-getting changes. As they were getting ready, none other than Ronald Reagan entered on his way to visit state legislators. The former president was applauded by many in the room, including a group of visiting schoolchildren. The ACT UPpers pointed at Reagan and chanted, "Murderer! Murderer!" apparently startling him. "His face dropped," said one witness.[142]

In addition to the disruptive tactics, ACT UP/LA members coordinated with the LIFE Lobby, a lesbian and gay rights lobbying group, and visited California state legislators' aides, among them, the aide to State Senator Ed Davis, the former LAPD police chief who sponsored a bill that would have created criminal penalties for HIV-positive individuals who engaged in sex without informing partners of their HIV status. They also visited with the aide to State Senator Robert Presley, who was working on a bill restructuring the prison health system to give each prison's chief medical officer control over healthcare decisions (as opposed to the warden). Not surprisingly, the second legislative aide was reported to be much more sympathetic to his visitors' concerns.

THE SUMMER OF 1991: ONGOING CONCERNS AND NEW MONEY

After their successful spring actions, ACT UP/LA was largely in planning mode during the summer of 1991. Members continued to work on prisoner's issues; they planned fundraisers; they sold t-shirts, pins, and stickers at lesbian and gay pride parades and festivals; and they networked with local groups bent on social justice. The County of Los Angeles continued to be a target of the group's wrath, as the public health establishment still fell short of promises made to the community about AIDS care. ACT UP/LA member Jeff Neff spoke at the

---

[141] Merkin, ibid.
[142] Merkin, ibid.

dedication of the new freestanding County AIDS Comprehensive Outpatient Clinic on June 3, 1991, as ACT UP/LA members distributed a leaflet entitled "This Clinic Is Built on a Fault."[143] In the leaflet, ACT UP/LA took the County public health officials to task for unconscionably long waiting times for appointments, for delays in establishing the clinic, and for continuing staffing problems at the twenty-bed dedicated AIDS ward at the County/USC hospital.[144] Fueling ACT UP/LA's ire about the County's foot-dragging was the fact that the June "dedication" of the clinic was actually *not* the opening of the clinic to patients. Ty Geltmaker, who had been attending AIDS Community Advisory Council meetings, reported that the clinic would probably not receive patients for another month due to contractor delays and the need for a state inspection. Geltmaker also reported that the dedicated AIDS ward at the County/USC hospital was in trouble; the number of available beds had been cut due to staff shortages, and the nurse manager at the ward had conceded that "AIDS hysteria has made it harder to recruit" staff for the ward.[145]

Sometime in the middle of 1991, ACT UP/LA and other ACT UPs received a new source of funding: monies began coming in from the AIDS charity "Red Hot + Blue." The first Red Hot + Blue album was one of the first benefit albums in the music industry designed to raise money for AIDs organizations. The album consisted of Cole Porter songs covered by contemporary recording artists, as Porter was in the process of being reclaimed as a gay icon.[146] According to a February 1991 report to the ACT UP/LA GB by Mark Kostopoulos, anti-AIDS activist groups were promised something between $300,000 and $600,000 (or about a third of the profits) from the first Red Hot + Blue (RHB) album.[147] Kostopoulos reported on discussions being held among AIDS service organizations, activist groups, and the Red Hot organization regarding how to split the monies raised by the sale of the album; these discussions generally focused on whether to consider regional AIDS case loads in distributing funds or whether another metric, like size of membership, should be considered. Kostopoulos pointed out that whatever the agreed-upon distribution, decisions would have to be made about what constituted a qualifying group. ACT UP/LA would receive some money; Kostopoulos estimated that, depending on what was decided, the group would see anywhere from $4,000 to $40,000 from the proceeds.

---

[143] Minutes, General Body meeting, June 3 1991. Collection of the author.

[144] ACT UP/LA "This Clinic Is Built on a Fault," Leaflet dated June 3 1991; ONE Collection.

[145] Ty Geltmaker, "Hospital Update," June 10, 1991, report to the General Body. Collection of the author.

[146] The Red Hot organization continued to produce other benefit albums (Marco R. della Cava, "Red, Hot + Blue Stays on Its Mission," *USA Today*, February 23, 2009, http://usatoday30 .usatoday.com/life/music/news/2009-02-23-red-hot-blue_N.htm accessed March 25, 2013; see also www.redhot.org.)

[147] Mark Kostopoulos, "Red Hot and Blue," February, 11, 1991. Collection of the author.

The RHB monies represented a major influx of resources for direct action anti-AIDS groups – after all, they were being considered for funding along with AIDS service organizations – but figuring out how to distribute the monies was a challenge for the loosely organized network of anti-AIDS organizations; the ACT UPs' decentralized structure was not conducive to making a decision about how to take a large sum of money from a benefactor. In April 1991, ACT UP/NY activists Eric Nowlin and Ann Northrup sent a packet of information to other ACT UPs about the RHB money in which they detailed what they knew about Red Hot from their meetings with the producers. The packet contained Kostopoulos's discussion of the pros and cons of the various distribution schemes and his questions about how to actually make a decision that was democratic and fair.[148] Nowlin and Northrup seemed aware of the democratic challenge that the money presented and argued that the monies should be dispersed with "the full involvement of every ACT UP/AIDS activist organization involved." They also told other ACT UPs that the only reasons that they were writing about the Red Hot money was because the album's producers contacted them, and they stated that "(u)ltimately we must collectively agree to a process that will work for us all."

In July 1991, Kostopoulos and representatives from ACT UP/New York, ACT UP/San Francisco, and ACT UP/Golden Gate wrote a letter to "all ACT UPs and AIDS activist organizations in the US" advocating the formation of a "Red, Hot and Blue" committee that would "consider all existing and future proposals submitted by the chapter for the distribution of Red Hot and Blue funds, and . . . formulate a final proposal . . . which would then be submitted to all the chapters in the US" in August.[149] The minutes of an ACT UP Network conference call suggests that RHB monies were available to ACT UPs after September 15, 1991, which means that the money was used to send activists to a series of actions deploring Bush and advocating for universal healthcare in Washington, DC, in September and October of 1991.[150] It is likely that ACT UP/LA received this initial and subsequent infusions of monies from the Red Hot project because the organization spun out new albums that continued to sell. As I discuss in Chapter 5, early concerns about the potentially disruptive effects of the Red Hot money were eventually borne out, at least for ACT UP/LA; as ACT UP/LA demobilized, the group later came to reject much needed Red Hot money because of feelings that decisions about distributions had been made undemocratically.

In the summer of 1991, ACT UP/LA continued to work on two issues – one national and one local – that would unexpectedly intertwine in the fall: the

---

[148] Eric Nowlin and Ann Northrup, "Red, Hot and Blue Letter to All ACT UPs," April 14, 1991, Collection of the author; Unsigned, "Proposed Response to RHB Letter," c. February 1991, ONE Collection.

[149] Mark Kostopoulos et al., "Creation of a 'Red Hot and Blue' Committee," Letter dated July 12, 1991, ONE Collection.

[150] Amy Meyer, "ACT UP Action Network Conference Call," July 10, 1991, ONE Collection.

October Washington, DC, protests against President Bush's inept leadership on AIDS and for universal healthcare, and the potential passage of California Assembly Bill 101 (AB 101), a measure designed to deal with discrimination against lesbians and gays. Planning for the universal healthcare rally began with conference calls between members of ACT UPs from fourteen different cities of the ACT UP Network. ACT UP/LA's Mark Kostopoulos was a point person in planning the rally, which was scheduled in coordination with actions by ACT UP/NY and ACT UP/DC.[151] Actions also needed to dovetail with the Second AIDS Treatment Activist Conference (also known as ATAC 2).[152] ACT UP/LA members had a prominent part in planning what would end up being five days of conferencing and activism (with up to 200 activists there for ATAC 2 alone).[153] While attending ATAC 2, Kostopoulos was quoted by a *Washington Post* reporter about the tension between those who counseled "time and patience" in dealing with Congress and those who wanted immediate change; Kostopoulos told the reporter that "[w]e've worked for three years to help change the way AIDS is thought about, but all our successes haven't changed the fact that people continue to die."[154]

The DC rally brought out the efforts of ACT UP/LA members dedicated to broader questions of healthcare provision and social justice. Kostopoulos, Gunther Freehill, Tony Arn, Saundra Johnson, Lamar Pugh, Don Rhine, Bill Flanagan, and Ferd Eggan put together a twenty-page "Handbook for Activists" around the universal healthcare demand.[155] The handbook, edited by Freehill, was a healthcare policy wonk's dream document. It detailed the ACT UP Network's demands, but also contained articles on the US's private/public health insurance system, recent Congressional proposals to deal with the healthcare system, a comparative view of "national health care systems in the industrialized world," and a glossary of the terms used. Any activist who read the handbook would have been well prepared to face reporters' or bystanders' questions.[156]

As ACT UP/LA planned for Washington, the effort to pass AB 101, which began in early 1991, continued into the fall. At the end of September, California

[151] Mark Kostopoulos, Letter to ACT UP/Network Members, July 13, 1991, ONE Collection; Amy Meyer, "ACT UP Action Network Conference Call," minutes, July 10, 1991; ONE Collection: "Time to Become an AIDS Activist," Flyer from ACT UP/DC c. September 1991; ONE Collection.

[152] "The 2nd ATAC 72 Hrs of AIDS Treatment Activism." Flyer from ACT UP/NY, c. September 1991; ONE Collection.

[153] Karlyn Barker, "Taking AIDS Battle to Capitol Hill," *The Washington Post*, September 29, 1991; ATAC 2. "About the Strategy Sessions." Flyer c. September 1991; ONE Collection.

[154] Barker, ibid.

[155] ACT UP Network. "Universal Health Care: A Handbook for Activists." October 1991. Collection of author. Many of the articles in the handbook also appeared in ACT UP/LA *News* 4:4 (September/October 1991).

[156] With updated statistics, the handbook would be useful reading for anyone seeking clarity in the 2009–2010 battle over the "Patient Protection and Affordable Care Act" (i.e., "Obamacare").

Governor Pete Wilson vetoed the bill, and widespread protest broke out; these protests had ramifications for ACT UP/LA as the group absorbed a new cohort of angry lesbians and gays who were new to direct action protest (see Chapter 4). All through the summer of 1991, ACT UP/LA members could find materials about AB 101's progress through the legislative process in Sacramento on the literature table, and updates about the bill were given at GB meetings. Several members of ACT UP/LA, notably Connie Norman, worked directly with the Life Lobby, which had an actual office in Sacramento and lobbied to get the bill through the legislature.[157] ACT UP/LA members were provided with talking points and a letter-writing template so that they could contact legislators. A rally was held in Los Angeles in mid-June to protest the imminent death of the bill, which had been placed in a "suspense file" pending the approval of a state budget.[158] Even QN, a group not known for their electoral efforts, goaded the community with a flyer headed by the question "do you care enough about your rights to make a few simple phone calls?"[159] Part of the outrage expressed by lesbians and gays when Wilson vetoed the bill was generated by expectations on behalf of many in the lesbian and gay community, including ACT UP/LA members, that AB 101 would become law.[160]

ACT UP/LA AND THE CATHOLIC CHURCH: LOCAL REVERBERATIONS OF ACT UP/NY'S STOP THE CHURCH CONTROVERSY

The latter half of 1991 saw a flare-up of the bad blood between ACT UP/LA and the local Catholic Church as a result of actions taken by ACT UP/NY. The Los Angeles Archdiocese tried to stop public television station KCET from airing a documentary entitled *Stop the Church*, which chronicled a December 1989 protest at Saint Patrick's Cathedral coordinated by ACT UP/NY and Women's Health Action and Mobilization (WHAM) against the Church's opposition to safe sex and abortion.[161] ACT UP/LA had struggled with the LA archdiocese over its opposition to safer sex education and the distribution of condoms, and there had been local protests that took place in tandem with the better known New York action.[162] ACT UP/LA picketed four Catholic

---

[157] The Life Lobby existed from about 1985 to 1998, was bipartisan, and was linked to other more "mainstream" lesbian and gay activist organizations. See http://lgbtpov.frontiersla.com/2011/02/24/eqca-history-part-3-life-lobby/ for a brief history.

[158] "AB 101 Letter Writing Guide." Handout c. June 1991. Collection of author. Flyer, "Rally A.B. 101," June 1991. Collection of author.

[159] Queer Nation. "Do You Care Enough About Your Rights to Make a Few Simple Phone Calls?" Flyer c. May 1991. Collection of author.

[160] For a general discussion of how the AB 101 demonstrations changed the landscape of lesbian and gay Los Angeles, see Kenney (2001) and Faderman and Timmons (2009).

[161] See Carroll (2015: 155–161) on the "Stop the Church" controversy in New York City.

[162] On the protest at St. Patrick's Cathedral, see http://www.actupny.org/YELL/stopchurch99 .html.

churches on a Sunday morning and distributed "health literature and condoms" to churchgoers.[163] ACT UP/LA members were especially galled by Cardinal Roger Mahony; Mahony was a popular figure in LA and liberal on many issues, but he was active in the National Council of Bishops who opposed safer sex education and condom distribution in schools.

National PBS had planned to screen *Stop the Church*, made by video artist Robert Hilferty for $4000, as part of its *POV* series; but, fresh from a controversy earlier in the year over airing Marlon Rigg's documentary on male black gay sexuality, *Tongues Untied*, they canceled the scheduled broadcast of Hilferty's documentary.[164] KCET actually went against the national decision and opted to show the film, in part due to considerable pressure it was receiving from the local lesbian and gay community; ACT UP/LA, QN, and Gay and Lesbian Alliance Against Defamation (GLAAD) were all planning to "zap" (tie up) the station's phone lines during its pledge drive if the documentary was not shown (Bullert 1997: 132).[165] KCET's executives decided to strategically package the video as part of a planned discussion of the controversy.[166] This move defused the phone zap threat but did not mollify the Archdiocese. When the station's compromise was made public in late August, the local Catholic Church was outraged and refused the station's invitation to be part of the broadcast (Bullert 1997: 134). The broadcast was delayed as the Church tried to stop it; at the same time, ACT UP/LA and other gay and lesbian groups lobbied the station to include filmmaker Hilferty as part of the broadcast. ACT UP/LA and others protested outside KCET's offices in Hollywood on August 27, the original date of the broadcast. On September 5, Cardinal Roger Mahony called a press conference denouncing KCET for Catholic-bashing and accusing the station of caving into "blackmail" from the lesbian and gay community.

Mahony and the Church took out ads in the *Los Angeles Times* and the *Los Angeles Daily News* urging KCET viewers to re-evaluate their relationship with the station; one KCET board member resigned, taking nearly $100,000 in pledges with him (Bullert 1997:135). *Current*, a magazine devoted to public broadcasting issues, reported that Mahony's anti-KCET campaign was like "a rhetorical H-bomb" fired at KCET.[167] ACT UP/LA countered the cardinal's

---

[163] ACT UP/LA. "ACT UP Attacks Archbishop's Reversal on Safe Sex Education," Press release dated December 8, 1989; ONE collection.

[164] For a detailed examination of the *Stop the Church* controversy see, B. J. Bullert, 1997, *Public Television: Politics & the Battle over Documentary Film*, New Brunswick, NJ: Rutgers University Press, chapter 6.

[165] ACT UP/LA, "What Does It Take to Make You Angry?" Flyer, c. August 1991, ONE Collection; Terri M. Ford, "'Stop the Church' – Stop the Censorship," *Frontiers* September 13, 1991, p. 27.

[166] Sharon Bernstein, "'Stop the Church' to Be Part of KCET Special," *Los Angeles Times*, August 21, 1991.

[167] Steve Behrens. 1991. "Cardinal Blasts Airing of Documentary: Like Some Viewers, He's No Fan of Point-of-View Shows." *Current*, originally published September 9 1991, accessed online March 21, 2013, at http://www.current.org/wp-content/themes/current/archive-site.

press conference with a press release of its own that chided the Church for having the temerity to criticize the lesbian and gay community for engaging in pressure tactics to get the video shown while the Church used the same pressure tactics to stop the broadcast.[168] KCET did air *Stop the Church* on September 6, packaged with a panel discussion about the controversy; no one from the Church participated, and ACT UP/LA urged others in the anti-AIDS community not to participate because of KCET's failure to invite Hilferty.[169] KCET actually showed taped footage of the Mahoney press conference as part of their broadcast. While the KCET package was eventually shown on WNET/ New York and other public television stations late at night, after prime time (Bullert 1997: 140), KCET lost more than $50,000 in contributions from the board member who resigned, and three hundred subscribers cancelled their subscriptions.[170]

The lesbian and gay press covered the *Stop the Church* controversy, as did the *Los Angeles Times*. The *Times* printed thirteen letters to the editor about KCET and the controversy surrounding *Stop the* Church, including two from ACT UP/LA members Jim McDaniels and Mark Kostopoulos.[171] The *Times* also printed a co-authored op-ed piece by Gunther Freehill and AIDS Healthcare Foundation personnel director Eliseo Acevedo Martinez, in which Freehill and Martinez urged Cardinal Mahony to "admit that the Church is not doing all it can to stop the AIDS epidemic." They criticized the Church's contradictory stance of preventing safer sex information from getting to parishioners and, at the same time, running hospices for PWAs. Notably, Freehill and Acevedo Martinez were critical of ACT UP/LA for making the protest against the Church unduly personal and warned activists that "being offensive is not necessarily being effective."[172]

---

[168] ACT UP/LA, "ACT UP/LA Condemns Cardinal Roger Mahony's Censorship," Press release c. August 1991 and distributed at the August 19 General Body meeting; ONE collection.

[169] ACT UP/LA. Letter dated September 2, 1991 from ACT UP/LA; ONE collection.

[170] Sharon Bernstein, "KCET Pays Price in Flap with Church," *Los Angeles Times* October 10, 1991, pp. F1, F10. ACT UP/LA received at least one letter refusing to donate to the group on the basis of its support for showing Stop the Church (Yolanda Arias, Letter to ACT UP/LA, September 13, 1991, ONE Collection).

[171] "Letters to the Times: Controversy over ACT UP Film," *Los Angeles Times* September 13, 1991.

[172] Gunther Freehill and Eliseo Acevedo Martinez, "Blasphemy, Lies, Videotape: The Encounter Over AIDS: Public TV: Cardinal Mahoney, Gay Activist and KCET Are All Less Than Honest in Their Positions on 'Stop the Church,'" *Los Angeles Times*, September 13, 1991. The *Times* later published pieces by Alexander Cockburn and ACT UP/NY's Spencer Cox that defended the protests against the church and by George Weigel and Cardinal Mahony that defended the church's actions. (Alexander Cockburn "Unchallenged, the Censors Will Prevail," *Los Angeles Times* September 20, 1991; George Weigel, "KCET's Action: The Antithesis of Freedom," *Los Angeles Times* September 20, 1991; "Commentary: Catholic Policy on AIDS Programs: Acts of War or Love?" *Los Angeles Times* October 5 1991, p. F14.)

CONCLUSION: REFLECTING BACK ON FOUR YEARS
OF CONTENTION

By the fourth anniversary of ACT UP/LA's founding in December 1991, its members were beginning to look back to assess their accomplishments. In fundraising letters, the group emphasized its commitment to direct action and listed evidence of its effectiveness in getting authorities to address all areas of the AIDS crisis, from public health provision, to housing, to basic research, to PWA care provision and education in LA schools.[173] The December 1991/January 1992 issue of ACT UP/LA *News* featured a joint interview by Jim McDaniels of "three active members who were present at the very first meeting: David Lee Perkins, Mark Kostopoulos and Peter Cashman."[174] The three veterans stressed ACT UP/LA's accomplishments. Kostopoulos told McDaniels that:

> Our accomplishments are both tangible and intangible. I frankly think the intangible are more important. We've made AIDS a political issue and certainly the way the Gay and Lesbian community thinks about AIDS is very different now than four years ago. … There are concrete accomplishments too. The whole drug approval process has been completely revamped … there's an AIDS ward and outpatient clinic at County Hospital.

Perkins shared his view about the tangible accomplishments of ACT UP/LA:

> There's the West Hollywood HIV Clinic which would be run by the Gay and Lesbian Services Center had we not put pressure on the county Health Department. In Frontera … we have gotten an HIV doctor for the women who didn't even have a competent doctor in the first place, and even an AIDS library at the prison. We have been instrumental in forming ACT UP chapters in the Central Valley, Orange County and Long Beach.

And Peter Cashman, a native of Tasmania, stated that "even in Sydney Australia we were very instrumental in the formation of ACT UP."

But even as they lauded ACT UP/LA's accomplishments, the three men's responses to the question of whether they were themselves – all three were HIV-positive – living longer because of their involvement in ACT UP/LA reflected three different assessments of the personal consequences of activism and highlighted how a diversity of politics within the group was managed. Cashman stated that, despite some breaks in his involvement with the group, "I always feel better when I'm around ACT UP." Perkins attributed his continued good health to his rejection of denial around his HIV status and the opportunity for action that ACT UP gave him. Kostopoulos, who would be dead in half a year, told McDaniels that

---

[173] Richard L. Beeker and Joshua Wells, "Dear Friend," Letter, September 1991. Beeker and Wells were co-facilitators of the Fundraising/Finance committee; ONE Collection.

[174] Jim McDaniels, "Interview with Three Founding Members of ACT UP/LA," ACT UP/LA *News*, 4:5 (December 1991/January 1992), pp. 6–7.

some say that AIDS activism is killing me. . . . I think the reality is that it doesn't matter. The point is the quality of my life. Certainly the activism I've engaged in has made for an amazing four years. I would not trade them away for anything. That's the point.

From 1987 on, ACT UP/LA had given direct action anti-AIDS activists in Los Angeles a community with whom to fight. Started by elements within the lesbian and gay progressive community in coalition with others, ACT UP/LA's general body plus committee structure was designed to maximize participation and generalize decision-making while accommodating differences in interest. Participants avoided formalization of any aspect of the group, especially of leadership, but they could not prevent the existence of charismatic informal leadership, such as the kind provided by Mark Kostopoulos. ACT UP/LA members worked on an ambitious membership-driven agenda and oscillated between ongoing local struggles with homegrown adversaries and nationally coordinated actions.

Conceiving their unity as a result of coalition of those in the anti-AIDS community with different interests, ACT UP/LA began to face the internal challenge posed by members who wished to organize on the basis of an ascribed identity – that of women. Beginning in mid-1990, the ACT UP/LA Women's Caucus, a part of and apart from the GB, organized to put women's AIDS issues on ACT UP/LA's agenda. In the next chapter, I examine the formation of ACT UP/LA's Women's Caucus and show how the WC's founding members used the WC to make women's AIDS issues visible to the rest of the group. The WC, which faced endemic problems as women working in a male-dominated organization, always needed the support of men from the GB to achieve its aims. With the next chapter, and Chapter 4, which examines intersectional crises of heterogeneity in ACT UP/LA, I begin to tell a story about the group's trajectory as influenced by structural inequalities that activists confronted as they struggled together against AIDS.

3

Battling for Women's Issues and Women's Visibility in ACT UP/LA

Women in this male-dominated society sometimes have the sensation that they are invisible, that they exist in the shadows while men take center stage – at work, in politics, in science, in the media, and even in our minds.

– Gina Corea (1992)

It [ACT UP] was really exciting ... the thing that was a bit intimidating is that it was, you know 98% men ... and that there were hardly any women. But the women were very incredibly inspiring ...

– Judy Sisneros[1]

WHY FORM A WOMEN'S CAUCUS? THE CONFLUENCE OF INTEREST AND IDENTITY

In late January/early February of 1990, the question of sexism within the AIDS Coalition to Unleash Power, Los Angeles (ACT UP/LA) showed up as an agenda item at General Body (GB) meetings. An unsigned position paper was distributed entitled "SEXISM IN ACT UP/LA."[2] The authors of the paper stated that

[w]e, as women, want to continue with our commitment to ACT UP/LA, its philosophy and its goals. We are, however, concerned that unless we, as an organization, tackle the problem of sexism, that ACT UP may be affected in a serious and detrimental way.

A list of examples of sexism followed, including the group's failure to address matters involving women and HIV/AIDS; tokenism in assigning tasks; personal attacks on women; and what the authors described as "(p)assive acceptance of sexism," which was defined as the acceptance of sexist behavior by others. Mark Kostopoulos responded to the position paper, airing his concerns that

---

[1] Judy Sisneros, interview with author, 2000.
[2] "Sexism IN ACT UP/LA." Unsigned document c. late January 1990; ONE collection.

"conscious efforts to place women in positions of visibility and authority" not be taken as tokenism.[3] Kostopoulos agreed that ACT UP/LA's women were doing a disproportionate amount of the work on women's AIDS issues, stating that "[w]omen historically have done the nuts and bolts work that keep society going while men were given the more flashy roles."

Kostopoulos's favorable reaction to women organizing as women within ACT UP/LA was not universally shared. Diversity within a social movement organization is generally seen as a challenge by participants (Agustin and Roth 2011), and without a self-conscious, deliberate, and concrete organizational approach to the making of "inclusive solidarity" (Ferree and Roth 1998), social movement organizations run the risk of fracture and factionalization. As noted in Chapter 2, ACT UP/LA had been able to capture the energy of lesbians and gays who wanted to take direct action against AIDS by emulating ACT UP/NY's committee structure, a structure built on the interests and experiences of participants. The interest-based committee structure was also a porous one; individuals could move from committee to committee. But, somehow, a women's caucus challenged ACT UP/LA's interest-based committee structure in way that the already existing People with Immune System Disorders (PISD) caucus did not.

Although the women who formed the Women's Caucus (WC) were dedicated to the GB even as they were frustrated by the sexism they found there, their loyalty to the GB was questioned. Jeri Deitrick, a highly active ACT UP/LA participant who helped organize the WC, saw it as a way to "be as powerful as the men's group" and "have a women's take on everything."[4] She remembered that forming the WC – and designating it as women's space– caused "a lot of animosity between" the WC and the GB, with some men calling the women "supremacists."[5] This name-calling drove Deitrick "crazy" as she tried to maintain her close ties with ACT UP/LA men and accommodate lesbian separatists who wanted to do anti-AIDS work.

Deitrick wasn't imagining male displeasure at the WC's formation. In his interview in 2000, Gunther Freehill, another highly active ACT UP/LA participant, stated that while he identified as a feminist, he was wary of the formation of internal caucuses of any sort:

I think that part of problem that I had with the Women's Caucus politically was my commitment to the room ... in the early days of ACT UP, the room was all powerful ... having people walk in the room and having equal vote and having equal say. ... Part of the problem I had with the Women's Caucus was that they would like go off by themselves and make decisions and then they weren't subject to discussion. ... And depending on your view of the politics of it, that's either okay because that puts women in charge of their destinies or it's not okay, because it cuts

---

[3] Mark Kostopoulos, "Sexism Discussion." Document dated February 5, 1990; ONE collection.
[4] Interview with author, 2000.
[5] Interview with author, 2000.

the power of the room. And I think we never had a really thorough balance of those two issues.

Freehill is right that the WC would go off and make decisions by themselves that weren't subject to discussion; the WC women were accorded a great deal of deference by the larger and mostly male GB. However, there were reasons that ACT UP/LA men deferred to WC women. The WC represented the confluence of identity difference and interest difference; the WC women asserted a set of different interests *based on* their gender identity. In a group where "solidarity [was] based on emotional experiences of identity in the sense of a 'sameness of selves' and feeling 'at home'" (Ferree and Roth 1998: 628), the WC's assertion of difference was disruptive, and both WC and ACT UP/LA members struggled with the meaning of the internal boundary that the WC created.

In this chapter, I examine the gender politics that were involved in the formation and maintenance of ACT UP/LA's Women's Caucus. I examine how feminist women in ACT UP/LA, a "feminist-friendly" organization (Roth 1998) organized. The WC had some strong successes in ACT UP/LA, but maintaining a feminist women's voice was a continuous struggle. In examining the WC members' attempts to create a women's voice in ACT UP/LA. I extend Taylor and Whittier's (1992: 111) concept of "boundary-making," the process by which a dominated group sets itself apart from the mainstream, to dynamics internal to ACT UP/LA. The WC's boundary-making efforts were legitimized by ACT UP/LA's feminist-friendly political stance, and the creation of the caucus itself allowed feminist women to draw on (and draw out) the support of actively feminist ACT UP/LA men. I argue that the boundary that WC members drew between themselves and the rest of the organization had the effect of moving them closer to the organization's center, but that this process was nonetheless fraught and that maintaining a boundary was never easy. I explore how WC members maintained boundaries between the GB and themselves by using a "policy" of the WC as women's space, as well as interactional strategies of "counting men" and reminding men that there were "women present." WC members became legitimated in the group as ACT UP/LA's "official women"; this ultimately resulted in the unintended outcome of "compartmentalization," the process by which ACT UP/LA's official women took on an increasingly larger share of the burden of representation of and activism on behalf of women. Ultimately, the WC reshaped the trajectory of ACT UP/LA as a group; while WC members couldn't accomplish large parts of their agenda without the larger (male) group's help, at the same time, the formation of the WC represented the point in time after which it would become impossible for ACT UP/LA members to take actions without thinking about gendered politics.

LAYERS OF WOMEN'S (IN)VISIBILITY IN THE AIDS EPIDEMIC
AND THE ANTI-AIDS MOVEMENT

> Being a lesbian is therefore a cultural struggle to break through silence and invisibility: we have ourselves only as battering rams. For many of us being out is high risk activity. Measure that against the public profile of gay men.[6]

> "Sam" mentions that *The Advocate* is now calling itself a gay *and* lesbian magazine. "That's right," Maurice says, "lesbians have earned the right to be on the masthead . . . that's what I heard them [friends working at the magazine] say."[7]

In 1990–1991, women made up approximately 40% of AIDS cases worldwide; some estimated that the figure would be 60% by the year 2000.[8] Although the statistics themselves were subject to contestation by feminist anti-AIDS activists, the demographics of the US epidemic were quite different. In 1990, women accounted for approximately 11% of all AIDS cases, with a disproportionate number of those affected being women of color.[9] Feminist activists were challenged by several visibility problems in their fight to have others recognize women as people living with AIDS at a time when all anti-AIDS activists were fighting to make AIDS visible as a health crisis. Anti-AIDS activists drew contrasts between media neglect of AIDS and the tremendous amount of media coverage other health crises like the Tylenol poisoning scare of 1982 received. As Corea (1992: 16–17) has noted, by the time of the October 1982 Tylenol scare, which claimed seven lives, more than eight hundred people were officially dead from AIDS, deaths that were marked in the pages of the gay and lesbian press and virtually ignored in the mainstream press and major wire services.

Beyond the invisibility of the AIDS crisis, a second layer of invisibility descended on women in the United States dealing with HIV disease. By 1991, the Centers for Disease Control (CDC) estimated that about 100,000 women in the United States were HIV-positive (Corea (1992: 327–328, note 3). Activists argued that since the CDC definition of the opportunistic infections and other symptoms associated with HIV disease did not include female-specific ones, there were more women's deaths from AIDS than were officially counted. Activists argued that researchers only paid attention to women as "vectors" of HIV transmission – to men and to babies – and did not to see them as people with AIDS (PWAs) in need of treatment themselves. Women who were HIV-positive were stigmatized as prostitutes – and prostitutes were further stigmatized as AIDS carriers (Alexander 1994). Because most HIV-positive women were heterosexual, they lacked the support of the increasingly well-organized lesbian and gay male

---

[6] N. Field, 1990, "Picturing Safer Sex for Lesbians," *Square Peg*, p. 29, cited in Altman (1994:48).
[7] Author's field notes, "Women and AIDS," Teach-in, November 17, 1990.
[8] Corea 1992:327–328, note 3.
[9] Anne C. Rourke, "Research Office for Women's Health Answers Complaint of Bias in Research," *The Los Angeles Times*, November 11, 1990, pp. A1, 40.

community and were even more closeted – even more invisible to the general public and to the AIDS community – than HIV-positive men (Corea 1992: 59; see also Mitchell 1992; Scharf and Toole 1992). Feminist anti-AIDS activists began battling for recognition of alarming trends in women's relationship to HIV because, by 1990, AIDS was spreading among women at a faster rate than among men (Schneider and Stoller 1994: 7).

The lack of visibility of HIV-positive women and female PWAs had real consequences for their treatment or, more accurately, their non-treatment. Women's lack of visibility led to a consequent lack of resources to help women who were HIV-positive, both from government and other establishment sources, and from organizations within the AIDS service community (Scharf and Toole (1992). Women of color – who had (and have) poorer access to healthcare generally – were disproportionately affected by the disease; 21 percent of women dying of AIDS were Latinas, and 53 percent were African American, with the death rate from the disease nine times higher among African-American women than among white women (Schneider and Stoller 1994: 7). Congruent with the "woman as HIV vector" approach, research done on women with HIV/AIDS was done on pregnant women, with "virtually nothing known medically about AIDS in nonpregnant women" (Schneider and Stoller 1994: 8). It was not until 1993 that the CDC listed female-specific infections as part of the definition of AIDS after much intensive activism on the part of ACT UP women and other women's health activists (Schneider and Stoller 1994: 8).

Another layer of invisibility for women in the AIDS crisis involved the role of lesbians as activists in the anti-AIDS movement. Visibility has been both a central metaphor and a central demand in gay and lesbian activism (Adam 1987: Armstrong 2002; Crimp 1990; Ghaziani 2008) as the gay liberation/gay rights movement sought to bring homosexuality "out of the closet." Lesbians and gays sought the privileges of full "sexual citizenship" (Seidman 2005); that is, the recognition of lesbian and gay experiences and the conferring of a full array of long-denied civil rights. Because of the demographics of the US AIDS epidemic, making AIDS visible was inextricably linked to making gay and lesbian lives visible. For most anti-AIDS activists, including those in ACT UPs, responding to the epidemic meant changing governmental and drug company priorities and removing the stigma that attached to homosexuality. Many ACT UP actions were directly aimed at making demonstrators visible to a general public beyond targeted authorities, therefore countering the heterosexual neglect that rendered gays and HIV-positive persons invisible (Gamson 1989).

Within the (activist) lesbian and gay community, however, lesbian invisibility had been a continuous source of tension (Adam 1987; Phelan 1989: 37; Stein 1992). Lesbian feminist identity in particular was subject to different forces than gay male activist identity. For example, as Second Wave radical feminism expanded the pool of women open to their lesbianism (Stein 1992), some lesbian feminist women became concerned with maintaining the boundaries of their community (Taylor and Whittier 1992). Some white lesbian feminists took a separatist turn, which of necessity resulted in some alienation from gay men and from organizing with gay men (Adam 1987:94; Phelan 1989; Duggan 1992; Stein 1992). While some have argued that AIDS brought lesbian women back into relationships with gay men as they cared for gay men and struggled beside them against the neglect of the epidemic (Hollibaugh 1994; Stein 1992; Mitchell 1992), others have asserted that lesbians were part of community debates about AIDS from the beginning of its emergence as a disease (Brier 2009; Stockdill 2003; Winnow 1992). Lesbian activists like Cindy Patton were among the first to discuss how the lesbian and gay community should respond to the AIDS crisis in Boston's *Gay Community News* in 1983 (Brier 2009: 11). Jackie Winnow (1992: 69), looking back on her activism in the early days of epidemic, wrote that she began work against AIDS

when AIDS hysteria endangered our civil rights, increased anti-lesbian/gay violence, divided our community over the bathhouse and sexuality issues, and increased discrimination ... it was clear that large number of gay men were getting it, and that our survival as a people depended on our response.

Despite lesbian activism, the demographics of the early US AIDS epidemic, coupled with the legacy of tension between lesbians and gay men, led to the idea in many quarters that lesbians were unaffected by AIDS. Many gay men saw lesbians as "uniquely free" of the HIV virus (Altman 1994: 47–48, 156), a position that had the practical consequence of consigning lesbians to secondary, supportive roles in anti-AIDS activism. Gay men's "epidemiological pre-eminence" (Altman 1994: 72) as PWAs cast women's and lesbian women's efforts as merely supportive, obscuring the real impact of AIDS on lesbians and all women and forcing lesbian women to clarify their reasons for activism against AIDS. In some ways, the position of lesbian women in the early anti-AIDS movement paralleled that of women activists in the anti-draft movement of the 1960s and early 1970s. As Thorne (1975) has argued, women in draft resistance were unable to participate in some forms of protest (e.g. burning draft cards), which created a separation between those activists who were seen as putting themselves on the line – men – and those who could merely lend support – women.

As feminist activism around AIDS continued, lesbian activists increasingly asserted a logic of self-interest as their reason for fighting the disease. They focused on how AIDS affected women as women and lesbian women as lesbian women, and thus gay male "epidemiological pre-eminence" became subject to dispute. For example, Lurie (1990: 211) stated that, as a lesbian activist, she "reject(ed) the analysis that I might be doing AIDS activism out of some altruistic or maternal sense. I am fighting for my own life." The self-defense argument for activism was made plausible by the general lack of knowledge about how HIV was spread to women and by women to other women. In 1989, the rate of "unknown" transmission of HIV was four to

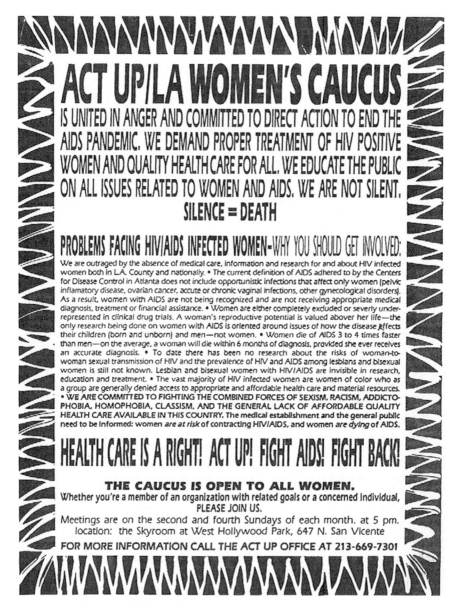

ACT UP/LA WOMEN'S CAUCUS

IS UNITED IN ANGER AND COMMITTED TO DIRECT ACTION TO END THE AIDS PANDEMIC. WE DEMAND PROPER TREATMENT OF HIV POSITIVE WOMEN AND QUALITY HEALTH CARE FOR ALL. WE EDUCATE THE PUBLIC ON ALL ISSUES RELATED TO WOMEN AND AIDS. WE ARE NOT SILENT. SILENCE = DEATH

PROBLEMS FACING HIV/AIDS INFECTED WOMEN—WHY YOU SHOULD GET INVOLVED:

We are outraged by the absence of medical care, information and research for and about HIV infected women both in L.A. County and nationally. • The current definition of AIDS adhered to by the Centers for Disease Control in Atlanta does not include opportunistic infections that affect only women (pelvic inflammatory disease, ovarian cancer, accute or chronic vaginal infections, other gynecological disorders). As a result, women with AIDS are not being recognized and are not receiving appropriate medical diagnosis, treatment or financial assistance. • Women are either completely excluded or severly underrepresented in clinical drug trials. A woman's reproductive potential is valued abover her life—the only research being done on women with AIDS is oriented around issues of how the disease affects their children (born and unborn) and men—not women. • Women die of AIDS 3 to 4 times faster than men—on the average, a woman will die within 6 months of diagnosis, provided she ever receives an accurate diagnosis. • To date there has been no research about the risks of woman-to-woman sexual transmission of HIV and the prevalence of HIV and AIDS among lesbians and bisexual women is still not known. Lesbian and bisexual women with HIV/AIDS are invisible in research, education and treatment. • The vast majority of HIV infected women are women of color who as a group are generally denied access to appropriate and affordable health care and material resources. • WE ARE COMMITTED TO FIGHTING THE COMBINED FORCES OF SEXISM, RACISM, ADDICTO-PHOBIA, HOMOPHOBIA, CLASSISM, AND THE GENERAL LACK OF AFFORDABLE QUALITY HEALTH CARE AVAILABLE IN THIS COUNTRY. The medical establishment and the general public need to be informed: women *are at risk* of contracting HIV/AIDS, and women *are dying* of AIDS.

HEALTH CARE IS A RIGHT! ACT UP! FIGHT AIDS! FIGHT BACK!

THE CAUCUS IS OPEN TO ALL WOMEN.
Whether you're a member of an organization with related goals or a concerned individual,
PLEASE JOIN US.
Meetings are on the second and fourth Sundays of each month. at 5 pm.
location: the Skyroom at West Hollywood Park, 647 N. San Vicente
FOR MORE INFORMATION CALL THE ACT UP OFFICE AT 213-669-7301

FIGURE 3.1: Flyer, ACT UP/LA Women's Caucus c. 1990.

five times higher for women than for men, prompting "safer sex" forums specifically aimed at lesbians (Corea 1992: 195). The idea of lesbian women's activism as simply "doing for others" – as activism solely on behalf of gay men – was rejected by many activist women, and, accordingly, women in ACT UP's largest chapter, ACT-UP New York, began a series of demonstrations in the late 1980s regarding issues involving women and AIDS (ACT UP/NY Women & AIDS Book Group 1990). In 1990, The ACT UP/NY Women & AIDS Book Group published a collection of writings called *Women, AIDS and Activism*, whose contributors ranged from well-known lesbian-feminist anti-AIDS activists to pseudonymous female PWAs. The effect of the book's publication on ACT UP/NY and nationwide is reminiscent of the effect that watershed Second Wave feminist collections like *Sisterhood Is Powerful* or *The Black Woman* had on feminist organizing. Feminist activists against AIDS insisted that making women visible in the AIDS epidemic made the case for AIDS as a *pan*demic. It is this larger national (and eventually global) context of women's invisibility that feminist anti-AIDS activists in Los Angeles confronted when they organized, but they confronted the problem of gay male epidemiological pre-eminence in its localized, embodied form as they made choices about how and when to organize with men.

ACT UP/LA'S WOMEN'S CAUCUS AND THE PROBLEM OF NUMBERS

> ACT UP is a boy's club, and they are all boys ... and when I started there was one woman in, one or two women ... and then all the time these boys were making these jokes "oh you've got enough for a women's caucus now" and it was totally a joke ... and then finally one day, I just said, "okay yeah."
>
> – Jeri Dietrick[10]

On June 3, 1990, several women involved in ACT UP/LA, along with many others, called for the creation of an ACT UP/LA Women's Caucus as an explicitly feminist entity that would work on issues involving women and AIDS. The WC's initial meetings were advertised to the broader community beyond ACT UP/LA; twenty-one women reportedly came to the first meeting.[11] That initial WC, many of whom were not "ACT UP/LA" women, immediately formed internal subcommittees to research the availability of services and treatment for HIV-positive women in the LA area and to publicize information about women and AIDS. The next month, twenty-nine women came to the WC meeting. By late 1990, the average number of women at WC meetings was consistently under fifteen, and most often under ten, and the majority of WC members were rooted more firmly in ACT UP/LA proper.

When I came to my first WC meeting in November of 1990, having seen a flyer for the group's meetings in my West Hollywood neighborhood, I was surprised to see men in attendance:

---

[10] Interview with author, 2000.
[11] Judy Sisneros, 1990. "Women's Caucus Report," p. 15 in ACT UP/LA *Newsletter* 3:4 (August/September).

There are about an even number of men and women in the room, which puzzles me, although I don't ask about it. The men and women seem to know each other well, and make jokes about who was seen with whom at what bookstore.[12]

Without my asking, the anomaly of men attending a WC meeting was explained to me by "Carolyn," one of the WC's founders. She told me that ACT UP/LA was planning two major actions around women's issues – a local "Week of Outrage" and a nationally coordinated set of demonstrations at the CDC in Atlanta – and men were at the meeting to help with coordinating the two actions. In the same conversation, Carolyn stated that the rationale for the WC came from the fact that women were only 10 to 20 percent of the GB; often "women didn't feel that they had a voice" there, and many felt that the GB did not address itself adequately to women's HIV-related needs.[13] Less than a week later, I attended my first WC event during the "Week of Outrage," a "Teach-In" on issues involving women and AIDS, attended by both women and men. At the Teach-In, I spoke briefly to "Andrea," who was active in both the WC and the GB:

I say goodbye to Andrea [and tell her] I was actually thinking of going to a General Body meeting. "Oh," she says, and rolls her eyes. "Why?" I respond. "Are they a real event?" "Well, they're a bit overwhelming," she says, "kind of the dating game." This is said with a bit of a smirk on her face. . . . I ask her how many men attend the GB meetings. "About 150," she says, "but we're getting more women to go."

During the time that I participated, the WC had men in attendance more than half the time it met on its own, in part because the "caucus" turned into a "committee" during GB "working" meetings that took place twice a month, and no men were ever told to take their chairs and leave the circle. Men attended WC-initiated actions and indeed were crucial to the success of these actions, and men were almost always present in greater numbers than women. What did it mean for women in ACT UP/LA to organize around women's issues within an organization that was overwhelmingly male, at a point in the history of the AIDS epidemic when those dying from the disease were overwhelmingly male? As Judy Sisneros and Jeri Dietrick stated in the chapter's epigraphs, feminist anti-AIDS activists in ACT UP/LA found themselves greatly outnumbered by

---

[12] Author's field notes, WC meeting, November 11, 1990.

[13] During 1990 and 1991, 80 to 220 people attended Monday night GB meetings. In previously published work (Roth 1998), I estimated that ACT UP/LA had a female membership of about 10 percent in those years. Women made up a larger percentage of the group at times when the group was smaller, at its beginning and toward its end. Faderman and Timmons (2009: 406–407, note 58), quoting Judy Sisneros, argue that ACT UP/LA was 15 percent lesbian. Leaving aside the conflation of lesbian and female, given ACT UP/LA's informal membership, one can only guess at the number of women active in the group at any one time; in any case, the difference between my estimate and Faderman's and Timmons's translates to two to three women. The more important point is that those activist women were always vastly outnumbered by men.

men. For some women, this was not a problem, and not all women in ACT UP/LA worked closely with the WC. Terri Ford, for example, sometimes went to WC meetings but characterized herself as a participant in the "mainstream" of ACT UP/LA, in part due to her work in hospice care, where she was "taking care of men and women."[14] But even some men saw the formation of a woman's caucus as inevitable, as Dietrick implies. Guther Freehill had reservations about caucus formation; at least in hindsight, another male activist, Wendell Jones, saw the WC's creation as an inevitable expression of ACT UP/LA's politics of self-determination, even though he seldom worked directly with the caucus. Jones, interviewed in 2011, recalled feeling that ACT UP/LA was at once a conducive and challenging place for women's anti-AIDS activism:

> Consistently people in ACT UP respected the women and let them make the decisions . . . but I will still say that there were unconscious ways men would dominate things or not be as respectful as they should to the women . . . and I don't mean just with the women's things, [but] the ways that people would compete with each other.[15]

Other former ACT UP/LA activists remembered moments where men's sexism led them to be "not as respectful as they should be to the women." Helene Schpak, who was a leader in ACT UP/LA, a participant in the WC, and a chief proponent of a more universal, integrative set of actions around women and health, remembered the controversy created by some men's depiction of women:

> SCHPAK: I remember at one meeting in particular, you know sometimes we do fun things, but a couple of the guys staged a small performance thing and they dressed up as women and they enhanced their features and there were some women who thought it was just wonderful and hilarious and some of us who thought that was insulting and degrading.
> ROTH: Were they being drag queens?
> SCHPAK: Uh huh [yes], but not even a kind of respectful drag queen. It was just so horrible and I thought "how can you do that with women sitting here?"[16]

Schpak recalled that, at the time, she made it clear that she thought the performance was "hugely insulting," but that not all the women agreed with her, and that this "caused a huge rift among the women."

Another central player in the WC who was also very active in the GB, Jan Speller, confirmed that the WC never drew all ACT UP/LA women into its fold but that, nevertheless, it was the WC's job to inject the larger group with a shot of real commitment to women's issues:

> [A]s much as I can admire ACT UP for having, having or trying to, maintain a feminist perspective in their work, the fact is they were men, and a lot of them were white men, . . . I wanted to discourage that sort of "remembering women" or doing women's

---

[14] Interview with author, 2012.
[15] Interview with author, 2011.
[16] Interview with author, 2011.

work in name only in order to attract supporters in coalition work … but to really do women's work.[17]

Speller connected the problems of women's visibility within ACT UP/LA with larger questions of lesbian visibility in the gay community, arguing that any number of community organizations simply added "lesbian" to their titles and literature and felt that was enough. Speller instead felt that what was needed was "a fundamental shift in … thinking" about feminist and women's issues and that the WC was a step in bringing about that shift.

Judy Sisneros, who, like Speller and Deitrick, considered herself both an ACT UP/LA and WC activist, integrated her participation in the WC with her commitment to the larger group – the "room" as Freehill referred to it. Sisneros saw the WC as another venue for her considerable activist energies:

The very first or second General Body meeting that I went to, I was handed a flyer by Jeri Dietrick, saying that the Women's Caucus is starting, come to the meeting. … I don't really think of it [going to the WC] as a transition from one group to the other … because I fully participated in the Caucus but also in the General Body. I was agitating/legal [committee] co-facilitator with someone else for the General Body at one point. … We were a very action-based organization, so depending on whether I was involved in a specific action or not, that kind of set the tone for what I was doing within the organization.[18]

Sisneros felt that the WC was more than just another place for her to work as an ACT UP/LA activist, but she also cited the problem of numbers as a reason for the WC's importance. When I asked her whether the WC was an important place for her, she answered: "Oh God, yeah. Oh yeah, I loved it. It was great. I mean, you know, we weren't outnumbered there by men – there were no men." This was interesting, given that men were at the meetings, as I pointed out to her. She explained: "Yes, there were men at the meetings. But let's face it, the overpowering … the … attitude of the group is that it's a women's place … for women and for lesbians."

For some WC members, the WC was the way into ACT UP/LA and into anti-AIDS activism from outside the group. Mary Lucey, who was HIV-positive, came to the initial WC meetings to learn about her disease. She and her partner, Nancy McNeil, played key roles in the WC and in ACT UP/LA, and both Lucey and McNeil eventually took jobs within the paid AIDS work sector (see Chapter 6). Lucey was working as an AIDS policy analyst for the City of Los Angeles when I interviewed her in 1999. She told me that, after testing positive in April of 1990, "we had called all the AIDS agencies in Los Angeles … and every time we kept saying 'well I've already tested positive' and they'd say, 'well there's really nothing we can do … you are kind of a lost cause here.'" MacNeil knew some people in ACT UP/LA and told those people how "pissed off" she

[17] Interview with author, 2000.
[18] Interview with author, 2000.

and Lucey were about their inability to get information about Lucey's disease. According to Lucey, these ACT UP/LA activists told MacNeil "well you should really come and talk to us, because we really like pissed off people." Lucey also recounted that, in the early days of her participation in the WC, she had to make herself, a seropositive lesbian, visible to the well-intentioned feminist activists who attended the first few WC meetings:

So I remember the Women's Caucus was meeting on a Sunday, in Silverlake . . . there was probably about fifteen women there and Nancy and I were sitting in the back of the room kind of quiet, you know, and they were talking about, "well have you ever seen an infected woman, have you ever met an infected woman, how do we reach these women, how do we help these women" . . . and Nancy and I just kept looking at each other, thinking "oh my God, they don't think any of us are here." . . . [S]o then I stood up and said, "well, you know, I'm infected." You know, it was dead silence, because I'm not quite sure they knew what to say . . . it wasn't fear. I didn't sense fear at all. I sensed a "oh we really should do something" . . . . It wasn't a threatening situation. And I didn't feel . . . I didn't feel any sense of discrimination or anything like that . . . it was just dead silence.[19]

When I asked Lucey about other HIV-positive women in the group, she indicated that Connie Norman, a transwoman, was also HIV-positive. Norman did not come to WC meetings, and, according to one interviewee, Wendell Jones, was actually involved with the local all-male Radical Faeries group, where her transgendered presence was controversial.[20]

Thus the problem of male epidemiological pre-eminence in the AIDS pandemic translated into a male-dominated ACT UP/LA, which then translated into locally outnumbered female anti-AIDS activists. These women, prompted by moments of sexist display and seeking a way to work on women's AIDS issues, formed the feminist WC. Once formed, the boundary invoked by WC members between the WC and the GB became a continuously contested, unintentionally compromised, and ultimately permeable border.

THE MAKING OF AN INTERNAL GENDER BOUNDARY AS A MEANS OF INCREASING WOMEN'S VISIBILITY

The members of the WC of ACT UP/LA wanted to increase the visibility of women dealing with AIDS by putting a woman's face on AIDS. Sometimes they did so literally. In preparation for an upcoming demonstration at the HIV prisoners ward at the Frontera Women's Prison in Chico, California, and national actions at the CDC in Atlanta in late 1990, the WC worked with members of the GB to decide on what kind of graphics to use at the different actions. Male members of the GB came to a WC meeting to discuss four different graphics that would be used for the demonstrations. There was

---

[19] Interview with author, 1999.
[20] Interview with author, 2011.

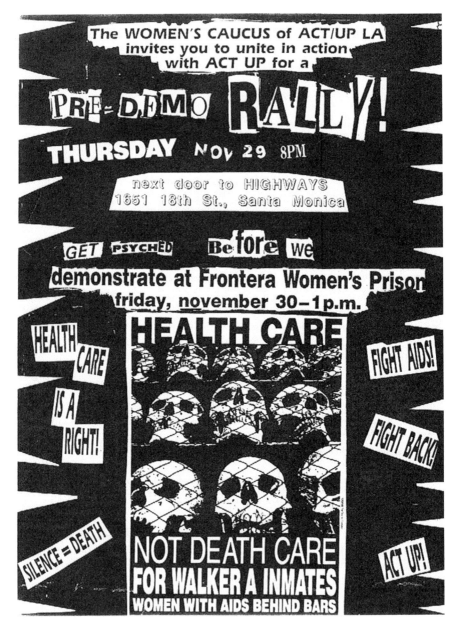

FIGURE 3.2: Flyer, Pre-demonstration rally, November 1990.

much discussion of the graphics, which were ultimately seen as relying too heavily on skull imagery. The WC members wanted the focus to be on the women of Frontera and on women with AIDS in general. Although some skull imagery prevailed in the end, the debate that took place at the meeting over women's visibility was only one instance of the WC's constant battle to address interrelated visibility burdens in fighting for women with AIDS. They needed to make themselves visible as lesbians to the heterosexist public and political establishment, they had to become visible as lesbians to a gay male community, and they had to make visible the needs of HIV-positive women to all of the above. But in order to embark on the visibility agenda, WC members had to become more visible to their fellow activists. They did this by forming the caucus, a politically acceptable means of organizing identity in ACT UP/LA, a group that already had a PISD caucus for HIV-positive activists. By forming a feminist women's caucus, WC members set themselves apart from ACT UP/LA's General Body and increased their visibility within the group's internal political landscape.

WC members' setting up a feminist group within a group was also legitimated by ACT UP/LA's feminist-friendly identity. Like other ACT UPs, ACT UP/LA "officially" saw itself as a feminist organization; Altman (1994: 72) characterized ACT UP nationally as "clearly one of the organizational forums where a feminist analysis of AIDS has been able to have some impact." ACT UP/LA was thus characterized by an explicit openness to feminist politics, going beyond the "post-feminist" piecemeal acceptance of feminist stances that characterized some individuals and organizations in the 1980s (Rapp 1990; Stacey 1990; Stein 1992). Members of feminist-friendly organizations go beyond a tacit or "taken for granted" (Rapp 1990) incorporation of some feminist attitudes or beliefs into their personal consciousness to a public stance of being open to feminist identities and ideas; they close the "distance" (Stein 1992: 52) that post-feminists have taken toward feminist politics. On the local level, the first meeting of ACT UP/LA in December 1987 was endorsed by groups such as "Lesbian Nurses," the San Fernando Valley Branch of the National Organization for Women; "Wholistic Health for Women"; "Women's AIDS Project"; and the Women's Building, a lesbian feminist art and community space.[21] Individual endorsers of the initial ACT UP/LA meeting included Betty Brooks, a local feminist educator and leader, and Jinx Beers, the publisher of *Lesbian News*. In March 1988, three months after ACT UP/LA's founding, information on events concerning women and AIDS had made it into meeting minutes at least.[22] The ACT UP/LA newsletter reported on the demands for action on women's HIV issues made in "*Le Manifeste de Montreal*/Declaration of Universal Rights and Needs of People Living with HIV Disease," presented

---

[21] ACT UP/LA, Flyer, December 1987. "Bring the Spirit of Washington Home," ONE Collection.
[22] ACT UP/LA meeting minutes. March 14, 1988; ONE collection.

by activists at the Fifth International Conference on AIDS in Montreal.[23] Although overwhelmingly made up of men, ACT UP/LA had a feminist-friendly track record.

Obviously, being part of a feminist-friendly organization would be good for women and even better for feminists. The WC came to be seen as the body within a body tasked with the role of keeping ACT UP/LA feminist by "confronting sexism in the (G)eneral (B)ody."[24] Keeping ACT UP/LA feminist came to be one of the WC's tasks, but it was not members' motivation for forming the WC. WC members were self-interested; they formed the caucus to increase their ability to work on what they saw as women's AIDS issues, and, in doing so, they were able to draw upon the energies of men and non-WC women. Forming a caucus created a boundary between the WC and the GB of ACT UP/LA, which in turn created the conditions under which the feminist members of the WC could be more visible within the larger organization and organize their interests as members of a specific gendered social identity. In boundary-making, movement members "mark the social territories of group relations by highlighting differences between activists and the web of others in the contested social world" (Taylor and Whittier 1992: 111). Boundary-making increases the visibility of historically dominated constituencies. Although the effort of boundary-making has been considered by social scientists as a way that activists make themselves visible to a larger public (Jenson 1987; Molotch 1979; Snow and Benford 1992), boundary-making can also raise the internal visibility of historically dominated groups outnumbered within an organization. For feminist WC members, forming a caucus was virtually the only avenue open to them if they wanted to stay in ACT UP/LA *and* pursue a "women and AIDS" agenda; that is, if they wanted to organize based on their interests as women.

But in order to be effective, ACT UP/LA's WC needed help from men. The WC was never an autonomous organization, and the larger numbers seen at the initial meetings held in Silverlake didn't last. The WC quickly devolved into a small group, and its female members took on a large umbrella agenda of women's AIDS issues. Given their small numbers and their ambitious agenda, the WC needed men to support their actions. The formation of the WC allowed for two kinds of male support: the solidarity shown by men in the GB and the active support of a small but crucial group of feminist-identified men who worked closely with the WC when permitted. Many, if not most, men in ACT UP/LA identified as feminists, but only a small group of men worked directly with the WC, drawn to the group by their interest in WC issues, just as they were drawn to other committees by their interests in agitating, AIDS treatments, or fundraising. These men were in effect male WC members, although never

---

[23] Mark Kostopoulos, "Montreal AIDS Conference," ACT UP/LA *Periodical* [newsletter] 2:3 newsletter pp. 10–11; ONE collection.

[24] Handout, "Attention New Members," March 1991. Author's collection.

defined as such. As I discuss next, the men's work and their very presence were constant concerns for female WC members who wanted to maintain "women's space" within ACT UP/LA.

FEMINIST FRIENDLY MEN WITHIN FORMALIZED WOMEN'S SPACE

> There were some extremely supportive men. If it had been turtles getting AIDS, they would have wanted to support us turtles, you know? Because that's the kind of people they are.
>
> – Mary Lucey[25]

Feminist-identified men who worked closely with the WC aided with a variety of tasks. They helped staff WC actions, they provided refreshments, they helped sell Tupperware as a fundraiser for the WC, they offered transportation and accommodation for a speaker for the Teach-in on women and AIDS. One male ACT UP/LA member, "Dylan," coordinated a "Safe-sex Vending" event that took place in late 1990 at a number of West Hollywood (women's and mixed) bars as part of a "Week of Outrage" focused on women's AIDS issues. Men attended WC meetings during GB working meetings every other week on Monday nights; they attended the separately held WC Sunday night meetings often, although their presence was a subject of explicit debate among WC members.

With men in attendance at WC events and actions, and participating in most WC meetings, the focus on women and AIDS was subject to "slippage"; that is, a shift from a focus on women's AIDS issues – a focus that would broaden the spectrum of who the epidemic affected – to a sole focus on men's AIDS issues (Roth 1998). Slippage was evident at the WC-sponsored "Women and AIDS Teach-in" in November 1990, where attendance was about 50 percent male. Two hours into the Teach-in, I noted the following:

"Don" speaks, asking Anna with regard to the undocumented women's health care, couldn't she put pressure on the Catholic Church and Catholic hospitals to open up to helping Latina women ... he is the first man to actually ask a question about women so far.

With the exception of Don and his lover, "Sam" – two men who worked closely with the WC – ACT UP/LA men at the Teach-in continually asked speakers about gay male issues, and WC members countered by asking questions about women and AIDS to refocus the discussion. "Anna," a Chicana researcher/activist with a Southern California-based project looking at heterosexual transmission in Latino couples, was peppered with men's questions as to the sexual lives of the secretly bisexual husbands, the need for the Latino community to have its own "Rock Hudson moment" to focus its awareness on

---

[25] Interview with author, 1999.

AIDS, the possible sources of HIV infection of a local activist priest who was then ill with (and has since died from) AIDS, whether the Latino community was embarrassed by its "gay problem," and possibilities for educational campaigns on AIDS in the Latino community. Only the WC women – and Don and Sam – focused the discussion back on its intended topic, Latinas with AIDS.

In the following example of slippage, Anna has been recounting her experience with one couple whom she names "Jose and Maria," where the secretly bisexual HIV- positive Latino immigrant Jose has promised God to keep his wife safe if she tests negative. Anna told the Teach-In audience that the couple had stopped having sexual intercourse. One of the male ACT UP/LA attendees, "Brad," addressed Anna after hearing this:

Brad jumps in. "So are you saying that Jose and Maria have not had sex all this time?" Anna answers, nodding, and says "that's right." Brad follows this up with a query about how Jose feels about it. Anna answers that the situation is a "relief" for Jose, since he is primarily worried about infecting Maria. Brad keeps following up, asking why Jose sees it as a relief. Lester chimes in, saying to Anna "you mean, he's no longer guilty about having gay sex?" Anna nods, and says "yes that's part of it too." Brad then addresses Anna and says, "*that's* not what I meant" rather testily, and then asks Anna if Jose is relieved to not be having sex with Maria. Anna answers perhaps, she doesn't know.

Brad's aggressive questioning – his concern with Jose's sex life – continued until one of the women in the audience changed the subject back to women and AIDS. Other men at the Teach-in, with the exception of Don and Sam, followed Brad's lead of changing Anna's subject to that of gay Latino men; some were even less civil than he. In short, in "the audience versus Anna," the battle was one of where to focus. Anna wanted to talk about the specific problems of Latinas *and* Latinos confronting AIDS, while some male members of the audience were much more concerned with the plight of gay Latinos:

Sam asks Anna about what ACT-UP can do to help, since it's a white gay male organization? Anna says that ACT-UP has to find "the Latina voice in the community," and get more Latinas involved in the Women's Caucus. Brad then asks Anna is the problem that the Latino community is uninformed or embarrassed by its "gay problem?"

Moments after this exchange, a WC member spoke up:

Trina addresses Anna. "I just want to say that the Women's Caucus is here for you." She asks Anna to let the WC know if there's anything they can help with. Anna answers by saying "please be patient with us."

The exchange among Anna, WC, and ACT UP/LA men showed how hard it was to refocus male activists' concerns about who was actually affected by HIV/ AIDS. The Teach-in battle thus exemplified slippage, the way that focus on women's AIDS issues could be taken off women by (usually) well-meaning men. Slippage like that at the Teach-in could occur at any WC event with male attendance and therefore remained a concern as long as men outnumbered women both in the organization and at women's events.

In order to prevent slippage, WC members had enacted a policy of provisionalizing men's attendance at meetings and formalizing women's space by designating Sunday night WC meetings as women's space. On December 23, 1990, right before Christmas and after major local and national actions on women's AIDS issues that men helped plan and participated in, a discussion took place in the Women's Caucus, prompted by a request by Dylan to keep attending WC meetings. The WC members went back and forth about the wisdom of letting Dylan attend; one spoke about how the WC meetings were "women's space, without men period"; another stated that the WC should be women's space because of the "safety factor" and the "stereotypical men/women thing, with men being all aggressive, etc." even while acknowledging that Dylan was not aggressive. Yet another WC member eschewed the use of the word "allowed" to describe men's presence in women's space and suggested that the group's policy of having men petition to attend requires men to "think ahead" about their reasons for coming to WC meetings. This policy had actually led to dissatisfaction among some GB men; one WC member, "Pippa," noted that the ACT UP/LA gossip sheet *Tiara* had an item with someone writing in and calling the WC "the whining caucus," partly on the basis of the group's supposed vacillation about letting men attend.[26]

The debate over male attendance at WC meetings shows that operating as a women's caucus in ACT UP/LA was complicated by the facts that (1) women needed men in order for their actions to succeed (and they liked some of the men a lot), and (2) some ACT UP/LA men wanted to work on women's issues, and the rest of ACT UP/LA was organized to facilitate members' working on what interested them. But, given women's small numbers in the group, the salience of the women's AIDS issues agenda was at risk. WC members were in the paradoxical position of needing male support to maintain their effectiveness but having to limit male presence in order to maintain women's space. ACT UP/LA's feminist friendliness gave the WC members the right to determine who came to meetings, thus empowering the women to invite men in or disinvite them as the women saw fit. In practice, considerable meeting time in the WC was spent reiterating the *formally* separate nature of the Sunday night meetings – as opposed to the times during working GB meetings, when anyone could attend.

It was the *formal* definition of the WC's meetings as women's space that mattered the most to WC members, even though this formal definition was always at risk of being undercut. If men had to petition to attend Sunday night WC meetings, then their presence did not technically detract from the formally separate nature of WC meetings; of course, their actual participation eroded the reality of women's space. Therefore, WC members officially saw male

---

[26] Author's field notes, Women's Caucus meeting, December 23, 1990.

attendance as provisional, and most ACT UP/LA men backed the WC members in this view.

While the formal separateness of WC meetings was upheld despite the presence of men, the reasons that WC members gave for the need for a women-only policy varied. One member, Carolyn, was concerned on principle with accommodating lesbian separatist women who wanted to act in concert with the WC against AIDS. In practice, the WC of ACT UP/LA would have been an impossible place for separatist lesbians to work. Other WC members were actually not very fussy about the rationale for keeping WC meetings formally separate from GB men or, at the very least, cared inconsistently about it. For example, in 2000, when I asked Jan Speller – who lived with male ACT UP/LA leaders Mark Kostopoulos and Guenther Freehill – about her feelings about the gender politics of ACT UP/LA and the WC, she responded that

I was sort of in a social milieu of Mark, Gunther, Tony [Arn], Peter [Cashman] ... frankly, the intelligentsia of the group, ... who had really good politics ... who were feminists, understood the critical nature of reproductive rights, knew how all those issues of ... and struggled with race issues, but how all those issues of gender, race, class, income and homosexuality all worked together to keep people out of power, and how it affected the AIDS epidemic. So I was satisfied.

At the same time, Speller also felt that ACT UP/LA was "basically a male movement. And so ... basically I was signing on and buying into ... a male movement. So I had ... you know, an internal ... I don't know what that word is, when things don't fit ... " I suggested the word was "dissonance," and Speller agreed saying "Right. Tons of dissonance."

In her interview in 1999, the late Stephanie Boggs recalled that, in reality, the policy of voting on male participation was constantly re-examined by the WC:

[Men] had to be specially voted in and there was always an exception and as a matter of fact, we would keep revisiting this, because we would find men ... coming to the General Body [working] meetings and they would want to work on some issues with us and they would want to become members of the Women's Caucus, and it would be put to a vote.

Boggs recalled a conversation with Jeri Deitrick about keeping the WC as space for women because in GB meetings, women were often silent and overly deferential to the men. Boggs felt that the group dynamic was different when women were predominant and agreed with Deitrick that quieter women were more likely to speak in an all-women setting. On the other hand, she also felt that some members of the WC sometimes used "gender like a weapon to beat people up over the head."

Boggs also recalled that the "women-only" policy had in part to do with the need for privacy when discussing gynecological issues, a rationale for women's space that was stated publicly at least once in front of the GB. In January 1991, a month after dealing with Dylan's request for attendance, WC members felt it necessary to restate the policy on male attendance at WC meetings for the entire group at a GB meeting. When this reiteration of policy was made, the rationale of providing space for women in order to counter male aggression was omitted and that of providing separatist accommodation was actually contradicted:

Pippa gets up to restate the WC position on male attendance. "Men are welcome at the working meetings," she says. "We are not separatists, as we've said over and over again. . . . We meet separately for privacy issues, to discuss gynecological treatment, for safety."[27]

Thus, the reasons for maintaining "women's space" varied over time, but the formally exclusive nature of the separate meeting was insisted upon as a means of maintaining the boundaries between ACT UP/LA and the WC. The WC was powerful to the extent that the boundary was maintained; being WC women bought members a good deal of control over their actions. But numbers trumped the boundary; three months after the January announcement on men's attendance, men were invited back to the outside meetings to help plan a May 1991 demonstration for prisoner rights in Sacramento.

WOMEN'S STRATEGIES FOR REINSCRIBING GENDER DIFFERENCE: COUNTING MEN AND CALLING OUT "WOMEN PRESENT!"

WC members used interactional strategies to make women more visible and to remind ACT UP/LA men about gender difference. Two key strategies for reinscribing gender occurred in two different sites: (1) at WC meetings, members "counted men," making everyone aware of male presence and thus not taking that presence for granted; and (2) at GB meetings, WC members let men know that there were "women present," so that GB members could not proceed without acknowledging gender difference.

Counting men – noting how many men were or would be at an event – was a frequent activity at WC meetings, and it was especially significant because the number of regular WC members was so small. Jan Speller recalled that

attendance was really an issue . . . we would bring issues to the larger group . . . but you know four or five or six or seven people who are already seriously involved in the larger body and doing all the other groups, in addition to whatever other activist or AIDS work they were doing. . . . I don't think we had a lot of energy or resources to accomplish a lot.[28]

How many men were or would be at an event was a frequent subject at WC meetings, as illustrated by the following example. At a WC meeting in December 1990, one member discussed having a video night as a fundraiser and asked about how a previous video fundraiser had gone; she was assured that "some men came, and that whole men and women thing was fine."[29]

---

[27] Author's field notes, General Body meeting, January 14, 1991.
[28] Interview with author, 2000.
[29] Author's field notes, Women's Caucus meeting, December 23, 1990.

Counting men led to attempts to control the number of men at WC events in order to keep a focus on women's AIDS issues. These attempts were primarily unsuccessful. For example, one WC member in November 1990 was concerned that male participation in the "Dance of Death," a guerilla theater event where the group, dressed as different types of everyday women, would "die" on the Venice Beach boardwalk and distribute information about women and AIDS, would change the focus of the event. She stated then that she "doesn't want more men [for the event]"; there were a few men in drag who were going to participate, but she did not want the whole group being dominated by that image.[30] At the following meeting, another WC member recapped the "Dance of Death," noting that there were more men than women at the event and that there were also more than a few men in drag there. This concerned WC members; they worried that the male images would obscure the one they wished to create of ordinary women being affected by AIDS.

WC members also felt the need to repeatedly remind GB men that women were present and that women's presence could not be taken for granted or ignored. One example of calling out "women present" took place on the way to an action in support of female HIV-positive prisoners at the Frontera women's prison AIDS ward in Chino, California. Of the 100 or so who demonstrated at the Frontera prison demanding better treatment for women on the AIDS ward there, approximately twenty were women. On the bus on the way to the protest, this moment occurred:

There are fifty or so people on the bus. People are playing with the p.a. system, making jokes about "on your flight this evening" … A youngish GB member gets up, takes the mike and says in a very campy way, "Alright, everybody, let's sing the theme song from the Brady Bunch!" Before he can start, Trina growls loudly from behind me, "Forget it! That show ruined my life."[31]

"Trina's" reaction to a 1970s television sitcom may not seem noteworthy, but she challenged the GB member's idea about what the show should mean to others in ACT UP/LA. She questioned the "camp" sensibility that dominated male GB humor by pointing out that the Brady Bunch was not the kind of cultural touchstone that everyone could share and safely mock together. Men could see the Brady Bunch as merely silly; a lesbian woman like Trina had a very different response to the show's rigidly traditional female stereotypes (stay at home mom, selfless maid, blonde girl children mostly involved with worrying about their hair and whether boys liked them). As when Helene Schpak rejected drag humor by ACT UP/LA men as disrespectful to women, Trina's rejection of camp humor signaled a moment when male definitions of what was culturally part of being gay was challenged.

---

[30] Author's field notes, Women's Caucus meeting, November 25, 1990.
[31] Author's field notes, Women's Caucus meeting, November 30, 1990.

Another example of the "women present" strategy was the WC's "WET Minutes" presentations made at GB meetings. The WC began presenting "WET (Women's Educational Thang) Minutes" during their reports in GB meetings in August of 1991. WET minutes were intended to inform the GB of specific problems confronting HIV-infected women. In giving GB men this information, WC members communicated that men's knowledge of the effects of HIV disease was not complete. In one instance, a WC member delivered a WET Minute on the gender-specific opportunistic infections that HIV-positive women suffered from – e.g., pelvic inflammatory disease and refractory vaginal yeast infections – about which the GB men were presumed to be ignorant. It is important to note that, first, presenting WET Minutes in some measure contradicted the WC's stated reasons for women's space being necessary for gynecological privacy and that, second, WET Minutes were a break with the de facto protocol for committee reports, which were almost never, in my experience, used to deliver strictly educational Teach-in-type information. The break with the de facto committee report format was never challenged by any of the men; on the contrary, several WET minutes were greeted with anticipatory applause by GB members.

On an informal level, WC assertions that there were "women present" were sometimes so subtle as to be covert, as when one WC member specifically designed an ACT UP tee-shirt for women's bodies instead of men's.[32] Other "women present" actions by WC members were less than intentional but more than unconscious. For example, rather than scattering or sitting with other committees of which they were a part, WC members tended to sit together at GB meetings, thus making a bloc of women visible to the rest of the group. In subtle, overt, and informal ways, WC members reinscribed gender difference as they counted and even tried to control men in attendance at events and as they reminded the GB men that there were "women present" in the ranks. Reinscribing gender served to reidentify the boundaries between the WC and the GB, highlighting and making visible the position and presence of women in ACT UP/LA but also highlighting the limits of lesbian and gay solidarity.

THE PARADOX OF BECOMING OFFICIAL WOMEN: DEFERENCE AND COMPARTMENTALIZATION

> I see Sam, who has been standing around in the back, on the right side of the room, passing out the pamphlets to everyone. He passes me by on the left side of the room as I am getting up ... "Andrea's bossing me around and making me hand these out," he whispers to me as he hands me a pamphlet.[33]

---

[32] The WC member/artist Trina told me that women's torsos were generally shorter than men's, which meant that graphics for a woman's tee-shirt need to be placed higher up on the shirt to be seen.

[33] Author's field notes, Teach-in, November 17, 1990.

> Don says he thinks that the Women's Caucus should be the one to make the decision and that the group is not under the obligation to poll every female member of ACT UP.[34]

> FDA Action proposed – Women's Committee proposes an action against the FDA to provide pregnant women access to drug trials, but doesn't have the resources to plan it. Someone please pick this up.[35]

As a result of the boundary-making strategies of the WC, and as a consequence of feminist-friendly politics within ACT UP/LA, the GB treated WC members as "official" representatives of women's interests in ACT UP/LA, despite the fact that not all women in ACT UP/LA came to WC meetings. Since ACT UP's committee structure gave WC members the opportunity to be visible in front of the GB at every meeting, WC members came to be seen as speaking for all ACT UP women. Certain decisions and tasks were considered to be under WC control, and WC members were accorded a certain amount of deference within the larger group. As Gunther Freehill suggested, this deference on the part of the GB toward one caucus or committee was unique.

The insistence by female WC members and the men who supported them on this deference – not that it is the word that anyone would have used – was respected even in situations where a male ACT UP/LA member was not particularly keen on working closely with the WC. When male GB members brought the graphics to the WC meeting for approval, there was some indication that they were not happy to be there.[36] But the WC was seen as being the ones who should make decisions about women's issues, and WC members generally had a free hand in making decisions about women's AIDS issues in the group even while they relied on men for support. WC members, for example, decided who got to go to conferences on women and HIV and were supported in these decisions by almost all GB men.

GB deference allowed WC members to act as official representatives of ACT UP women. The WC determined, in fact, what women's issues were discussed within ACT UP/LA because there were no obvious women's AIDS issues. As a result of being official women, the WC chose their own agenda; these choices and not those of other GB members guided their work. WC members chose to call attention to substandard conditions for HIV-positive women prisoners in California's prison system, they challenged the CDC definition of AIDS to include women-specific opportunistic infections and conditions, they criticized AIDS Clinical Trials Group drug protocols for women that were marred by the lack of informed consent, they agitated for the enrollment of women in drug trials where inclusion criteria unfairly excluded them, they even started a letter campaign aimed at asking drug companies to have labels placed on

---

[34] Author's field notes, Women's Caucus meeting, November 25, 1990.
[35] ACT UP/LA Minutes for General Body meeting, April 4, 1991. Author's collection.
[36] Author's field notes, Women's Caucus meeting, November 11, 1990.

newly released over-the-counter yeast infection remedies warning that recurrent yeast infections could be a sign of HIV infection.

The accomplishment of being official women needs to be understood in light of the fact that not all ACT UP/LA women came to WC meetings or even liked the idea of having a WC. Nonetheless, WC members insisted and were granted the right to represent:

Milly says that 2 airfares have been approved by the General Body to send participants to the conference. She recommends that two women from the women's caucus be sent, but it's an issue because not all women in ACT UP come to the Women's Caucus meetings. Trina says that that may be true, but that we want someone going who is "familiar with the women's issues and not just the AIDS issues." Don says he thinks that the women's caucus should be the one to make the decision, and that the group is not under the obligation to poll every female member of ACT-UP. Others nod in agreement.[37]

As a result of the deference that GB men showed to the WC, WC members spared themselves from having to take on a generic women's agenda, although, given ACT UP/LA's participant driven agenda and democratic structure, it is doubtful that an agenda could have been foisted on them. But the deference shown the WC led to some interesting choices about what a women's issue was. For example, the WC core members never put a lot of emphasis on pro-choice clinic defense, which was an important activity for many ACT UP/LA members. Geltmaker (1992: 636–637) cites clinic defense as the one "not specifically AIDS-related issue" that ACT UP/LA members supported consistently, arguing that clinic defense was an issue "where feminism, gay and lesbian activism and the politics of AIDS lock arms." Notably (and, in my view, accurately), Geltmaker did not characterize clinic defense as a WC project, and updates on clinic defense efforts were given only at GB meetings by the Agitating Committee. As such, the issue of clinic defense was recast by ACT UP/LA as not solely feminist but about the politics of AIDS healthcare. For example, when I asked Pete Jimenez in 2011 about his participation in clinic defense, he stated that the clinics provided more than reproductive care and abortions and that he had done clinic defense because one never knew if a woman might be entering a clinic to have an HIV test done.

By becoming ACT UP/LA's official women, the WC could count on the GB's deference and the more concrete contributions of feminist identified men, but they encountered the problem of needing to represent women in other ACT UP/LA spaces. While most WC members attended other ACT UP/LA committee meetings, to the extent that they represented women, the need to have them at committee meetings grew. The core members of the WC, never a group much larger than ten – were in high demand, and this became an ongoing problem for them. Moreover, despite the help of feminist-identified men, the WC never quite overcame the problem of the "compartmentalization" of women's

---

[37] Author's field notes, Women's Caucus meeting, November 25, 1990.

issues within ACT UP/LA" (Roth 1998). Compartmentalization was the tendency for GB men to delegate all responsibility for women's issues to the WC. Compartmentalization can be seen as the downside of the control that WC members were able to amass as official women; by being ACT UP/LA's official women, WC members ended up having almost all responsibility for ACT UP activism on women's issues delegated to them. Deference by GB men toward the WC could slip easily into ignorance of the WC's actions, a sense on the men's part that the women were taking care of women's things.

One member of the WC, "Milly," wrote a two-page letter in June 1991 accusing the GB of compartmentalization (although that is my term, not hers). In response to what she saw as the "rubberstamping" of a whimsical WC proposal changing a decision that the WC and GB had already made, Milly wrote

disregard is, in my mind, the worst kind of sexism. Whether intentional or not, when women's issues or proposals made by a working group of women are brought to the floor, and are treated differently than those brought forward by any other working group in ACT UP, the message sent to women is that women and the topic of women and AIDS is devalued in the organization.

Milly saw as worrisome the tendency of most men in ACT UP/LA toward pushing all concerns about women and HIV onto the WC, compartmentalizing those issues. In that sense, sexism was disguised as deference, and deference structurally sanctioned male ignorance of women's issues.

WC members were aware of the compartmentalization of their agenda, and they were at times resentful that they could not count on more men to be as active on behalf of women as WC members were:

Milly tells the WC that the Treatment Committee asked her to find a second woman to go to the ACTGs in March. She says that she finds it "patronizing" that the GB wants to send two women to the ACTGs. ... There is some discussion ... with Jill and Maggie asking why the second person can't be male. Milly says "there's no reason why a man can't look at women's issues at the ACTGs," but goes on to say that the fact is that the men don't do as good a job of reporting [women's] issues, and that the WC should send a second woman.[38]

Despite WC efforts, the compartmentalization of women's issues was an ongoing problem for the WC, as indicated by Millie's letter, and it proved extremely difficult for WC members to separate the positive effects of being ACT UP's official women from the negative ones.

CONCLUSION: OPPORTUNITIES AND CHALLENGES FOR FEMINIST WOMEN IN ACT UP/LA

To summarize, the women who founded the ACT UP/LA WC created a group within a group – engaged in internal boundary-making – in order to make

---

[38] Author's field notes, Women's Caucus meeting, January 27, 1991.

themselves visible to the GB. In doing so, they disrupted the interest-based committee structure of the organization by creating another identity-based caucus, and they proceeded to call on the active support of a few feminist-identified men and the more passive but still important support of men in a feminist-friendly organization. WC women, however, faced the constant possibility of slippage of their focus on women's AIDS issues as a result of being part of a male-dominated group. In order to bring visibility to women's AIDS issues and battle slippage, WC members formalized women's space. They used interactional strategies to reinscribe gender difference such as counting the number of women and men at meetings and actions and asserting that there were "women present" at those same events. The WC became ACT UP/LA's official women, who were deferred to by most GB members, but their issues were also subject to compartmentalization because the GB expected WC members to take care of women and AIDS issues for the rest of the group.

In discussing the organizational politics of gender in ACT UP/LA through the making of a women's caucus, I wish to show that first, and most obviously, there was group support for a feminist agenda, despite the numerical predominance of men in the group. Yes, a women's caucus formed, but no, it was never entirely independent of the GB. This interdependence – ACT UP/LA gets to work on feminist issues, and feminists in ACT UP/LA get more power over their actions, as well as support for their agenda – undercuts the uncomplicated and oft-repeated conventional wisdom that ACT UP demobilized because of divisions between the "drugs into bodies" and "universal health care" camps. In Los Angeles, there was for a number of years support and action on a feminist agenda, and the WC was able to lead the group into action on women's AIDS issues. WC members' constant demands that anti-AIDS politics be feminist politics was crucial for the direction that ACT UP/LA took and continuously underscored the coalitional basis of the oppositional direct action anti-AIDS community. The WC had successes, even as women's voices were perennially at risk of not being heard in ACT UP/LA; WC members' self organization did not change their minority status within the larger group.

It would be a mistake to think of battles over gender politics in ACT UP/LA as limited to the victories and frustrations of the WC. In the next chapter, I explore how the intersectional crises of heterogeneity within the group – increasingly divisive gender politics, but also the politics of race/ethnicity and the differences in political experiences of activists – affected ACT UP/LA's trajectory as an anti-AIDS direct action organization. The formation of the WC alerted ACT UP/LA members to the tensions caused by inequalities among them – in particular the antagonism between the goals of constructing community solidarity across difference and respecting rights to self-determination for members who were different from the (gay) white male norm. But gender politics within social movement groups – within any socially significant groups – are never limited to the explicitly stated. ACT UP/LA members continuously confronted gendered and raced questions of who their compatriots were, where the boundaries of their communities lay, and how to apportion attention to the many AIDS-related issues they confronted. These intersectional crises tested the coalitional strings of interest that held the group together and weakened solidarity, leading to ACT UP/LA's slow demobilization.

4

Intersectional Crises in ACT UP/LA

We weren't the only ACT UP that was having trouble with membership and internal conflict.

– Jan Speller[1]

I've heard people quoted as saying 'the women in ACT UP ruined ACT UP.'

– Judy Sisneros[2]

ACT UP/LA is a *programmatic*, not a *representational* organization.

– Wade Richards[3]

INTRODUCTION: INEQUALITIES, COMMUNITY BOUNDARIES, AND CONFLICT WITHIN ACT UP/LA

There was little consensus among ex-activists about what "killed" the AIDS Coalition to Unleash Power, Los Angeles (ACT UP/LA). One thing was for sure: those interviewed showed considerable reluctance to name gender divides as responsible for killing the organization. This was interesting to me as a researcher since the activists' reluctance to blame gender divides for the group's demise ran counter to scholarship and other statements that saw gender divisions in the anti-AIDS movement as leading to the movement's demobilization (Brier 2009; Gould 2009; Halcli 1999).

When I asked ACT UP/LA's Judy Sisneros about gender divides in the group, she responded with the comment quoted above – "I've heard people quoted as saying 'the women in ACT UP ruined ACT UP.'" Sisneros mocked the idea that

---

[1] Interview with author, 2000.
[2] Interview with author, 2000.
[3] Wade Richards, "Girl! Where in the World Did You Get That White Sheet? Or What Did Wade Really Say at the ACT UP/LA Retreat?" Two-page position statement, c. December 1990; ONE Collection. Emphasis in the original.

gender divides were consequential, suggesting that it was outlandish enough so that no one even directly said such a thing *to* her. At another point in her interview, Sisneros entirely dismissed the idea that women were responsible for ACT UP/LA's demise; at the same time, she frequently referenced acute gender tensions in the group and moments of gendered discord that threatened the unity forged among lesbian, gay men, and others fighting AIDS.

Looking back, how do we account for activists' experiences of tensions caused by structural inequalities? Certainly, participants in ACT UP/LA were conscious and aware of inequalities and the challenges they represented for creating unity. They perceived their group as a coalition, and they organized a structure – a General Body (GB) plus committees – to accommodate the differing interests. The structure was also used by those with specific identities to form caucuses. During much of ACT UP/LA's life, three caucuses – the People with Immune System Disorders (PISD) caucus, the Women's Caucus (WC), and the People of Color Caucus – met regularly and were at least partially open to anyone in the GB because the caucuses met as if they were committees during the time set aside for committee work at GB working meetings. As noted in Chapter 3, although working in a women's caucus within the General (male) Body of ACT UP/LA was a challenge for members of that caucus, ACT UP/LA as a progressive organization supported work by those with marginalized identities whose take on the AIDS crises might be different from that of others in the group.

Nonetheless, ACT UP/LA's structure could not forestall moments of what I call "intersectional crisis" – that is, a moment of gendered/racialized/ethnicized discord. In this chapter, I examine three quite different intersectional crises within ACT UP/LA: (1) the influx of participants into ACT UP/LA in late 1991 as a result of California Governor Pete Wilson's veto of Assembly Bill 101 (AB 101), a lesbian and gay rights bill, which challenged ACT UP/LA to accept new members not versed in the gender and racial/ethnic stances of the group; (2) disputes beginning in early to mid-1992 within ACT UP/LA about resources used for the needle exchange project and about efforts to move the Monday night GB meetings to different sites around LA in order to reach more people of color; and (3) local and negative reverberations about "competing" gendered national protest actions that took place in April 1993 during the March on Washington for Lesbian, Gay, and Bisexual Rights and Liberation. The first two crises were primarily about tensions that erupted in ACT UP/LA as the organization opened itself up in the wake of its perceived success as a militant anti-AIDS group; the last crisis, which focused on actions at the Washington, DC, march, was the one most explicitly seen as a gendered division at the time.

Before considering each of the intersectional crises in turn, I first briefly consider what scholars have had to say about the generative power of conflict in LGBT politics; namely, that conflict can be harnessed and managed in order to mobilize activists. I next briefly consider what ACT UP/LA activists thought about unity across differences within the group, specifically what they had to say about the politics of gender difference and racial/ethnic difference and whether ACT UP/LA had a responsibility to look like the epidemic – that is, whether the group had representational responsibilities in doing direct action. I then turn to analyses of three intersectional crises in ACT UP/LA, which I define as protracted moments of conflict that centered on problems created by structural inequalities. These intersectional crises, I argue, are crucial for understanding how inequalities play a role in activists' interactions with each other and thus need to be part of a story that accounts for the group's trajectory.

THE ROLE OF CONFLICT IN THE LGBT MOVEMENT

In his 2008 book, *The Dividends of Dissent: How Conflict and Culture Work in Lesbian and Gay Marches on Washington*, Amin Ghaziani asked if conflict within social movements was inevitably corrosive: "Are internal conflicts purely detrimental or can they have some positive repercussions for mobilization?" (2008: xiv). Studying the assembling of national coalitions that led to a series of marches for LGBT rights in Washington, DC, in the 1970s and 1980s, Ghaziani argued that "infighting" – which he defined as "the expression of a difference of opinion or the offering of a discrepant view that does not produce or occurs prior to an organizational defection or dissolution" (2008: 18) – allowed activists to reflect on the "state of the movement" and thus could be "generative" – that is to say beneficial – for movements.

In Ghaziani's view, infighting helped locally focused lesbian and gay rights groups of the 1960s and 1970s coalesce to stage nationally coordinated events (2008: 55). Ghaziani distinguishes infighting from factionalization and other forms of schism. As he sees it, defections are evidence of activists' failure to resolve conflict; it is hard to argue with such a common sense assertion (2008: 12). A more intriguing finding about infighting in the LGBT movement is the way that infighting was a process all but planned because of the desires on organizers' parts to be as inclusive as possible. March planners wanted diversity in coalition, especially of the regional kind; they wanted lesbians and gays from the "hinterlands" to be heard alongside the voices of those from New York and San Francisco, and the organizers of the first march in 1979 created an inclusionary template for future marches, one in which "dissent was perceived as welcome through 'openness norms'" (2008: 98–99).

As discussed in Chapters 1 and 2, the 1987 National March on Washington for Lesbian and Gay Rights was crucial to the spread of the ACT UPs, as ACT UP/New York's template for anti-AIDS direct action – a coalition of activists with various interests and identities – inspired activists in other cities. The participatory structure of a GB coupled with committees (and sometimes surrounded by affinity groups) was readily copied. But infighting at the local level *within* organizations among individuals is a different animal than interorganizational conflict. ACT UP/LA was conceived as a coalition of individuals, a structure that doesn't quite make sense in social movement theory, which treats coalitions as formed among groups. After all, organizations can leave coalitions and remain as organizations; within discrete organizations, activists can go back to organizing on the basis of "exclusive solidarity" (Ferree and Roth 1998). If individuals leave organizations, they leave and are presumably no longer available to the organization.

After a number of years of whirlwind anti-AIDS activity, ACT UP/LA members began to be confronted with the fruits of its success when more people were attracted to it. The members of the group had to decide just what kinds of representational tasks it could take on in addition to its programmatic aims, to use Wade Richards's words. The question for ACT UP/LA was just how much difference could be accommodated within the organization's boundaries.

In ACT UP/LA's earliest years, when the group was small, differences among activists were minimized. For example, Helene Schpak remembered that ACT UP/LA in its early years transcended potential gender divisions through action:

We had had a very tight insulated group for quite a while ... there was a point in time where you knew everybody, we were focused, we would do actions and our kind of signature post action would be sitting around a table and we would pass the kiss. ... It was very sweet. But it was that kind of a close connection which we all felt, and at that time, there wasn't the distinction of male/female. We really felt there was a single focus of what we needed to do and that we were the people willing to risk whatever it was that we thought we were risking to do it.[4]

As ACT UP/LA grew and differentiated in terms of projects and interests, gender divisions came to play a greater role in internal conflicts, as the WC formed and created space for feminist women to control a women's AIDS agenda (see Chapter 3). While the WC challenged the men in the GB to live up to anti-sexist ideals, it also drew on male support, and its "important women leaders" were trusted by the GB.[5] In short, while the WC members were not always happy about gender politics within ACT UP/LA, the discussion of gender *as* politics was legitimized within the larger group, and actions on women's AIDS issues were a key part of the group's agenda.

In contrast, ACT UP/LA had more trouble integrating people of color into the group, and debates about the organization's responsibilities to communities of color were more fraught. As a progressive organization influenced by the racial/ethnic self-determinist politics of the 1960s and 1970s, ACT UP/LA's members were conscious of racial/ethnic oppressions. One of ACT UP/LA's first actions was protesting the Immigration and Naturalization Service (INS)'s policy of requiring HIV tests for visitors and the INS's efforts to retroactively apply the policy to undocumented immigrants seeking amnesty under the 1986

---

[4] Interview with author, 2011.
[5] Ferd Eggan, Interview with author, 1999. Ty Geltmaker (1992) also felt that ACT UP/LA's gender relations were relatively good compared to other ACT UPs; in his 2011 interview, he described the men in ACT UP/LA as "probably the most feminist group of men I had run into."

Immigration Reform and Control Act.[6] The position paper listing ACT UP/LA's demands of the INS specifically noted that the INS and amnesty policies requiring testing disproportionately affected the Hispanic community. From its inception, ACT UP/LA maintained a variety of coalitional links with groups from communities of color, and, only a few months after the group's founding in December 1987, its newsletter featured articles about people of color's AIDS issues in the context of seeking to educate readers about how AIDS was affecting different constituencies, including women, students, and prisoners.[7]

Some people of color within ACT UP/LA felt marginalized and, along with white members, made efforts to extend ACT UP/LA's reach into the LA metroscape of segregated diversity. Efforts to reach out to racial/ethnic communities beyond the boundaries of West Hollywood actually began in July 1989, when a "Latino Outreach" subcommittee of the Networking/Outreach committee formed.[8] That subcommittee eventually became the People of Color Caucus (alternatively known as the POC or POCC) by 1991.[9] Writing about the efforts of the Networking/Outreach committee to help Latinos deal with AIDS, ACT UP/LA's Joseph Malagon expressed complex feelings of being Latino in a predominantly white group. Malagon described ACT UP/LA as having a "discriminatory past" and noted that, in racial/ethnic communities, there were rumors of ACT UP/LA's " 'white male fraternities,' racist attitudes and policy exclusions." Malagon started going to ACT UP/LA meetings anyway to help break down barriers among communities, even while he was dismayed by the lack of people of color in the room. He was less than hopeful about the possibilities for cross-racial/-ethnic direct action organizing against AIDS, although he prescribed possible solutions, most of which involved white people's active engagement in learning about people of other racial/ethnic communities.

Like the WC, ACT UP/LA's POC was always small, and, like the members of the WC, POC members networked nationally. Mark Simmons was the co-chair of the POC and attended two national conferences of ACT UP activists of color as an ACT UP/LA representative. Simmons described the first conference, the ACT UP/New York-sponsored People of Color Activist Conference, as

---

[6] ACT UP/LA, "The New INS vs. Lady Liberty," unsigned position paper, c. January 1988; ONE Collection; Jim McDaniels "Interview with Three Founding Members of ACT UP/LA," ACT UP/LA *News*, 4:5 (December 1991/January 1992), pp. 6–7.

[7] Randy Schultz, "AIDS and People of Color," ACT UP/LA Newsletter 1:3 (April/May 1988), p. 5; Michael Puente, "AIDS in the Latino Community," ibid., pp. 5–6. Schultz is identified as a member of "Black and White Men Together"; Puente, whose article appears in both English and Spanish, is identified as the assistant director of "Cara a Cara," a Latino community AIDS service project.

[8] ACT UP/LA meeting agenda, July 31, 1989; ONE Collection.

[9] Mark Simmons and David Brown, "ACT-UP/Los Angeles' Network & Outreach Six Months Goal Setting Strategy," distributed at General Body meeting, July 1, 1991. Collection of author.

"empowering."[10] The activists at the conference specified that communities of color did not have access to early drug intervention treatments, to alcohol and substance abuse programs, to adequate healthcare, or to clinical trials and basic information about HIV. When people of color were enrolled in drug trials, those trials had considerable problems in their design, neglected giving informed consent to patients, and relied on placebo-controlled studies among vulnerable populations who could only associate placebos with notorious episodes like the Tuskegee syphilis experiment. A few months after this conference, in November 1991, Simmons and other unnamed members of ACT UP/LA's POC attended a national conference for anti-AIDS people of color in Seattle.[11] Simmons reported back to the GB that the Seattle conference had "both good and bad points"; he criticized what he saw as the conference organizers' lack of new information about the scope of the epidemic in communities of color. He bemoaned the way that repeated discussions about basketball great Magic Johnson's recent disclosure of his HIV status had hijacked discussions of the issues and concluded that Johnson's announcement would make work in communities of color harder, not easier.

While many ACT UP/LA members were uncomfortable with the "all white" image of the group, it was never easy for members of ACT UP/LA to even discuss what to do about the relative lack of people of color in the group. Discussions could devolve into white activists attacking other white activists for not being racially sensitive. For example, Wade Richards, a person with AIDS (PWA) and a central participant in the Treatment and Data committee, was taken to task for the purportedly racist contents of remarks that he made at an ACT UP/LA retreat in February of 1991.[12] In response to those remarks, another ACT UP/LA member anonymously put a flyer on the table at a GB meeting comparing Richards to a member of the Ku Klux Klan. In response, Richards wrote an open letter to the GB in which he broached questions of how or whether ACT UP/LA could or should "represent all the diverse communities affected by AIDS." Richards recalled only having voiced concerns at the retreat about whether ACT UP/LA could meet the needs of people of color with HIV, that is, whether or not it could be a representative organization. The idea of ACT UP/LA as programmatic organization – a term that Richards attributed to fellow activist Cat Walker – made sense to Richards even while he argued that people of color's AIDS issues needed to be of concern to all members. Not surprisingly, Richards noted that a tactic like leaving an anonymous flyer on the

---

[10] ACT UP/LA General Body meeting minutes February 25, 1991, collection of author; Mark Simmons, "People of Color AIDS Activist Conference," ACT UP/LA News, 4:3 (June/July 1991), p. 8.

[11] Mark Simmons and "Members of ACT UP's People of Color Caucus," "Report from Seattle," c. December 1991, ONE Collection.

[12] Wade Richards, "Girl! Where in the World Did You Get That White Sheet? Or What Did Wade Really Say at the ACT UP/LA Retreat?" Two-page position statement, c. February 1991; ONE Collection.

literature table comparing a member to a Klansman did not encourage any "real discussion of race."

In my own interviews with former ACT UP/LA activists, recollections of racial/ethnic political divides were much less salient than those of gender divides. This lack of retrospective concern about race is almost certainly a result of who was interviewed: twenty-two out of the twenty-six interviewed were white (with six identifying as Jewish); three interviewees identified as all or part Latino; one identified as African American. Phill Wilson, the only African American I interviewed, felt that his presence in early ACT UP/LA was welcomed, especially for what it signified about the group's desire to be multiracial; however, Wilson was active only in the early days of ACT UP/LA.[13] The late Pete Jimenez, who identified as Latino, stated in his interview that he very much resented claims that ACT UP/LA had been only composed of white gay men and that such claims, made right to his face, had angered him.[14] In contrast to Wilson, Jimenez's activism in ACT UP/LA started much later and lasted through the years of the group's demobilization, when the group again became a smaller and more unified entity.

As I hope to show in the rest of this chapter, the politics of gender and racial/ethnic divide were very much internal conflicts about where the boundaries of the ACT UP/LA community were and what kind of responsibility the group had to that community, however defined. Was ACT UP/LA's community the lesbian and gay community? Was it a community of those who shared a particular view of how to confront authority about the AIDS pandemic? Was the community composed of everyone who was actually affected by the pandemic? These questions were part of the intersectional crises that developed in ACT UP/LA as the organization lost its early insularity and developed a reputation for effective and militant action. It was that reputation that drew new participants to the group in the wake of the veto by California's Republican governor of a lesbian and gay rights bill, Assembly Bill 101 (AB 101), in the fall of 1991.

INTERSECTIONAL CRISIS 1: AB 101 AND CHALLENGES TO ACT UP/LA'S VISION OF ANTI-AIDS ACTION

On September 29, 1991, Republican Governor of California Pete Wilson vetoed Assembly Bill 101. AB 101 would have prevented discrimination against lesbians and gays in areas such as employment and housing. In a four-page letter to the legislature that was made public, Wilson stated that he vetoed the bill because he felt that it would have had a negative impact on small business and that sufficient protections were already in place to prevent discrimination

---

[13] Interview with author, 1999.
[14] Interview with author, 2011.

against lesbians and gays. He also stated that he regretted that his veto might give "false comfort" to anti-gay bigots.[15]

The governor's veto generated outrage among gays and lesbians in California, who responded with an explosion of street demonstrations and marches statewide. Vigils were held in Sacramento; a "near riot" was reported in San Francisco.[16] On October 10, according to the *Sacramento Bee*, downtown Sacramento saw "thousands of angry and defiant protestors" taking over the area for four hours, "blocking traffic, smashing car windows," and surrounding the state capitol building.[17] The *Bee* estimated the crowd at close to 4,000, although the newspaper undercut the significance of the number, suggesting that the organizers had wanted a turnout of twice that. *The San Francisco Chronicle* described the state capitol protest as "the most turbulent Capitol demonstration since the Vietnam War."[18] The *Chronicle* writer thought the crowd may have been as many as 6,000, and noted that it included "bare-breasted women and leather-clad men." The *Chronicle* writer estimated that the protests in Sacramento had caused hundreds of thousands of dollars in damage to public property.

In Los Angeles, "angry and disappointed gays and lesbians demonstrated in West Hollywood" within hours of the veto, "blocking traffic and burning the California State flag."[19] Demonstrations continued the next day in both downtown LA and in West Hollywood, with demonstrations in the following days held in Beverly Hills, Silverlake, the San Fernando Valley, the Los Angeles International Airport, and even Anaheim in Orange County.[20] ACT UP/LA, Queer Nation, and the Gay and Lesbian Community Services Center worked together to organize the protests, even though many of ACT UP/LA's most active members were in Washington, DC, attending a nationally coordinated set of actions for universal healthcare when the veto came down. Those ACT UP/LA members returned from several intense days of direct action in DC to find that their community had taken their example of militant disruptive protest to heart – and then some.

ACT UP/LA participant Wendell Jones recalled that the protests against the AB 101 veto changed his life. He and other ACT UP/LA members had been in DC demonstrating for days without sleep and returned to Los Angeles while the

---

[15] M. R. Covino, "Veto Counter to Poll," *Vanguard News and Reviews*, 11:15 (October 4 1991), p. 1.

[16] Keith Clark, "Near Riot in San Francisco," *Vanguard News and Reviews*, 11: 15 (October 4 1991), p. 1.

[17] Andy Furillo, Robert Davilla, and Patrick Hoge "Downtown Engulfed by Gay Protest," *The Sacramento Bee*, Saturday October 11, 1991, p. 1.

[18] Robert B. Gunnison, "Gay Rights Protest at State Capitol," *The San Francisco Chronicle*, October 12, 1991, p. 1.

[19] Sandy Dywer, "LA Erupts in Protest," *Vanguard News and Reviews*, 11:15 (October 4, 1991), p. 14.

[20] Jeff Clark, "LA Streets Still Sizzle," *Vanguard*, 2:16 (October 18, 1991), p. 1. See also Faderman and Timmons. 2009. *Gay LA: A History of Sexual Outlaws, Power Politics, and Lipstick Lesbians*. Berkeley: University of California Press, p. 324.

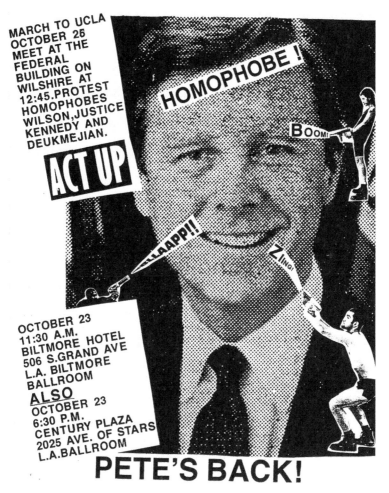

FIGURE 4.1: Flyer protesting California Governor Pete Wilson, early 1990s.

lesbian and gay community was erupting over the veto: "I went to bed, and I heard all this screaming outside and I ran down. … I lived close to Santa Monica Boulevard and there were all these people running in the streets and so I went down and I joined them."[21] Jones describes going down to "Boystown" – the west end of West Hollywood, especially the one-mile strip of Santa Monica Boulevard west of La Cienega Boulevard and east of Doheny Drive – and starting to march with "all these crazy gym boys" and ending up miles away, out of steam and near the point of collapse. Jones remembered being literally pulled into the safety of a neighbor's pickup truck when the driver had

[21] Interview with author, 2011.

happened to spot him in the crowd. The moment for him, while exhilarating, was one of literally "burning out."

Other stories of returning to LA after DC were just as dramatic. Walt "Cat" Walker was also in DC when AB 101 was vetoed, and he had been arrested as part of civil disobedience actions at the US capitol building; he was responsible there for helping civil disobedience neophytes block a doorway. He and others were waiting for their court hearings when word of the LA protests came to them:

So all hell broke loose here in LA and here we were in Washington DC and we kind of considered ourselves kind of the cream of LA gay activists at this point [laughs], and we were in DC. .... It's like when we first heard about the veto, we actually said things like "oh they'll probably have a big demonstration in San Francisco, but LA won't do anything, especially with us here." And then we heard that there were these great big demonstrations in LA and it like, blew our minds ... especially because the people who were leading and organizing these demonstrations were people who had not been involved in ACT UP, they were like a new group of people.[22]

Helene Schpak was also in DC and recalled that when she heard about Wilson's veto, she and another activist from San Francisco organized an impromptu action to break into a government building – she didn't recall which one – and steal the California state flag and burn it. Schpak returned to LA and participated in the many marches that protested the veto.

With or without the cream of the activist crop temporarily stuck in Washington, protests against Wilson's veto continued in Los Angeles; Kenney (2001: 157) referred to the AB 101 protests as "diffuse, decentralized, and somewhat rambling." Many of the protests took the form of marches, such as the one that brought Jones to his breaking point. I witnessed one of the early responses to the veto first-hand when a rowdy group of protestors swept down Santa Monica Boulevard while I and others watched through the picture windows of our gym. The marches themselves quickly became more organized; another on October 2 started at the Pacific Design Center in West Hollywood and "mushroomed into a march of thousands to the Hollywood Bowl, scene of a sold-out concert by Sting," covering a distance of four and a half miles.[23] By the ninth of October, protests had taken place for eleven consecutive days, and peaceful marchers had even gone down to the Los Angeles International Airport, where their mere presence was enough to disrupt operations.[24]

The LA protests received national attention, with *The New York Times* reporting that Wilson's veto had damaged a hard-won consensus about how

---

[22] Interview with author, 2011.
[23] Tracy Wilkinson, "Gay Republicans Say Wilson's Veto Betrayed Them," *The Los Angeles Times* (October 3, 1991), http://articles.latimes.com/1991-10-03/news/mn-4417_1_gay-republicans.
[24] Scott Harris, "Gay Protests Spreads to LA Airport," *The Los Angeles Times* (October 10, 1991), p. B1, B3.

to deal with the AIDS epidemic and rekindled views that saw some victims of AIDS as innocent and others as guilty of contracting the virus willfully.[25] While most of the marches proceeded peacefully under police escort, frustration at Wilson boiled over at a march to the Century Plaza Hotel on October 23 to protest a fundraising dinner for Wilson; that protest resulted in at least nine arrests as police on horseback tried to control a crowd of several hundred demonstrators. Wilson's speech inside the hotel was interrupted by two activists, one male and one female, who yelled that Wilson was "a bigot and a liar."[26] Several of the arrestees in Century City were ACT UP/LA members; they held a news conference the next day decrying the police response to the Century City protest as a police riot. Stuart Bailey from ACT UP/LA was quoted in *The Los Angeles Times*, describing the violence: "The cops came at us wielding their batons at whomever they could hit, attacking us on foot and charging into the crowd on horseback."[27]

As a result of lesbian and gay community anger about the governor's veto, attendance at ACT UP/LA's Monday night GB meetings easily doubled, from approximately one hundred to two hundred people or more. ACT UP/LA's openness – anyone who came to the GB meeting could vote – coupled with the fierce reputation the group acquired as the most militant game in town when it came to fighting AIDS, made it attractive to the newly enraged. But these new ACT UP/LA members were chiefly men, and, according to Jan Speller, they were not necessarily "AIDS" people. In my interview with her in 2000, Speller called the AB 101 protestors merely "reactive" to the veto – that is, not truly committed to a long-term, strategic, and leftist brand of activism. She described herself as feeling that all the marching after the veto was

... a waste of fuckin' energy ... and it was a party, too. I mean it was a huge party, in the way that some activism is ... but it was also kind of like, "okay, and now what?" You know, because we just knew it would be a matter of time before all those people would go back to the gym, right? *Walking* wasn't really what they wanted to do, you know.[28]

Echoing Wendell Jones' characterization of many of the marchers as "crazy gym boys," Speller described the marches as "strenuous," full of "all these buffed out white boys who could march really fast."

Speller's tongue-in-cheek complaint about the fitness of the AB 101 protestors indicated her concern at the time that the influx of men meant that ACT UP/LA women would need to start from scratch in educating men about women's AIDS issues. At the time of the long marches, Speller, a major

[25] Richard L. Berke, "AIDS Battle Reverting to 'Us Against Them,'" *The New York Times*, (October 6, 1991).

[26] Frederick Muir and Charisse Jones, "Police on Horseback Break Up Gay Protest," *The Los Angeles Times* (October 24, 1991), p. B1.

[27] David Ferrell, "Gays Decry LAPD's Behavior at Rally," *The Los Angeles Times* (October 25, 1991).

[28] Interview with author, 2000.

player in the WC and in the GB lived with male ACT UP/LA members, and the network that brought her and kept her in ACT UP/LA was a mixed-gender one. She described herself as loving the way that lesbians and gay men interacted in ACT UP/LA for the most part since, prior to joining, she had been living in conservative Orange County, where as she put it "women had to really, really struggle to have a voice" in what were often entirely gay male spaces. Speller also felt that her best contribution to ACT UP/LA was going to "the General [Body] Meetings and bringing a feminist perspective and a lesbian perspective to the larger group." But the newly active AB 101 people hadn't had experience dealing with activism within mixed-gender groups because they hadn't had experience with activism, period. They didn't easily make the links among general discrimination against lesbians and gays, and women's and men's AIDS issues that members of the WC tried to push ACT UP/LA participants to make.

Speller was not alone in her assessment of the lack of political education of the AB 101 influx. Mark Simmons, co-facilitator of the POC of ACT UP/LA, wrote in the newsletter that since the AB 101 veto, he had been "inundated with photos ... and comments of the upheaval caused by Governor Pete Wilson's veto of AB 101," but that for him "[s]everal things are missing. The absence of people of color in the demonstrations is a significant mirror of the gay and lesbian movement in Los Angeles."[29] In his full-page, prominently featured opinion piece, Simmons continued:

It's not surprising that the vast majority of the protestors are white. It's not surprising that the vast majority of protestors are not AIDS activists. It's also not surprising that the vast majority of protestors are what I would term "closet activists." By becoming galvanized overnight, these protestors are either middle-class or upper-middle-class gays and lesbians who have the most to lose. These are the affluent members of our community who have finally been put in the position of being discriminated upon, not because of race or gender but because of sexual persuasion. ... These recent protests have also grimly shown the reality of where the gay and lesbian community lies in its response to discrimination of people of color communities and HIV/AIDS. As long as ACT UP/LA has been in existence, we have never managed to have standing-room-only crowds at our Monday night meetings. ... I have yet to see these numbers at any AIDS discrimination rally. In my own particular view of this ricochet of activism from a single veto, I'm not impressed. ... One friend asked me why he hadn't seen me at recent protests. I simply commented that I'm in this fight every second of every hour of every day. My fight is about who I am as a black gay male.[30]

Simmons's dismay at the lack of diversity in the anti-veto marches was echoed in the wider gay press by Mario Solis-Marich, who wrote in the *Vanguard* that, despite the contribution of lesbians and gays of color to the

[29] Mark Simmons, "AB 101, Race and AIDS," *ACT UP/LA News* 4:5 (December 1990/January 1991), p. 3. Author's collection.
[30] Ibid.

movement, he had not seen "them leading our rallies and on my TV set."[31] Solis-Marich argued that lesbians and gays of color were people with long histories of activism in a variety of movements but that, in Los Angeles, there had been "years of mutual non-recognition ... between 'established' lesbian and gay leadership and the 'emergence of empowered' people of color." Solis-Marich, like Simmons, reported seeing only a "smattering" of people of color at the marches and worried that the absence of gays and lesbians of color from the marches would mean that they would be shut out of any future decision-making as to the direction a new movement might take.[32]

The AB 101 influx can be seen as what Nancy Whittier has called a "micro-cohort" – a group of activists introduced into a social movement at the same time and who, as a result of their particular experiences, "construct a distinct collective identity" in movement politics (1997: 769). Whittier writes that

because collective identity is shaped by the changing contexts that prevail when activists first commit to the cause, long-lived social movements contain cohorts with potentially disparate definitions of the movement. As recruits enter, their redefinitions of themselves and the cause can reshape the movement. (1997: 775)

Differences among micro-cohorts in a movement can therefore generate not just change but real conflict, as activists who enter at different times focus on their own agendas and discount, wittingly or not, the concerns of the members of previous micro-cohorts.

Stretching Whittier's term, I would argue that the AB 101 influx was, because of its large numbers, a new *macro*-cohort engulfing an organization that was itself fairly new. The new macro-cohort could best be described as angry about anti-lesbian and gay discrimination and only minimally educated about what a progressive direct action stance on AIDS might look like. There is little doubt, though, that the AB 101 influx brought new members to ACT UP/LA just at the moment when other ACT UPs around the country were losing steam. Still, members of earlier micro-cohorts – activists already busy in ACT UP/LA when the AB 101 veto hit – expressed mixed feelings about what the new members had done for/to the group. As noted earlier, Simmons was critical of the new macro-cohort's lack of diversity and lack of political education about the lives of people of color living with HIV, and Speller lamented the way that new ACT UP/LA members diffused the hard-won focus on women's AIDS issues. But the most veteran ACT UP/LA members did not agree on whether or not the AB 101 influx was a good thing or a bad thing. In a joint interview conducted by Jim McDaniels for the December 1991/January 1992 issue of

---

[31] Mario Solis-Marich, "The New Movement Must Empower People of Color," *Vanguard* 2:16 (October 18, 1991): pp. 6–7.

[32] A group of lesbian and gay people of color, Colors United Action Coalition, formed as a result of activists of color feeling ignored by white leaders of the AB 101 protests. See Kenney, 2001, chapter five, pp. 159–162.

ACT UP/LA's newsletter to honor the four year anniversary of the group's founding, Peter Cashman, Mark Kostopoulos, and David Lee Perkins, all of whom had been at the December 4, 1987, founding meeting, disagreed about the changes that AB 101 had wrought.[33] Cashman felt that "we need to pull back from AB 101 and get back to AIDS Work." On the other hand, Kostopoulos immediately looked on the bright side of the influx – sort of:

If the reaction to AB 101 is not simply an anomaly, if in fact it's an increased radicalization within the Gay and Lesbian community, it might give us a more prominent leadership role in the Gay and Lesbian community. How we adapt to that will be difficult. It would be a mistake to reject our role as a leader in the Gay and Lesbian community and at the same time we have to remember our agenda is AIDS. That tension could define the coming period.

Kostopoulos was correct in his assessment that ACT UP/LA was moving into a position of leadership for the community. He was more optimistic than other activists who felt that the reaction to AB 101 created real problems for ACT UP/LA's anti-AIDS work. In an undated position paper that was clearly written shortly after the AB 101 veto entitled "Coalitioning," Doug Fuller and Tay Ashton wrote to fellow ACT UP/LA members that the coalition work that ACT UP/LA had been doing with other groups in the lesbian and gay community had raised "legitimate questions ... about our role in future non-AIDS demonstrations."[34] Fuller and Ashton were concerned, as Cashman was, with ACT UP/LA's need to continue doing anti-AIDS work; they wanted the group avoid a situation where anti-AIDS work became "merely one of a litany of issues" in multi-issue demonstrations and actions. Fuller and Ashton advocated that ACT UP/LA "take a step back now to examine our goals and motivations surrounding coalition work."

At least one ACT UP/LA member remembered the effects of the AB 101 influx as being positive. Judy Sisneros disagreed that the new members who came as a result of the veto had negative effects on the group, let alone that these effects were gendered or raced. She felt that getting new people "makes you start to think ... about getting out of any ruts, and ... just brings fresh thinking to the group."[35] Sisneros told me that it was her assumption that any negative characterization of the influx would be made by "older people," that is, members who had been in ACT UP/LA longer. But Sisneros *was* one of the older people, from the standpoint of how long she had belonged to the group. Sisneros and Speller were roughly contemporaries and thus part of the same pre-AB 101 micro-cohort.

[33] Jim McDaniels, "Interview with Three Founding Members of ACT UP/LA," *ACT UP/LA News*, 4:5 (December 1991/January 1992), pp. 6–7. The actual joint interview was conducted on December 4, 1991.

[34] Doug Fuller and Tay Ashton, "Coalitioning." Undated position paper, c. November 1991; ONE Collection.

[35] Interview with author, 2000.

Within a year or so, the swollen numbers at GB meetings dropped. In 1993, John Kimball, who was active in the Treatment and Data Committee of ACT UP/LA, wrote an "opinion piece" addressing what he called "The Trouble with ACT UP/Los Angeles."[36] In it, Kimball argued that the influx of new members in late 1991 diffused the group's focus just at a time when AIDS was becoming a more complex issue and that disruptive direct action was getting harder to stage in a media-friendly manner. Nevertheless, Kimball wrote that the AIDS community was becoming broader and that ACT UP/LA needed to "embrace the entire AIDS community":

We cannot risk the danger of fighting exclusively for our issues, and ignore the fact that other communities are just beginning to fight battles that we thought were behind us. . . . I'm not saying that we have to stop to wait for other groups to "catch up" to us. What we must do is make our agenda bigger, in order to include these issues and make them our issues and fight them with all the vigor, anger and energy that have been the hallmarks of our battles and the badges of our victories.

As disagreements among activists suggest, it is an open question whether or not the AB 101 influx hurt ACT UP/LA as an organization or helped it. In any case, the influx represented an intersectional crisis for the group. It changed the group's gender/racial/ethnic balance in numbers but also in political understanding. The influx increased the group's numbers but also increased diversity in the group regarding *political education* because new members knew less about the politics of AIDS than older ones. The AB 101 macro-cohort fundamentally challenged the grounds on which solidarity had been built among ACT UP/LA's members, and ACT UP/LA's informality, its openness, and the direct action example it set made it difficult for the group to manage the energy literally marching its way. Having positioned itself as a direct action leader within the lesbian and gay community, ACT UP/LA could not protect itself from the larger community's gendered and raced understandings about political priorities.

INTERSECTIONAL CRISIS 2: CLEAN NEEDLES NOW AND THE BOUNDARIES OF COMMUNITY

> I'm against spending activist money on needle exchange, you know . . . you need to push the Feds, and everybody else who has all the AIDS money, like AIDS Project Los Angeles . . . to do that, to offer the infrastructure to do that.
>
> – Mary Lucey[37]

A significant and protracted intersectional crisis within ACT UP/LA occurred when members of Clean Needles Now (CNN), originally a subcommittee of the

---

[36] John Kimball, "The Trouble with ACT UP/Los Angeles." Undated position paper (c. June 1992); ONE Collection.

[37] Interview with author, 1999.

Treatment and Data Committee, began running an illegal needle exchange
program (NEP) in 1992. The question of whether ACT UP/LA could provide
social services – and, if so, for whom – became linked to questions of who was
part of the ACT UP/LA community, who could lead ACT UP/LA projects, and
whether the group could become more diverse. Ultimately, most ACT UP/LA
members rejected the idea of becoming a "hybrid" organization (Whittier 2011)
that could provide the *service* of needle exchange as a form of direct *action*.

In the early years of AIDS social service provision, there was little doubt that
providing services to people with AIDS was seen as a form of activism; Brier
(2009: 4), for example, argues that "AIDS workers" did not draw "a sharp
distinction between 'AIDS activism,' defined as direct action targeted against
the state and industry and 'AIDS service,' defined as entities that developed to
provide the actual 'services' to people with AIDS." Her definition of "AIDS
work" and "AIDS workers" thus collapses the distinction between service and
activism. But, by the early 1990s, activists in ACT UP/LA did make a distinction
between what their group did and what AIDS service organizations did, even
though many ACT UP/LA activists did AIDS work in service groups as well.
Debates in ACT UP/LA over needle exchange brought out members' opinions on
precisely what the difference was between direct action and service provision.
The debate also raised questions about what it would mean to provide services to
the AIDS community. Did ACT UP/LA owe its energies to members of the
lesbian, gay, and queer community, or to all those affected by HIV/AIDS?
These were overlapping but in no way identical communities. The latter – those
affected by HIV/AIDS – included intravenous (IV) drug users, people of color,
women, and straights. Ideologically, ACT UP/LA members were in solidarity
with all those affected by the HIV/AIDS pandemic, but ACT UP/LA was situated
in a communal space bounded socially and spatially by the contours of the lesbian
and gay community (Kenney 2001). Was it ACT UP/LA's job to organize outside
the lesbian and gay community? Was needle exchange the right project with
which to start reaching out to other HIV/AIDS affected communities?
The debates around needle exchange brought up these questions, and members
confronted their not always explicit assumptions about the politics of gender,
race/ethnicity, and sexuality in ACT UP/LA.

THE ORIGINS OF CLEAN NEEDLES NOW

CNN grew out of discussions held at ACT UP/LA's Treatment and Data
Committee meetings in early 1991. Needle exchange was first raised as an issue
at a GB meeting in 1991, when Treatment and Data committee members reported
on their concerns about IV drug use as a "growing route of transmission of
HIV."[38] Several Treatment and Data Committee members – Bill Flanagan,

---

[38] Treatment and Data committee report, "Current Scope of Need," January 4, 1991, p. 2.
Author's collection.

Connie Norman, and Brett McGuire – described their goal as providing "the knowledge and means for injection drug users to protect themselves from HIV transmission, and to get timely drug treatment."[39] Needle exchange as a topic continued to appear from time to time on GB meeting agendas, but did not receive a lot of attention even at Treatment and Data committee meetings. For example, in the almost three-inch thick "ACT UP/Los Angeles Treatment and Data Committee Treatment Primer" that I received when I briefly joined the committee as a representative from the WC, needle exchange was scarcely mentioned, with the primer including only a copy of a *Los Angeles Times* article about needle exchange and a checklist from a Seattle needle exchange resource manual.[40]

The political context for introducing a NEP in Los Angeles in the early 1990s was not encouraging. Throughout the late 1980s, the LA County Board of Supervisors, the five-member body responsible for making decisions on public health programs in LA County, was a conservative body, with a three-to-two conservative majority. The Board continuously ignored the advice of its own County AIDS Commission, which had been urging the County to take the minimal step of distributing bleach and condom kits to IV drug users as the City of Los Angeles had been doing.[41] The replacement of conservative supervisor Pete Schabarum by liberal Gloria Molina in 1991 shifted the dynamic on the Board, and, in March of 1991, the Supervisors agreed to spend approximately $40,000 for the distribution of bleach and condom kits.[42] The amount was paltry, but also reflected the fact that, in the early 1990s, no one really knew how extensive the spread of HIV was among IV drug users in the county.[43]

In August 1991, a few ACT UP/LA members joined other ACT UP activists from around the state for a meeting with California state health officials about the need for needle exchange as part of a "continuum of care" for IV drug users.[44] In a report given to the GB after the state meeting, Connie Norman argued for cost-effectiveness as a reason for the state to get behind needle exchange, pointing out "the hypocrisy of denying subsidies to AIDS drugs because of financial constraints while simultaneously refusing to adopt needle exchange – which will save the state money by reducing the numbers of new infections." Norman was quite comfortable using the language of cost-benefit

[39] "Needle Exchange Program," c. March 1991. Author's collection.
[40] "ACT UP/Los Angeles Treatment and Data Committee Treatment Primer" table of contents, c. December 1990. Author's collection.
[41] Bruce Mirken, "Needles as an A.I.D.S. Tack," *Los Angeles Reader* (March 22, 1991): 8.
[42] Bruce Mirken, "Needle Vote Nettles Antonovich," *Los Angeles Reader* (March 29, 1991); 5.
[43] Mirken, ibid., reported that in March 1991, there were an estimated 125,000 IV drug users in LA County, with perhaps 10% of them HIV-positive.
[44] "ACT UP/LA Treatment & Data Committee Treatment Issues Report," Number 8, August 19, 1991: 2. Author's collection. This report focused chiefly on a meeting with the California Department of Health Services, p. 2.

analyses to California state health officials, but arguments about cost and benefits of a NEP in ACT UP/LA were only partly about the rational use of resources. As discussed later, many members were reluctant to start a NEP; they were skeptical about whether or not ACT UP/LA could serve the communities, largely communities of color, where IV drug use was spreading the virus. Yet, in another way, the idea of running a NEP was in keeping with ACT UP/LA's militant identity since it meant practicing civil disobedience: needle exchange was not legal in Los Angeles County. By March 1992, CNN was listed on GB meeting agendas as a separate committee,[45] and, by April of that same year, CNN formulated a "Policy Statement," a version of which was published in the ACT UP/LA newsletter, that strongly advocated that ACT UP/LA follow the lead of ACT UP Seattle and work with local government to institute a NEP in Los Angeles.[46]

THE PALLADIUM FUNDRAISER: MORE MONEY, MORE PROBLEMS

CNN members argued strongly that a NEP should be funded with the proceeds of an extremely successful fundraiser that several committee members helped to produce. On April 4, 1992, a rock-and-roll concert/fundraiser took place at the Hollywood Palladium on Sunset Boulevard with proceeds going to ACT UP/LA and the Magic Johnson Foundation.[47] The line-up included the Red Hot Chili Peppers, Jane's Addiction, Fishbone, Primus, the Henry Rollins Band, Porno for Pyros, and The Beastie Boys. The concert was first announced to ACT UP/LA in a GB meeting in February 1992 by Lee Wildes, one of CNN's co-facilitators. He told the GB that the Palladium fundraiser would probably raise about $65,000 and that the money would be split with the Magic Johnson Foundation. Wildes stated that he hoped that some of the money would go to CNN's legal defense fund and that some would go toward scholarships that would allow activists to attend the upcoming Eighth International AIDS Conference in Amsterdam, but no formal proposal regarding spending was made.[48] The minutes describe the discussion about the fundraiser as "lengthy" and note that "further discussion was postponed until the next meeting."

By the time the concert/fundraiser took place, produced by Goldenvoice Productions, a punk/alternative rock concert promotion company active in Southern California, the event was explicitly billed as helping to promote needle exchange and the rights of drug users to be free from HIV disease:

---

[45] "ACT UP/LA General Meeting, Monday March 2, 1992" agenda. Author's collection.

[46] CNN/Clean Needles Now (ACT UP/LA) "Policy Statement on Needle Exchange, Harm Reduction and Treatment on Demand." Unsigned article *ACT UP/LA News* 5: 1 (March/April 1992), p. 9. Other versions of the statement are similarly unsigned, although contact people are listed.

[47] Press Release, "A Goldenvoice Concert to Benefit ACT UP/LA and the Magic Johnson Foundation." Author's Collection.

[48] Minutes of the General Body meeting, February 17, 1992; ONE collection.

Clean Needles Now, CNN, asserts that drug users have the right to be given information and equipment that can save their lives. By providing injection drug users with consistent access to bleach kits, sterile syringes and information that clearly defines drug-using behaviors and HIV transmission routs, CNN can help injectors modify their risky behaviors. ... This concert makes it possible for CNN to distribute drug treatment and safe(r) sex information, bleach kits, as well as to initiate a needle exchange program in Los Angeles. With 150,000 dead from AIDS and over a million people living with HIV, ROCK IS NOT ENOUGH: ACT UP! FIGHT BACK! FIGHT AIDS![49]

The Palladium concert/fundraiser was a success. The best estimate for the amount of money raised, after expenses and the split with the Magic Johnson Foundation, was a little over $63,000, a tremendous amount of money for ACT UP/LA.[50] But some members were uncomfortable with being allied in any way with the Magic Johnson Foundation. Johnson's announcement of his HIV-positive status in November 1992 and the incredible amount of publicity that the announcement received created consternation among many in the AIDS activist community. As noted earlier, ACT UP/LA's Mark Simmons felt that the Johnson announcement of his HIV status had hijacked the agenda of the People of Color conference that he had attended. Back in Los Angeles, someone left an anonymous flyer on the literature table at a GB meeting after Johnson's announcement, showing 1,782 small unsmiling face icons arrayed in rows, and captioned "[i]f you were to photocopy this page 841 times, you would get an approximate idea how many people have been infected by the HIV virus in the United States before Magic Johnson."[51] And, in an article for ACT UP/LA's newsletter, Richard Iosty took Johnson to task for trying to distance himself from the gay community by telling talk show host Arsenio Hall that he, Johnson, was "about as far from a homosexual as you can get." Iosty wrote that

[a]t a moment when Johnson might have challenged the inscription of homophobia within AIDS, he instead chose to be complicit with that homophobia, forcefully reinscribing the notion that only certain lives matter in this epidemic. It was 24 hours after his first press conference, and any hopes engendered by the straightforward assertions of that first performance that Johnson might be a spokesperson for HIV-positive persons was undercut by his queer bashing and willful participation in a media spectacle that constituted him as a hero, that located the site of all loss, grief, and hope in his figure.[52]

In ACT UP/LA circles, Johnson was no hero. And even though sharing monies from the Palladium fundraiser did not involve any real affiliation with his foundation, many ACT UP/LA members were profoundly uncomfortable with even a brief, instrumental connection.

---

[49] CNN Press Release, March 23 1992; ONE collection.
[50] Minutes, April 20, 1992 General Body meeting; ONE collection.
[51] The number comes out to a bit more than 1.5 million.
[52] Richard Iosty, "Magic Johnson and the Spectacle of Male Heterosexual Sentimentality," ACT UP/LA *News*, 4: 5 (December 1991/January 1992), p. 4.

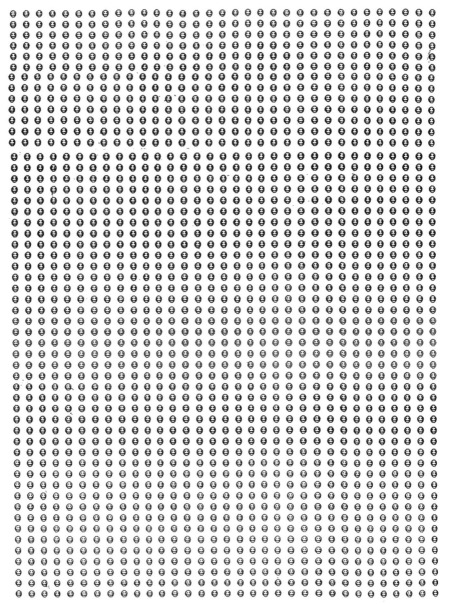

If you were to photocopy this page 841 times, you would get an
approximate idea how many people have been infected by the HIV
virus in the United States before Magic Johnson.

FIGURE 4.2: Flyer in response to Magic Johnson's announcement that he was
HIV-positive, 1991.

The money raised at the Palladium concert generated disputes in the GB about how to spend it. Within the next few weeks, serious disagreements emerged about spending the money solely on a NEP. ACT UP/LA's Agitating/ Legal Committee suggested that $10,000 from the fundraiser go to the overall – not just CNN – legal fund because the fund was very low and because it was anticipated that the CNN's proposed needle exchange activities, still illegal, might "quickly drain the legal fund."[53] Over the course of the next few meetings, ACT UP/LA discussed a "detailed budget" presented by CNN for a NEP for the coming year.[54] CNN proposed spending approximately $50,000 during 1992–1993 to conduct a NEP in South Central Los Angeles, including tracing the spread of HIV among IV drug users by collecting the "points" of used syringes and testing the blood on them by means of polymerase chain reaction (PCR).[55] The idea of collecting used needle points was deemed important by CNN members because they felt that if they could document a lowered infection rate among users, they could support a "necessity" legal defense" for their illegal actions if they were arrested and prosecuted. CNN asked for "a one year commitment from AU [ACT UP/LA] to program as [the] only way [the] program can be productive"; CNN promised to eventually apply for funds from grant-making institutions.

CNN's projected budget for its NEP was a huge amount of money for ACT UP/LA to devote to any one project, and it represented the lion's share of the Palladium fundraiser monies. The budget was discussed extensively at the April 20, 1992, GB meeting. At that meeting, CNN members argued that its proposed budget represented "four months of research, networking and interviews with needle exchange activists and drug treatment workers throughout California and across the country."[56] CNN stated that there was dire need for needle exchange in Los Angeles:

With an estimated 120,000 injecting drug users in Los Angeles, we will not be able to keep [up] with the demand for clean syringes and drug treatment information. Even at maximum efficiency, our NEP [needle exchange program] can only serve approximately

---

[53] Minutes for General Body meeting, April 6, 1992, and April 13,1992; ONE Collection.
[54] Minutes for General Body Meeting, April 13, 1992; ONE Collection.
[55] I found two versions of the CNN projected budget for 1992–1993 in ACT UP/LA's papers at the ONE Archive. It is likely that one of these versions was presented to the General Body at the April 13, 1992, meeting, with discussion tabled until April 20. However, I do not know how closely either draft conforms to what ACT UP/LA members heard then from CNN. One budget was for $51,117 and one was for $47,367 – with this figure written rather than typed in – although the figures in this latter budget actually add up to $53,642. The biggest item in both budgets by far was for PCR tagging and testing of needles ($15,000). The next highest item of $10,400 in each budget was for "104,000 Insulin Needles and Syringes"; after that, more than $6,000 in each budget was slated for 25,000 bleach kits and $4,240 for the purchase and distribution of 80,000 condoms. ("CNN Needle Exchange Budget Expenditures – 1 Year of Distribution: May 1, 1992–May 1, 1993." Two unsigned documents; ONE Collection.)
[56] "CNN Needle Exchange Budget," ONE Collection.

1% of all IVDU's [IV drug users] in Los Angeles. Our intention is to set up a pilot needle exchange program that will serve as a model and that we can use as an example to pressure local government to fund and legalize our program or to force Los Angeles officials to create one based on ours.[57]

In a statement that accompanied the budget, the CNN committee maintained that its work would " blur the line between direct-action politics and lifesaving AIDS defiance of state and local laws, therefore, it will function as a kind of day-to-day demo until local law authorities choose to make examples of us and arrest us."[58] CNN member Henry Chang wrote a separate statement for the GB characterizing CNN's proposed work as community-based activist science.[59] Chang acknowledged that what CNN was asking for was unusual for ACT UP/LA, but he also insisted that the NEP had to be funded as CNN envisioned:

[W]e must ask ourselves whether we want a (would be) poorly-executed, somewhat-blinded NEP where its efficacy cannot be ever determined or evaluated, or a PCR-based evaluation of NEP for its ability to link the mechanics of needle-exchange directly to the level of infection of circulating needles. I would vote for the latter without any reservations. People want to hear what they want to hear. However, the main idea here is that, whenever possible, we should all *let the needles do the talking!*"[60]

The April 20 meeting was apparently a very contentious one. The minutes for the meeting, taken by Cat Walker, succinctly summed up the outcome of the contention – ACT UP/LA's conditional support of CNN's efforts – because the GB decided to give CNN only some of the money they asked for and asked CNN not to move money "among categories in the budget."[61]

THE DEBATES ABOUT THE (PERSONAL) POLITICS OF CNN

After the April 20 meeting, discussions about the wisdom of a CNN NEP carried on. Some ACT UP/LA members expressed anger about the decision to fund CNN's NEP through the means of the group's gossip sheet *Tiara*; significantly, many of these reactions were anonymous. The angry responses centered not just on the kinds of requests that CNN made but also on how CNN members purportedly behaved toward the rest of ACT UP/LA.[62] One contributor, "Sign me Pissed!" accused CNN of "separatist politics," describing members of the committee as having a "super-secret 'Don't ask me

---

[57] "CNN Needle Exchange Budget," ONE Collection.
[58] "CNN/Clean Needles Now" statement, Unsigned. c.4/92; ONE Collection.
[59] Henry Chang, "Let the Needles Do the Talking." April 20, 1992; ONE Collection.
[60] Chang, emphasis in the original.
[61] Minutes, General Body meeting April 20, 1992; ONE Collection.
[62] The denouncements of CNN appear in the *Tiara* issue dated April 27, 1992. In stark contrast, the previous week's *Tiara* (April 20, 1992) had only one mention of CNN, praising their "devotion and hard work" and noting how much money the Palladium concert had raised for the group; ONE Collection.

what I'm doing 'cause I'm not telling you 'cause you're not part of the way-cool in-crowd, the inner circle of CNN'" attitude. "Sign me Pissed!" was especially angered that several of the CNN leaders left the GB meeting after their proposal had been voted on. Another *Tiara* contributor vented about his or her feelings of being made to feel bad because of opposition to the CNN, having been called a "murderer" for questioning the group.[63] An unsigned cartoon appeared in *Tiara* that used the characters of Dagwood Bumstead and his boss, Julius C. Dithers (from the cartoon strip "Blondie") to argue that not enough time had been devoted to discussion of the CNN proposal and that members had forgone having their questions answered in order to simply ratify CNN's request. One *Tiara* contributor who supported CNN and who signed her name – Terri Ford – even expressed her unhappiness that many CNN members, including co-facilitators Lee Wildes and Renee Edgington, had walked out of the meeting after their proposal had passed.

The *Tiara* contributors played up their disappointments with the personal attitudes of some CNN leadership. Others took more political views about CNN. In my interviews, only one former ACT UP/LA member, Geneviève Clavreul, cited opposition to needle exchange per se as a reason for challenging CNN's actions, and she stated that she *never* voiced this opposition publicly when she was in ACT UP/LA.[64] Activist Peter Cashman saw needle exchange as a bad fit for ACT UP/LA:

The whole thing was to run some sort of a study to validate needle exchange. Our point was that's all well and good but no one is going to accept your study. You know these studies have to be done at a very high level and that this is a big waste of money and what is the point? ... If that's going to be done, it has to be done by someone else.[65]

Cashman felt that ACT UP/LA couldn't do a community-based scientific study justice; another ACT UP/LA member, Mary Lucey, a self-described former "junkie," recalled feeling that the needle exchange/tracking project was likely to be funded by other entities and that ACT UP/LA should have concentrated on tasks that "never ever get money." James Rosen, who was active with the Treatment and Data Committee, stated in no uncertain terms in his interview in 2012 that he did not think that needle exchange was an appropriate project for the group: "I really was against it. I didn't think that was ACT UP's responsibility." But other ACT UP/LA participants had much friendlier feelings toward CNN; for example, partners Jeff Scheurholz and Pete Jimenez both recalled that they actively assisted CNN members with needle exchange, at one point helping to label used needles to assist with tracking points.

---

[63] Emphasis in the original.
[64] Interview with author, 2011.
[65] Interview with author, 1999.

Had the debates over CNN been strictly about its fit with the rest of ACT UP/LA, they may have still been fairly divisive, given how much money was involved. But gender, sexuality, and racial/ethnic politics were part of debates about CNN, which were at once about personalities *and* about ACT UP/LA's responsibilities. CNN's longtime co-facilitator was a married, straight white woman named Rene Edgington who was part of the alternative art world in Los Angeles and who had ties beyond the activist lesbian and gay community that proved useful to CNN (e.g., to Goldenvoice Productions). She was also distrusted by some in ACT UP/LA. Edgington was, in the words of the late Ferd Eggan who considered her a friend, regarded by many as "just this nasty bitch."[66] Eggan, the city's third AIDS Policy Coordinator, responded to my question about whether Edgington was "just this nasty bitch" or just this "straight nasty bitch," by acknowledging that Edgington's sexuality played a role in how some members related to her:

I think that there was a certain amount of straight-bashing of this straight woman and how could she conceivably understand … they [other members] did not have a universally positive feeling about this white straight woman who was leading work around needle exchange, which was largely needed to be developed in communities of color so it wasn't just … I mean … gender is always raced, and race is always gendered.

Jeff Scheurholz actively supported CNN and described himself as "so pro Renee," but he acknowledged that his feelings were not universal: "[a] lot of people had really bad things to say about her … and I never saw that side of her and I worked with her a lot when we both worked on Clean Needles." Pete Jimenez felt that some of the animus against Edgington was her devotion to a world outside of the regular experience of most ACT UP/LA members: according to Jimenez, Edgington "knew that there was this whole population that the rest of the group wasn't paying attention to ….helping with clean needles was another part of prevention and nobody was really focused on that." Neither Scheurholz nor Jimenez were willing to rule out the possibility that some of the hostility toward Edgington was based on her sexuality. Scheurholz felt that, like other explicitly straight female ACT UP/LA members – he named the late Stephanie Boggs and Cookie Pemberton – Edgington was sometimes ignored by the rest of the group, especially socially.

Edgington's visibility as a leader but also as an outsider – someone whose main ties were outside the lesbian and gay community, someone who was married and straight – helped at least a few former ACT UP/LA participants to misremember CNN's NEP as a divisive women-only project. In my 1999 interview with Peter Cashman, J. T. Anderson, and Stephanie Boggs, the three conflated the Palladium concert with another fundraiser, the Reality Ball, which took place two months later in June 1992. The Reality Ball was devoted to

---

[66] Interview with author, 1999.

women's AIDS issues and consisted of a set of performances by local and nationally recognized lesbian and gay performers, a dance, and a silent art auction. Renee Edgington played no part in the Ball's production, and CNN did not participate as a committee. The only connection between the Reality Ball and needle exchange was a mention of the latter in a list of government responses needed to end HIV disease.[67]

Stephanie Boggs, who had been part of the WC, told a story in her interview about how Edgington wanted money from the Ball to go to needle exchange. Boggs recalled that Edgington worked in concert with two members of the WC, Judy Sisneros and Helene Schpak, to try to divert the funds raised by the Ball, relating that Sisneros and Schpak came to the floor of a GB meeting asking that *all* the money raised by the Ball be turned over to the WC, with the implication being that Edgington would then be able to use the money for CNN. It's highly unlikely that such an agreement existed, and Bogg's claims are not supported by the archival record. The minutes for the June 15, 1992, GB meeting that took place five days before the Ball report that a proposal was made by the WC that "all profits from the Reality Ball be earmarked for Women and AIDS activities." This proposal, which passed by a two to one margin, also stated that the GB would still need to approve actual expenditures and that any committee could use the money, which would explicitly *not* be under the control of the WC. It does seem possible that the proposal that funds from the Ball be turned over to the WC had as its precedent the request by CNN to earmark the Palladium funds for needle exchange. In any case, the Reality Ball lost approximately $7,000.[68]

Boggs also recalled that the Reality Ball was videotaped – which it was – and that there were hopes that selling the video could help raise money for ACT UP/LA, but that one male ACT UP/LA member told her that he intended to "eat up" all the money from the Ball through the video's production "so you bitches don't get a penny."[69] Emblematic of activists' ambivalence about gender divides in ACT UP/LA, Boggs saw his remarks as just his individual expression and not a sign of collective male anger over who was getting what cut of fundraising monies. Given ongoing gender tensions in ACT UP/LA, given simmering disputes about ACT UP/LA's racial/ethnic composition (discussed later), and given Edgington's central, visible involvement with needle exchange, it remains a very open question as to how needle exchange was perceived by many in ACT UP/LA: was it a necessary project for ACT UP/LA's next step, or was it an inappropriate, gendered distraction from ACT UP/LA's real purpose?

[67] Press release "ACT UP/LA's 1992 Reality Ball," May 20, 1992; ONE Collection.
[68] Minutes, General Body meeting, September 21, 1992; ONE Collection.
[69] Interview with author, 1999. According to the General Body meeting minutes from July 20 1992, there was to be a screening of a "rough cut" of the video and a party for those who worked on the Ball at a local club. Terri Ford, who I interviewed in 2011, provided me with a copy of part of the video. I do not know if it was actually ever sold as a fundraiser.

ACT UP/LA'S RACIAL POLITICS, RODNEY KING,
AND THE BOUNDARIES OF COMMUNITY

CNN garnered ACT UP/LA's conditional support for its NEP, but local conditions for the launch of an ACT UP/LA-sponsored project in communities of color could not have been less auspicious. Less than two weeks after the April 20, 1992, GB meeting that funded CNN, the Rodney King riots/civil unrest/rebellion broke out, causing at least fifty-one deaths and billions of dollars of damage to property, especially in areas of LA City where CNN had hoped to operate.[70] At approximately the same time as the CNN debates and the Rodney King unrest, ACT UP/LA's POC committee presented the GB with a "working document ... intended to provide the framework for discussion regarding issues that the Racism Committee believes to be fundamental in how People of Color exist as an entity within ACT-UP Los Angeles."[71] The authors of the unsigned working document asserted that there were circumstances preventing people of color from participating in the group – a question of representation – and that ACT UP/LA committees were not following through with agendas that met the concerns and needs of PWAs of color and their communities – a matter of programming. The document's authors were concerned about the representation of people of color in different parts of ACT UP/LA, asking that the Treatment and Data Committee make sure that POC representatives were sent to AIDS Clinical Trial Group meetings in Washington, DC, and to International Conferences on AIDS, that the Media Committee distribute the newsletter in communities of color, and that the Networking/Outreach committee translate all outreach material into Spanish. The authors told the WC to give the GB more information about the effects of AIDS on women of color.

Given LA's metroscape of segregated diversity, the matter of attracting more people of color to ACT UP/LA inevitably became a discussion about geography: where should ACT UP/LA hold its Monday night GB meetings? In June 1992, discussions began about moving the site of GB meetings from West Hollywood's Plummer Park to other sites. At the June 15, 1992, meeting, two POC members – Steve Corbin and Lee Wildes, both active in the CNN as well – broached the topic of rotating meetings as "an outreach tool to other AIDS affected communities."[72] Corbin, who was African American and Wildes, the CNN co-facilitator, specifically suggested rotating meetings among West Hollywood, Silverlake, and South Central sites. Their proposal unleashed a torrent of alternative suggestions about where to meet that were linked to discussions of how (or whether) ACT UP/LA could change to meet the challenge

---

[70] Marc Lacey, "Riot Death Toll Lowered to 51 after Coroner's Review," *The Los Angeles Times.* August 12, 1992.
[71] People of Color Committee working document. Unsigned, dated April 6, 1992; ONE Collection.
[72] ACT UP/LA meeting minutes, June 15, 1992; ONE Collection.

of the changing demographics of the AIDS epidemic. The GB charged Corbin, Wildes, the POC, and the Networking/Outreach committee with coming back the next week with a more concrete proposal. They did so – sort of. Wildes and Corbin submitted a signed, four-page proposal about the pros and cons of moving meeting sites. They sought agreement from the GB on the principle of rotation, putting off a decision about the specifics of new sites and asking that the POC and the Networking/Outreach committee be empowered to make more specific decisions about the rotation subject to a later vote by the GB. Corbin and Wildes, in other words, didn't really take the GB's request for specifics to heart. Instead, they took the opportunity to make an extensive case for rotating meetings as a means of expanding ACT UP/LA's social base from mostly gay, mostly male, mostly white West Hollywood to what they called other "target communities."[73]

Clearly, Corbin and Wildes were seeking to extend the discussions that were opened up by the CNN about broadening ACT UP/LA's purpose as an organization; just as clearly, many members wanted to respond somehow to the collective trauma of the Rodney King rebellion. Wildes's and Corbin's proposal about rotating meetings explicitly referenced the politics of race/ethnicity in the group because they acknowledged the segregated landscape of Los Angeles – which included the segregation of the visible lesbian and gay community. Wildes and Corbin wrote that they assumed "that current ACT UP members support the notion that our constituency is and should be all those affect by AIDS." If their assumption was correct, then it was reasonable to suggest that it was a problem for ACT UP/LA that "membership demographics in no way reflect AIDS demographics." At the same time, Wildes and Corbin seemed to know that not all members thought ACT UP/LA *should* move into other communities to organize. And it is striking how Wildes and Corbin used the language of social work to make their argument to other members of ACT UP/LA; they continuously referred to communities of color as "target communities," "target populations," "target area residents," and they argued for ACT UP/LA's need to engage in "aggressive incorporation of the target communities." Equally striking was their dismissal of members' fears of encountering homophobia in sites outside of West Hollywood; they argued that "as usual we'll just have to do some educating – just as these new members will have issues we'll have to learn about. *As a democratic coalition we assume that ACT UP wants new members specifically so that we can deal with their issues with authority.*"[74] It is unclear when and in what form Wildes' and Corbin's rotation proposal was voted on; in any case, Monday night GB meetings continued to take place in Plummer Park.

[73] Lee Wildes and Steven Corbin, "ACT UP – Get Moving!" Proposal to General Body, June 23, 1992 (one day after the June 22 General Body meeting); ONE Collection.
[74] Emphasis in the original.

While ACT UP/LA debated on whether to meet in communities of color; CNN actually began its NEP in those communities.[75] Edgington reported to the July 13 GB meeting that CNN's NEP was "working" and that the group had been able to retrieve 10 percent of the program needles they had distributed for PCR tracking.[76] But backlash toward CNN's NEP within communities of color was immediate. At the July 27 GB meeting, Edgington reported that CNN had *stopped* distributing needles, having felt "forced to do so" after meeting with the Watts Health Foundation, the Minority AIDS Consortium (MAC), and Rue's House (a shelter for PWAs). These community groups all objected to CNN's lack of consultation; the Watts Health Foundation, for example, was distributing bleach kits in the same park as CNN.[77]

CNN members began to lose other ACT UP/LA members' support, which had always been conditional. For one thing, the IV drug users in the "target communities" that CNN wanted to serve were mostly heterosexual; Cat Walker recalled that

(i)t seemed to a lot of us that it [needle exchange] wasn't ... it was outside of the gay community, for one, and the intravenous drug using community ... kind of felt sketchy to some of us, so we didn't feel entirely comfortable with it ... at the same time I understood what they [CNN] were doing, and I did think it was important ... it was another way to prevent AIDS and to help the situation, so I supported what they did, I just didn't feel like doing it myself.[78]

There were other ACT UP/LA members who, in contrast to Walker, did feel like doing needle exchange themselves, but they increasingly did so as non-ACT UP/LA activism. Jeff Scheurholz and Pete Jimenez both participated in CNN's NEP and were thus keenly aware that CNN had more or less "split off" (in Jimenez' phrase) from ACT UP/LA. According to Scheurholz, CNN's understandable need for secrecy led to ACT UP/LA members' equally understandable questions of "who are these people and what are they doing and how come you keep needing more money?"[79] ACT UP/LA members were not strangers to illegal actions, but it seems that some members were reluctant to support *strangers* conducting illegal actions with ACT UP/LA money.

An illegal, ongoing action was a different challenge for ACT UP/LA than a one-time act of civil disobedience. If CNN members were arrested, the work

[75] "Minutes from Super Sunday" [i.e., Coordinating Committee meeting], July 5, 1992; ONE Collection.

[76] Minutes, General Body meeting, July 13, 1992; ONE Collection.

[77] Minutes, General Body meeting, July 27, 1992; ONE Collection. *The Los Angeles Times* reported that even Diane Watson, the African-American California state senator who had sponsored a bill for a pilot needle exchange program, was concerned that CNN's efforts would muddy the delicate waters of getting a sanctioned pilot NEP in place; Watson had apparently asked CNN to stop. (Amy Pyle, "Clean Needles Put Into War on AIDS." *The Los Angeles Times*, September 9, 1992, pp. B1, B4.)

[78] Interview with author, 2011.

[79] interview with author, 2011.

would stop, and thus they continuously asked the GB for more control over their actions:

Renee [Edgington] expressed concern about confidentiality due to an article that appeared in the *Vanguard* concerning CNN's alleged needle exchange program in South Central LA. She was also concerned about ACT UP/LA's demand for more information on CNN. Renee felt that CNN's program depends on confidentiality due to questions of legality.[80]

In August 1992, CNN put forth a proposal at the meeting that "any information related to an upcoming covert action should be confidential to the greatest degree possible." This proposal failed.

In October 1992, CNN told ACT UP/LA's GB that it was postponing further needle exchange efforts until January 1993.[81] At the same time, CNN did come to an agreement with the Minority AIDS Consortium about needle exchange and began to publicize its NEP more widely, apparently changing course on the question of secrecy.[82] Greater visibility generated more community backlash; Ramona Hall, of the LA Center for Drug and Alcohol Abuse, was quoted in an article in the alternative paper *LA Weekly* as asking "[i]f distributing clean needles is such a good idea, why is ACT UP doing it here instead of Silver Lake or West Hollywood?"[83] The same *LA Weekly* article quoted CNN members as admitting that they should have spent more time trying to enlist the support of community organizations before starting their NEP. CNN's Steven Corbin characterized it as bearing the brunt of years of systematic abuse of the African-American community, which he described as "extremely paranoid, even of well-meaning white people."[84] Renee Edgington was quoted to the effect that CNN was, despite backlash, in the best position to "do something" about needle exchange because its members were best informed about NEPs.[85]

By late 1992, the initial grumbles about CNN's commitment to the rest of ACT UP/LA were very audible. The following is an excerpt from the minutes for the GB meeting of December 21, 1992; the minutes-taker noted that the following occurred:

Paul D. began a discussion between the general body and the members of CNN by proposing three questions to CNN:

1. Why don't members of CNN come to general meetings?
2. What has happened with the testing and evaluation of [needle] points for HIV?
3. What about finances?

---

[80] Minutes, General Body meeting, August 24, 1992; ONE Collection.
[81] Minutes, General Body meeting, October 19, 1992; ONE Collection.
[82] Minutes, General Body meeting, October 26, 1992; ONE Collection.
[83] Gloria Ohland, "The Eye of the Needle," *LA Weekly* (September 4–10, 1992): pp. 14–15.
[84] Ohland, p. 14
[85] Ohland p. 15

A lengthy discussion followed in which people expressed praise for CNN's work and the desire to keep CNN as a vital, active, and integral part of ACT UP/LA. Members of CNN answered many questions clarifying their work and wondered why there was no money to finance CNN's work when CNN raised over $70,000 this year. No testing of the collected points for HIV has been done, but the points retain HIV for up to a year. CNN is having difficulty finding a testing facility. If anyone has contacts in the medical community who can offer a testing facility, please contact CNN. However, there is not enough money to do an evaluation right now even if a testing facility were located.

Two months later, in February 1993, ACT UP/LA decided not to disburse any more money to CNN, and the relationship between what were now two separate entities was "under review."[86] That review took place on March 8, 1993; CNN members gave a report to the GB and then answered questions, many of which focused on CNN's growing relationship with the American Civil Liberties Union (ACLU), which was counseling CNN not to risk arrests by doing exchanges because continuing civil disobedience was unlikely to be worth the costs of arrests.[87] The anonymous minutes-taker for the March 8 meeting noted a strong sense in the GB that CNN was not really a part of ACT UP/LA anymore.[88] The minutes-taker editorialized his or her summary of the meeting, writing a "transcript" of questions from the floor and answers from a not believably flip, collectively voiced CNN:

Q. Why has CNN met twice previously on Monday nights, almost simultaneously with but separate from ACT UP/LA's meetings?
A. Because those two Monday nights were the most convenient night for committee members.
Q. Why do members of CNN attend only CNN meetings and not general-body ACT UP/LA meetings?
A. Some CNN members feel uncomfortable at ACT UP/LA meetings, because they may not understand what ACT UP/LA is discussing, and meetings can sometimes be unfriendly.
Q. Why is there an "us vs. them" attitude between ACT UP/LA and CNN?
A. Who knows? . . .
Q. Is CNN beginning to think of itself as a service organization (since it *does* serve approximately 500 clients a week in its exchanges) rather than a direct action group?
A. Needle exchange groups normally start in ACT UP-like organization but eventually are not contained by them.[89]

---

[86] J. T. Anderson, February 8, 1993. "Report from the Minutes for January and February 1993." ONE Collection.
[87] Minutes, General Body meeting, March 8, 1993; ONE Collection.
[88] Minutes, General Body meeting, March 8 1993; ONE Collection.
[89] Minutes, General Body meeting, March 8, 1992; ONE Collection. Emphasis in the original.

Despite misgivings, the GB voted at the March 8 meeting to fund CNN through May 1993 and to help it become a non-profit 501c-3 organization, thereby putting a de facto end date to the relationship between the two entities. Sporadic accounts of CNN's activities continued to appear in ACT UP/LA agendas and minutes through 1994, but under the heading "needle exchange" and not as committee reports. ACT UP/LA supported CNN and the ACLU when those organizations asked Los Angeles Mayor Richard Riordan to issue a "medical state of emergency" and thereby preclude the LAPD's attempts to break up the NEP that CNN was running in Hollywood.[90] But, just as in South Central, CNN's Hollywood NEP generated community backlash from landlords, residents, and the Guardian Angels, who somehow appeared on the scene in order to capitalize on the neighborhood dispute.[91]

The CNN committee, arising as it did from within ACT UP/LA and attracting others to the group who wanted to do work outside the lesbian and gay community, opened up debates about ACT UP/LA's focus as an organization. Gender, race, and sexuality politics were embedded in discussions about that focus, especially, but not only, in discussions about how, or really whether, to expand the organization's boundaries. CNN sparked an intersectional crisis for ACT UP/LA because the issue of doing service work for IV drug users in communities of color was a complex one that opened up questions without simple answers but with intersectional implications: Would ACT UP/LA be a programmatic or representative organization? If it was representative, could it really represent others – IV drug users, people of color, heterosexuals – "outside" the lesbian and gay community? Was social service really direct action? Even if it was, should ACT UP/LA be doing social service as direct action? How independent could committees be from the GB? Who could be a leader in ACT UP/LA? How single-minded was that leader allowed to be?

CNN outlasted ACT UP/LA – but the latter group was left weaker as a result of the intersectional crisis the former caused.[92] The last moment of intersectional crisis I analyze, over supposedly "competing" actions at the 1993 March on Washington for Lesbian, Gay, and Bi Equal Rights and Liberation, was the most explicitly gendered one at the time and, in a way, the simplest because it happened at a point in the organization's life when matters of gender inequality were made nationally visible.

---

[90] Minutes, General Body meetings August 1, 1994 and August 8, 1994; ONE Collection.

[91] Minutes, General Body meeting, August 15, 1994; ONE Collection.

[92] CNN likely lasted under the name "Clean Needles Now" until 2012, when it was absorbed by/transformed into the LA Community Health Project, a nonprofit that provides services for drug users. In 2012, CNN had an Echo Park address (now the LACHP office), a phone number, and a website (www.cleanneedlesnow.org, currently www.chpla.org) that listed weekly exchanges in downtown Los Angeles's Skid Row, Watts, and Hollywood. Prior to 2012, I had personally tried to contact CNN via phone and email and never received a response.

GENDER AND "COMPETING" ACTIONS AT THE 1993 MARCH
ON WASHINGTON

> There was this specific incident/issue that really was kind of the [last] straw ...
> which was the Lesbians and AIDS action ... during the March on Washington
> weekend ... that was one of the issues that put a split between several people that
> you know, women and several men that you probably remember too.
>
> – Judy Sisneros[93]

The third intersectional crisis in ACT UP/LA that I examine in this chapter
was at once the most overtly gendered and the most devoid of racial/ethnic
politics. Conflict erupted within the group in 1993 over "competing" anti-AIDS
events organized for the April 1993 March on Washington for Lesbian, Gay,
and Bi Rights and Liberation (MOW). National ACT UP networks including
ACT NOW and one made up of ACT UP women activists took the MOW as an
opportunity for action. ACT NOW organized a demonstration at the
Pharmaceutical Manufacturers Association (PMA) protesting the costs of
AIDS medication, drug companies' refusal to share proprietary information
on drugs, and what activists saw as the refusal of drug companies to develop
innovative therapies to combat the virus.[94] ACT UP women organized
a combination of a legal picket, "speak-out," and meeting with President
Clinton's Secretary of the Department of Health and Human Services
(DHHS), Donna Shalala, to raise awareness of issues involving lesbians and
AIDS.[95] It is important to note that these "competing" actions were planned so
as *not* to compete with one another. Both actions were scheduled well in
advance of the march; they were to take place two days before the actual
march, on Friday, April 23, 1993, and they were scheduled so as not to put
activists into a position of having to choose between them. The DHHS action
was to begin at 11 AM and be over by 1 PM, with the actual meeting with Shalala
scheduled for 11:30 AM; the ACT NOW PMA action was slated to begin several
Metro stops away at 2 PM.[96] Despite the care taken so that the actions did not
conflict, the planning, execution, and aftermath of the DHHS actions –
especially the meeting with Shalala – generated controversy that lingered in
ACT UP/LA.

Judy Sisneros was at the DHHS actions at Shalala's office. According to
Sisneros, several other ACT UP/LA women played an important role in

[93] Interview with author, 2000.
[94] "ACT UP Goes to Washington." Unsigned two-page introduction for activists, dated April 4,
1993; ONE collection.
[95] "Support Lesbians with AIDS." Multipage publicity/information packet on April 23, 1993,
Department of Health and Human Services action. April 1993; ONE Collection.
[96] "ACT UP Itinerary in DC." Undated, unsigned document c. April 1993, ONE Collection.
At least one press release by ACT UP/LA announced both actions as projects of the ACT UP
Network. ("ACT UP Marches on Washington," undated press release c. April 1993; ONE
Collection.)

Women who have sex with women are women of color, white women, sex workers, teenagers, mothers, wives, drug users, doctors, nurses, women in jail, homeless women, pregnant women, sexually active human beings, people living with AIDS/HIV. Women who have sex with women can identify as "lesbian," "gay," "bisexual," "asexual," or even "straight."

IF YOU ARE A WOMAN WHO HAS SEX WITH WOMEN, REGARDLESS OF HOW YOU IDENTIFY YOURSELF, YOUR HEALTH IS AT RISK

Join lesbian AIDS activists, the National Women's ACT UP Network, and our allies in a legal picket and speakout. We will be meeting outside the Department of Health & Human Services in Washington, DC on April 23, 1993 at 11:00am. This action will take place during the weekend of the March on Washington, and will focus on the invisibility of lesbians with AIDS/HIV. We are demanding that the US government recognize lesbians with AIDS/HIV; the FDA repeal guidelines which exclude women from clinical trials; a gynecologist be hired at all ACTG sites; the CDC collect accurate surveillance for women & lesbians with AIDS; and the NIH conduct comprehensive research into women-to-women transmission.

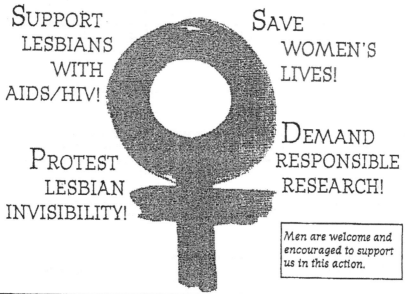

SUPPORT LESBIANS WITH AIDS/HIV!

SAVE WOMEN'S LIVES!

PROTEST LESBIAN INVISIBILITY!

DEMAND RESPONSIBLE RESEARCH!

Men are welcome and encouraged to support us in this action.

We will be meeting at HHS, located at 200 Independence Ave., SW (The Humphrey Bldg), 1 block from the Federal Center SW Metro stop, at 11:00 am. The speakout will begin at 12 noon. For more information, please call/fax The Lesbian Action Line ☎ (718) 965-4106, eastern standard time.

FIGURE 4.3: Flyer, Department of Health and Human Services Lesbian Visibility Demonstration, Washington, DC, April 1993.

planning the action, including Mary Lucey, Lucey's partner Nancy MacNeil, and Helene Schpak. Sisneros stated that the discussions within the ACT UP national women's network about the Shalala action were taking place roughly at the same time that members of ACT NOW "had started talking about the PMA."[97] Sisneros also described the national network of ACT UP women as keeping their plans under wraps; according to her, the women's network "kind of kept it within the group" for a while before sharing their plans with ACT NOW. Sisneros noted that when the plans for the Shalala meeting and actions became more widely known, "a lot of men ... were mad." Sisneros recalled that some of the men "started to treat us like traitors, like, you know, it's for women only, which is just crap. It was total crap ... it really brought out sexism in certain people who you know ... should be embarrassed about it. To this day." In any case, by March 1993, the ACT UP National Women's Network had begun advertising the DHHS actions, specifically stating that "we welcome everyone to participate in this action and we encourage all lesbian and bisexual women living with AIDS/HIV to speak out with us on April 23."[98] On the local level, one ACT UP/LA press release issued announced the DHHS actions and the PMA actions and urged attendance by all at both.[99] But another press release from ACT UP/LA announced only the DHHS actions and stated that men were encouraged to attend the DHHS lesbian and bisexual women's speakout, but were asked not to actually speak.[100]

The DHHS actions, designed by the national network of ACT UP women to raise awareness about issues involving lesbians and AIDS, were seen as a success. The meeting with Shalala was packed with activists who demanded that more research be done on woman-to-woman transmission of the HIV virus, that researchers explore how AIDS might develop differently in women, and that women-specific opportunistic infections be studied.[101] Activists wanted funding for prevention materials specifically targeted to women who have sex with women, better enrollment of women in clinical research trials, and mandated education for obstetricians and gynecologists. They also demanded HIV/AIDS services and programs that reached IV drug users and lesbians in prison.[102] Although the DHHS actions did not formally compete

---

[97] Interview with author, 2000.

[98] "Dear Friends." Flyer/letter, dated March 29, 1993, and signed by the "The New York Lesbian Caucus of the ACT UP National Women's Network." ONE Collection.

[99] "ACT UP Marches on Washington," press release, ibid.

[100] "ACT UP/Los Angeles to Demand Lesbians with AIDS Research at Health and Human Services." Press release, dated April 19, 1993; ONE Collection.

[101] "Support Lesbians with AIDS/HIV." Unsigned, undated informational packet, c. April 1993; ONE collection

[102] "Support Lesbians with AIDS/HIV." Unsigned, undated informational packet, c. April 1993; ONE collection. A photo-book on the MOW, *One Million Strong* (Cox, Means, and Pope 1993: 21–25) shows photographs of the DHHS action without naming it as an ACT UP-sponsored event, and the PMA action is nowhere to be found in its pages. The book's authors include coverage of the ACT UP-sponsored actions at the US Capitol demanding universal

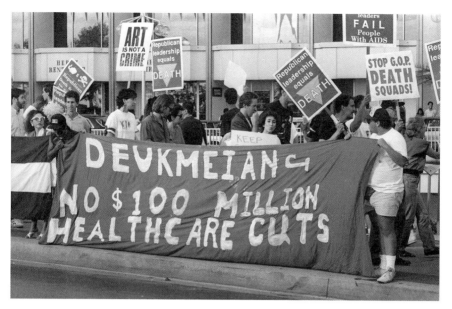

PLATE 1 ACT UP/LA demonstration at George H.W. Bush fundraiser, Century City, Los Angeles 1990. Photograph by James Rosen.

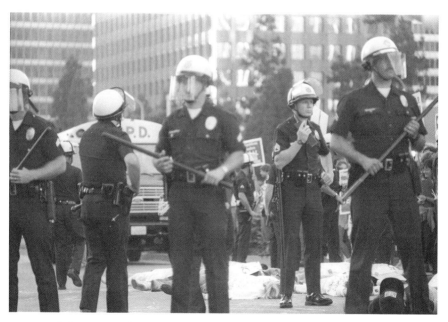

PLATE 2 ACT UP/LA "die-in" protest with police presence, Century City, Los Angeles, 1990. Photograph by James Rosen.

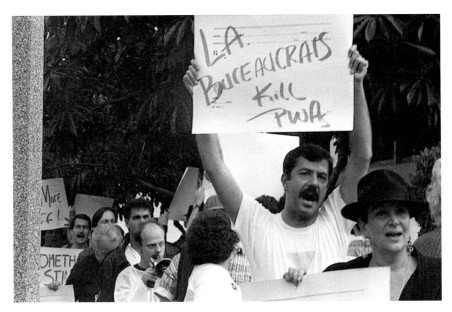

PLATE 3 ACT UP/LA protest against LA County, West Hollywood, April 1990. Activists protested long wait times for clinic appointments, short hours for pharmacy services and lack of medications. Photograph by James Rosen.

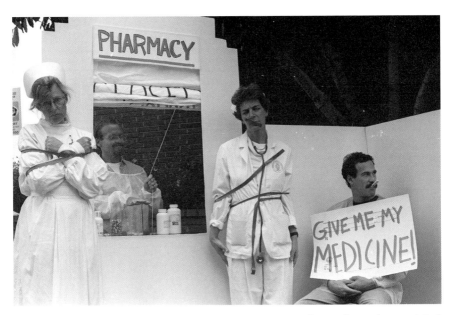

PLATE 4 ACT UP/LA protest against LA County, West Hollywood, April 1990. Mark Kostopoulos appears on the right holding sign. Photograph by James Rosen.

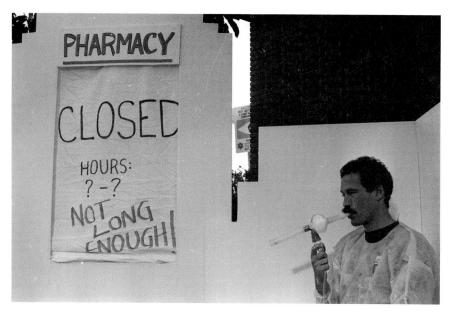

PLATE 5 ACT UP/LA protest against LA County, West Hollywood, April 1990 Mark Kostopoulos is "using" the inhaler. Photograph by James Rosen.

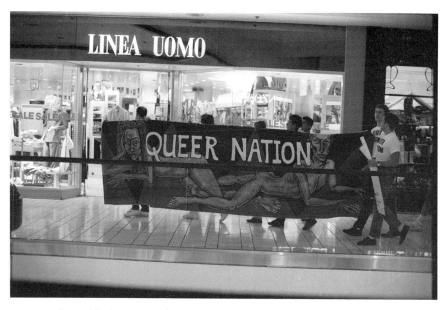

PLATE 6 Queer Nation protest/kiss-in, Beverly Center, Los Angeles, 1990. Photograph by James Rosen.

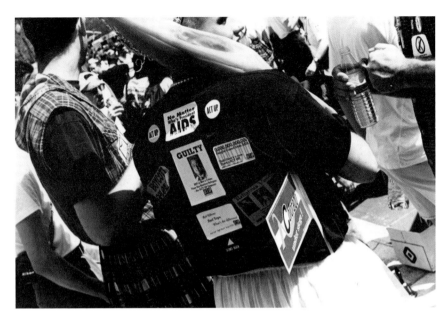

PLATE 7 Stickers on Pete Jimenez's shirt, ACT UP/LA action, c.1991. Photograph by James Rosen.

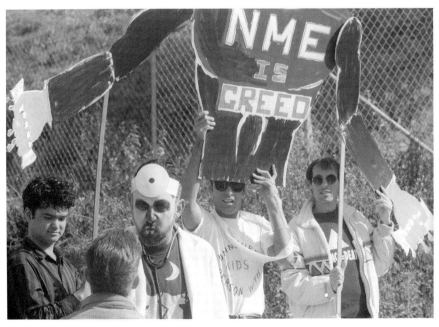

PLATE 8 ACT UP/LA protest against National Medical Enterprises (now Tenet Healthcare) for building private hospital adjacent to public LA County Hospital, May 1991. Wendell Jones is wearing face paint.

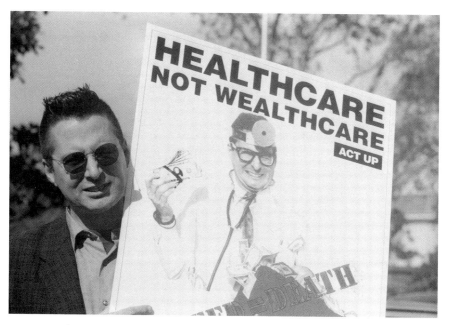

PLATE 9 Jake Epstine at ACT UP/LA protest against National Medical Enterprises, May 1991. Photograph by James Rosen.

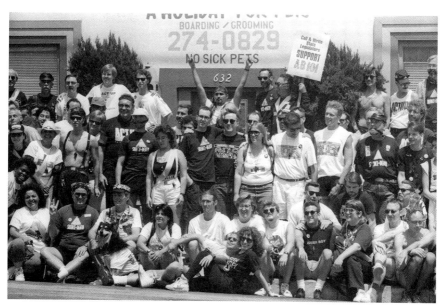

PLATE 10 ACT UP/LA at Christopher Street West celebration June 1991: Jeri Detrick is standing in the center of the photo wearing an "Action=Life" shirt; Mary Lucey can be seen sitting on the far left; Pete Jimenez is in the middle of the photo with arms raised in victory signs. Photograph by James Rosen.

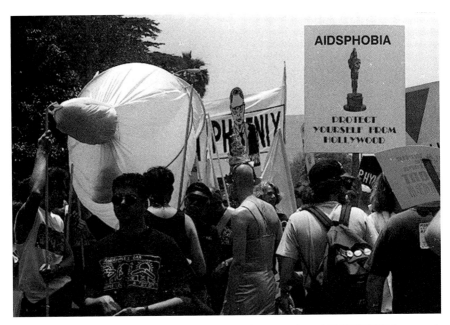

PLATE 11 ACT UP/LA at June 1991 Pride celebration: the "AIDSPHOBIA" poster is from the March 1991 Oscars' Action. Photograph by James Rosen.

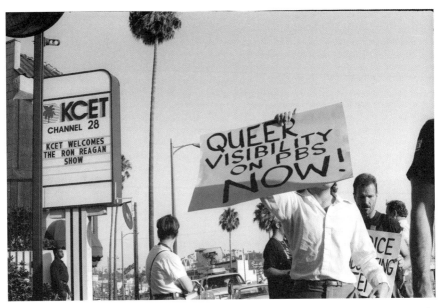

PLATE 12 ACT UP/LA protest against PBS station KCET for refusing to show the documentary "Stop the Church." August 1991. Photograph by James Rosen.

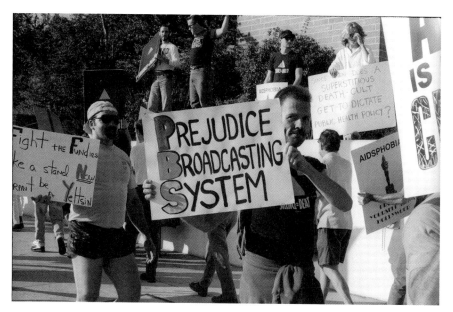

PLATE 13 ACT UP/LA protest against PBS station KCET for refusing to show the documentary "Stop the Church." August 1991. Photograph by James Rosen.

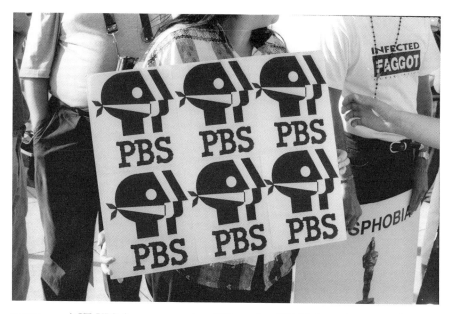

PLATE 14 ACT UP/LA protest against PBS station KCET for refusing to show the documentary "Stop the Church" August 1991. Photograph by James Rosen.

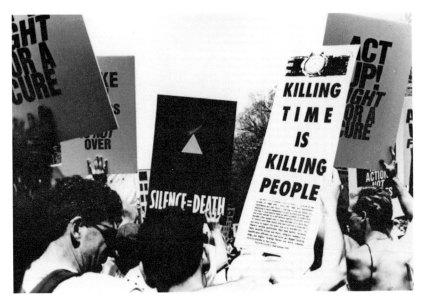

PLATE 15 ACT UP/LA, March on Washington for Lesbian, Gay and Bi Equal Rights and Liberation, 1993. Photograph by James Rosen.

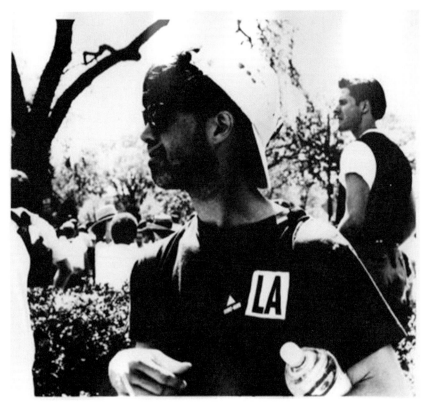

PLATE 16 Ty Geltmaker in ACT UP/LA tee-shirt at March on Washington for Lesbian, Gay and Bi Equal Rights and Liberation, 1993. Photograph by James Rosen.

with ACT NOW plans and were in line with ACT UP priorities nationally, the focus on lesbian issues made some ACT UP/LA men angry. Sisneros reported that, upon returning to LA, several male ACT UP/LA members stopped speaking to her, to Lucey, and to Schpak. Sisneros actually described the controversy about the Shalala and PMA action as being "the last straw" that divided ACT UP/LA women and men. When I asked Sisneros "what split ACT UP/LA and when?," her immediate answer was "I can tell you exactly when it was – April 25th, 1993."[103] According to Nancy MacNeil, the meeting with Shalala increased the "division between the women and men ... the men in ACT UP/LA felt betrayed, that they were maybe being placed second."[104] MacNeil recalled that some of the women involved in the national network who had planned the meeting actually had not cared about whether the meeting took place in ACT UP's name – an indication of gender divisions at the national level – but that she and her partner Mary Lucey felt that it was important that the meeting with Shalala "stay ACT UP affiliated":

Actually it was mostly Mary and I who said, "no," that we very much wanted to stay ACT UP affiliated. And that this [ACT UP] was our support network and these were the people who helped us when nobody else would help us ... and we had some loyalty issues. ... Of course the women counteracted ... that the men always overshadowed the women's issues ...[105]

The national and the local politics of gender divides in ACT UP and ACT UP/LA came together as female and male activists came away from the MOW feeling differently about the work they had done on the national level. It was clear that national ACT UP gender politics were becoming more fraught. If it is true that information about the women's DHHS actions was initially kept from ACT NOW, that initial secrecy might have been read into later efforts to actually coordinate actions at the MOW, which was shaping up to be a crowded weekend of actions, events, and demonstrations. ACT NOW seemed to be slipping away as a viable national network, and the actions it organized for the MOW did not seem to make the network stronger. Sisneros remarked at a GB meeting immediately after the MOW that she felt that "the status of the Network [ACT NOW] has been shaky since the meeting in

healthcare without referencing ACT UP's sponsorship; they nonetheless use a prominent photo of ACT UP/LA activists Jeff Scheurholz and Pete Jimenez at that action wearing ACT UP tee-shirts and stickers (see p. 150).

[103] Sisneros, although referring to the day of the DHHS and PMA actions, April 23, is actually giving the date of the MOW itself here.

[104] Interview with author, 1999.

[105] Interview with author, 1999. A brief summary of the meeting in Laurence and Weinhouse (1997: 160–161) puts fifteen women from ACT UP/NY and the ACT UP National Women's Network in the room with Shalala. The minutes of ACT UP/LA's May 3, 1993, General Body meeting, immediately following the MOW weekend, reported that the forty-five-minute "successful meeting with Shalala took place with fifteen HIV-positive women and "2 straight women" in attendance.

St. Louis in January [of 1993]. A split in the network has occurred due to problems about our actions in Washington."[106] Within ACT UP/LA, the WC members' involvement in planning MOW-related events seemed to be read locally as evidence that they were pulling away from ACT UP/LA men (despite MacNeil's statement to the contrary). Jeff Scheurholz, for example, recalled that ACT UP/LA women were busy as leaders at the MOW and that ACT UP/LA men were at different actions than the women. He speculated that the fact that so many ACT UP/LA women were involved in the planning of a "Dyke Visibility March" that took place the Saturday night before the MOW was something that "kind of separated us."[107]

The gender tensions present in ACT UP at the national level reverberated back to the local relations of the genders in ACT UP/LA in part because the organizers of the Shalala action did ask men to take a backseat not just in planning but also in participation. Despite the care taken to schedule the PMA and DHHS actions so that all activists could go to both, the press release issued by ACT UP/LA women did ask for men's silent support at the speak out, and this did not seem to go down well with some ACT UP/LA men. Men also were unhappy about being excluded from a meeting with a Cabinet secretary, since such a meeting was a rare event for AIDS activists.[108] J. T. Anderson expressed his feelings of outright displeasure at the idea that the Shalala action focused only on lesbians and AIDS. When I interviewed him in 1999, he quoted one of the organizers of the action as telling him that "[we] were all going to discuss with Donna Shalala women's issues ... period." While Anderson was sympathetic to the idea of focusing on women's issues, he also felt that a meeting with Shalala was too important to be only about women:

I can sort of understand ... at that time women's issues were not being discussed, but that tactic ... I mean ... I had had too many friends who had died from AIDS and maybe I don't think I knew of a woman who had died from AIDS, and to trivialize the deaths of my friends by saying we don't have any men's issues, we're only having women's issues, hurt me, although I understood the tactic, and I don't know that I disagree with it either.[109]

When I interviewed Cat Walker, who was present at the MOW, about the local effects of the "competing" DHHS and PMA actions, he answered with a somewhat different calculus about where the energy was in ACT UP/LA:

It did seem at that time that the Women's Caucus was trying to do stuff that just had to do with women. And they had good reasons for that too, I think. But I think that the men

---

[106] Meeting minutes, ACT UP/LA General Body, May 3, 1993; ONE Collection.

[107] Interview with author, 2011. The idea for a Dyke Visibility march was taken back to Los Angeles and incarnated as the Lesbian Love March through "Boystown" in West Hollywood in 1994: see Kenney 2001. On the 1993 Washington, DC, Dyke March, see Schulman 1994.

[108] "ACT UP/Los Angeles to Demand Lesbians with AIDS Research at Health and Human Services." Press release, April 19, 1993; ONE collection.

[109] Interview with author, 1999.

in the group felt like they were being excluded … and also felt like why … and I think that they felt that the group as a whole, its attention, was just suddenly being focused on women … and I think the reality was that it was because at that time, the Women's Caucus were the only ones who were really doing anything. … It was kind of like the men weren't really doing anything at the time but some of them would say, well why is the group doing women's stuff?[110]

It's easy to hear the ambivalence in both Walker's and Anderson's remarks about ACT UP/LA's increasing focus on women's issues. When I asked Anderson a moment later if the MOW actions were "a fatal blow" to ACT UP/LA, he replied "no," even though he described the MOW as "a bad moment" for ACT UP/LA.

Answering the question of why a weekend of national, successful, visible, well-coordinated, and well-attended anti-AIDS actions in Washington, DC, negatively affected ACT UP/LA can only be done if we understand the women's successes at the MOW as crystallizing ongoing gendered tensions in the group. By 1993, ACT UP/LA faced not only a threat to gay men's "desire … to stress their epidemiological pre-eminence" (Altman 1994: 72), but a possible end to gay men's pre-eminence in the group itself. And, as moments of solidarity among genders in ACT UP/LA became harder and harder to sustain, so did the group itself. As the last in a series of intersectional crises, the conflict around actions that were not meant to conflict at the MOW was explicitly experienced in gendered terms and represented one breaking point for ACT UP/LA from which the group never truly recovered.

CONCLUSION: THE ENERVATING EFFECTS OF INTERSECTIONAL CONFLICTS

In this chapter, I explored moments of intersectional crises in ACT UP/LA. These three moments – the influx of new "members" as a result of the AB 101 veto in 1991, the challenge represented by CNN and needle exchange in 1992 and 1993, and the rifts caused by actions at the April 1993 MOW – encapsulated implicit and explicit debates about what ACT UP/LA was, what its focus should be, and where its boundaries were. In contrast to the infighting that Ghaziani (2008) saw as generating a common culture around LGBT politics at the national level, conflict over inequalities within ACT UP/LA – inequalities due to gender, race/ethnicity and sexuality – were enervating. The macro-cohort of AB 101 who came to ACT UP/LA because of its fierce reputation required education about the complexities of gender and racial inequalities in doing anti-AIDS activism. The idea of generating the social service project of needle exchange from within the ranks of ACT UP/LA caused rifts among members who questioned the wisdom of the group's

---

[110] Interview with author, 2011.

engaging in social service, the idea that ACT UP/LA could or should serve communities of color, and the leadership of those who came from ACT UP/LA to lead within it. Lastly, gender solidarity was weakened as women in ACT UP/LA became increasingly vocal about women's AIDS issues and more successful at raising awareness about those issues at the national level in a way that made it seem that they no longer needed men to be successful

All activist spaces are continuously crosscut by large-scale, long-standing relationships of inequalities, making solidarity a similarly continuous challenge. The intersectional crises that ACT UP/LA members faced were not the only factors implicated in its trajectory as an organization, but the group's demobilization is unintelligible without a thorough understanding of how inequalities played out in interaction. In the next chapter, I look at other aspects of ACT UP/LA's long, slow demobilization, beginning in the last half of 1992. There is a story about the demobilization of the ACT UPs nationally that only partly explains ACT UP/LA's trajectory. Accordingly, I focus on local factors that demoralized group members, such as the deaths of leaders and the failure to achieve tangible success in battling local institutions, and I consider how the once generative oscillation between local and national actions that characterized ACT UP/LA's relationship to other ACT UPs in its period of mobilization fell apart. Ultimately, the group's numbers fell dramatically, and the few remaining members of the group could not sustain the ambitious umbrella politics of anti-AIDS action that had typified ACT UP/LA in its heyday. The last few members of ACT UP/LA disagreed about how the group ended, but by 1997 it was done; I explore what disagreements about the death of ACT UP/LA show about members' loyalty to a participatory and democratic vision of activism.

5

Demobilization: ACT UP/LA in the Years 1992–1997

We're all individually experiencing great frustration in ACT UP. I see burnout happening all around me. But I don't think it's so much from overwork as from a feeling of defeat ... we don't seem to be getting any closer to ending the AIDS epidemic ... we've gone as far as we can go with most of our old tactics. What worked in the past just doesn't seem to do the job anymore.

– Helene Schpak[1]

INTRODUCTION

In January 1992, the AIDS Coalition to Unleash Power, Los Angeles (ACT UP/LA)'s Public Policy Committee sent out a survey asking members to rank AIDS issues by their importance; they gave respondents choices such as "lack of research and access to AIDS drugs," "universal health care," and "safer sex education in public schools."[2] The wide-ranging, member-driven ACT UP/LA agenda that had characterized ACT UP/LA from its beginning was never set just by the Public Policy Committee, but from time to time the committee had established priorities for the group. But after more than four years of constant action, something was happening to the group; it was slowly demobilizing The influx of angry lesbian and gays who had joined ACT UP/LA as a result of California Governor Pete Wilson's September 1991 veto of Assembly Bill 101 (AB 101), had started to dissipate; Monday night General Body (GB) meetings at Plummer Park were getting smaller. The Public Policy Committee's attempt to gather information on members' interests and priorities was in line with helping ACT UP/LA continue to be a coalition of diverse individuals trying to do as much as possible on all fronts to stop AIDS.

---

[1] Helene Schpak. "Mark Kostopoulos October 26, 1954–June 20, 1992." ACT UP/LA News, 5:3, P.3.

[2] Unsigned. "Public Policy Survey," January 1992; ONE Collection.

In this chapter, I look at ACT UP/LA's demobilization, which took place roughly from the latter half of 1992 until the last few members of the group closed up shop in 1997. I discuss the local issues that led to demobilization. In addition to the internal conflicts driven by the intersectional crises that I discuss in Chapter 4, I argue that a confluence of factors demobilized ACT UP/LA. A leadership vacuum caused by the deaths of central participants combined with a sense of the intractability of problems and made it harder for activists to see themselves as effective, a sentiment echoed by Helene Schpak in the comment that opens this chapter. I also explore how the oscillation between the local and the national that had typified ACT UP/LA's activism proved less satisfying to the local group by exploring the fallout from the highly confrontational anti-AIDS protests at the 1992 Republican Party Convention in Houston. I look at the last few years of the much diminished group as ACT UP/LA's last few members rejected money that might have helped the group but that members felt came with strings attached that countered their vision of what a direct action anti-AIDS movement organization should look like. I conclude by exploring what it means that ACT UP/LA's last members disagree about how the group ended. The end in and of itself illustrates how loyal activists were to their vision of a democratic, member-driven ACT UP/LA, free of obligations toward any other entity.

In order to understand how this approach to the demobilization of ACT UP/LA compares with what have generally been seen to be the factors that contribute to the waning of militant anti-AIDS activism by the mid 1990s, I briefly consider what others have written about the movement's slow-down. Scholars have rejected the chronologically misinformed view that the advent of a new class of drugs – protease inhibitors – made the movement redundant; they have not been able to show evidence that the election of the presumably lesbian-and gay-friendly President Bill Clinton made a palpable difference in activists' feelings about protest; and they have questioned the "success kills" theory of movement demobilization. The argument that emotional shifts caused movement demobilization made by Gould (2009) is better supported by the case of ACT UP/LA, as is the idea of gender rifts being central to the downward trajectory of militant organizing. In the case of these last two explanations, however, considerable nuance given by attention to local factors must be added to the arguments in order to explain what happened to ACT UP/LA.

EXPLANATIONS FOR DEMOBILIZATION OF THE DIRECT ACTION ANTI-AIDS MOVEMENT

Scholars have written about the end of (most of) the ACT UPs and have posited a number of explanations about the phenomenon of these loosely connected grassroots groups dissolving at around the same time. These accounts do not agree on how many ACT UPs there actually were. Halcli (1999) estimated that the ACT UPs had decreased from about 113 in 1991 to just 8 by 1998, including ACT UP/LA's last few stalwart members. In their 2012 film, *United in Anger*, Jim Hubbard and Sarah Schulman list 143 ACT UPs worldwide (see http://www .unitedinanger.com) at the movement's height. Hubbard drew this list from existing lists used in previous documentaries.[3] When discussing the number of ACT UPs, it is wise to be cautious for two reasons: the informality of membership and the availability of the "brand name" ACT UP. Since membership in an ACT UP was informal, counting members in ACT UPs is a difficult if not impossible task. James Rosen, who was active in ACT UP/NY and ACT UP/LA recalled someone asking him and his partner Ty Geltmaker how to join ACT UP; they replied "you don't. Just show up."[4] While ACT UP/LA committees kept lists as needed (i.e., for fundraising, mailing the newsletter, or coordinating logistics for an action), names of participants were never taken at meetings, outside of the occasional sign-up sheet. While attendance made one a member, no one actively kept track of members. And the very name "ACT UP" was always available for use; it came to represent a brand of direct action. The groups who used the name "ACT UP" were only loosely connected to each other through the ACT NOW network or through networks of constituencies, such as women and people of color. Direct action anti-AIDS groups could adopt the name "ACT UP" in order to show what their vision of activism was, thus "branding" (Stride and Lee 2007) themselves in the process. But there is no way of knowing if those who took the ACT UP brand name were very active in their local fields, let alone if they actually adhered to the same sets of principles.

With the caveats about cataloging the number and membership of ACT UPs given, some explanations for demobilization are easier to dismiss than others. For example, the idea that the introduction of protease inhibitors, which were more effective and less toxic anti-retrovirals, made the ACT UPs irrelevant and led to demobilization is disputed by Gould (2009: 417). She notes that the introduction of protease inhibitors explanation for demobilization does not work from the simple standpoint of chronology. Protease inhibitors were introduced in 1995, at which point many ACT UPs were gone; certainly, ACT UP/LA was well past its peak period of mobilization by then. Gould also rejects both the idea that Clinton's November 1992 election as US President eliminated the desire by activists to continue doing direct action. The idea that Clinton's 1992 election raised lesbian and gay raised hopes enough to end anti-AIDS activism rests on the untested, often-used assumption that "success kills" social movements: supposedly, once movement actors get what they want, they stop. The premise that the ACT UPs were working to get Clinton elected is wrong;

---

[3] Personal conversation with author, Binghamton, New York, April 26, 2013.
[4] Interview with the author, 2012. Rosen recalled a conversation where someone had said to him and Geltmaker that they were "quitting" ACT UP: "we said, what do you mean, how can you quit? Whoever said you joined?"

some participants may have been, but there was quite a bit of political distance between many direct action anti-AIDS activists and the Democratic Party. If the ACT UPs were not collectively working to get Clinton elected, it is hard to see Clinton's election as much of a game changer. Many activists were distrustful of any elected politician. Clinton wresting the presidency from the Republicans would have been seen as a modest success at best, and the idea that his election led activists to abandon ACT UPs is implausible and, more importantly, unproved.

Kane (2010) has examined the confusion within social movement studies about the effects of "success" on movement mobilization, looking specifically at the legal achievements of the LGBT movement and consequences for mobilization in 1974–1999. She points out that movement theorists have come down on both sides of the question of whether "success kills," with some arguing that "success is necessary for a movement to grow, or even maintain its existing level of mobilization" and others arguing that movements that meet their goals lose momentum and decline (2010: 259–260). Kane's examination, conducted at the movement level and using the growth of social movement organizations as a proxy for movement mobilization, shows that the concept of success must itself be contextualized, and thus challenges previous assumptions about what happens to variegated social movements that have achieved some of their goals. As I discuss later, in the case of ACT UP/LA, the lack of success, particularly in the battles with LA County to provide adequately for public health, was a contributing factor to ACT UP/LA's demobilization.

Another possible explanation for the ACT UPs demobilization, and another variation on the "success kills" theme, is that of the institutionalization of activism: in this view, militant members left to take up positions in the AIDS service sector or government agencies thus decreasing their availability for direct action. This is an explanation that should be considered although, in the case of the militant anti-AIDS movement, concrete evidence for this view is lacking. While some former members of ACT UP/LA went on to work in institutional settings, some *came* from institutional settings to work in ACT UP/LA, and a few continued to keep a place in both ACT UP/LA and their place of AIDS work (see Chapter 6). There is no evidence of a wholesale defection of outsider activists moving to the inside from ACT UP/LA, let alone in the movement as a whole. In the case of ACT UP/LA, the vast majority of participants never were and did not become paid AIDS workers, so it is hard to see how such "defections" mattered. Rather than think of activists "abandoning" direct action, historian Jennifer Brier (2009: 4) has asked us to think about the porous boundaries between activist service provision and direct action, as she correctly cautions against narratives of anti-AIDS activism that envision sharp lines between direct action activists and activist service providers; in the case of Los Angeles, Kenney (2001) has argued that the lesbian and gay community had long seen the lines blurred between protest activism and activist provision of social services.

The most compelling recent explanation for the demobilization of the ACT UPs is Deborah Gould's (2009) argument that a shift of emotions or, more specifically, emotional *habitus* among activists contributed to the demise of direct action anti-AIDS protest. Emotional habitus is defined by Gould (2009: 10) as "socially constituted, prevailing ways of feeling and emoting, as well as the embodied, axiomatic understandings and norms about feelings and their expression." Gould argues that the blend of hope and anger that sustained ACT UPs was difficult to sustain over time. She puts special emphasis on the failure of activists to acknowledge the grief that they felt as the cascade of AIDS deaths in the community continued, arguing that unacknowledged grief was remade into despair. Although Gould maintains that despair need not lead to demobilization – that despair can be a "provocation" (438) to further activism – in Los Angeles, despair was not provocative – it was demoralizing.

Last, explanations for the demise of the ACT UPs on a national level have focused on rifts between white gay men, who sought a "drugs into bodies" approach to AIDS activism, and women and people of color on the other side, who wanted direct action efforts to focus on universal healthcare needs (Halcli 1999; Gould 2002, 2009; S. Epstein 1996; Gamson 1996; Leonard 1990). I think this explanation needs more nuance because the sides don't easily line up so well at the local level. But I do think that ongoing gendered and raced conflict – what I called "intersectional crises" in Chapter 4 – are part of the explanation for ACT UP/LA's downward trajectory.

There were several concrete and largely localized factors that led to demoralization in ACT UP/LA and therefore contributed to members' exiting. First, the death of leaders in the leaderless group, coupled with an inability to garner visible successes, led to "burnout" among many members. Second, the violence and arrests that met activists at the national actions that took place at the Republican Party's 1992 convention in Houston were more than LA activists bargained for, which led some to refocus their energies in a different direction. After serious drop-offs in numbers, a very small group of activists tried to keep ACT UP/LA alive, rejecting resources that may have saved the group but might have changed its identity as an autonomous, member-driven democratic entity. I conclude the chapter with a discussion of what it means that activists disagree over how ACT UP/LA ended and what the group's end meant to its last few participants.

FAILURE AND DEATH EXPERIENCED AS ONE: DEMORALIZATION IN ACT UP/LA

Contrary to the "success kills" explanation of social movement demobilization, it was successes that sustained ACT UP/LA. Success in changing AIDS policy or in increasing the resources spent on the care of people with AIDS (PWAs) was crucial to the esprit de corps of ACT UP/LA. In the group's earlier years, it could point to the opening of a dedicated AIDS ward at the County/USC public hospital, however delayed, as a success; it could point to the opening of the free-standing AIDS clinic, however overwhelmed it was; and it could rely on media coverage, some of it sympathetic, as it sought to raise the public's awareness about AIDS.

Successes proved more difficult for the group – one could argue that they were never easy to accomplish and always incomplete – and despair did demobilize it as activists dealt with the psychological toll of dealing with death – the death of loved ones, of leaders, and of members of the lesbian and gay community forgotten by their families and their government. These deaths seemed to confirm the belief among many ACT UP/LA participants that the group's best days as an effective organization were past. Put bluntly, deaths in and of themselves were seen as evidence of a lack of success.

Certainly, death was omnipresent in the lives of ACT UP/LA members. Activist Jake Epstine, a nurse at the Chris Brownlie Hospice, estimated that he "witnessed over five hundred people die there in a little over two years" and that the number of deaths drained him of energy and caused him to stop his ACT UP/LA participation.[5] And Cat Walker, who had been part of ACT UP/LA since its inception, remembered how managing his grief in the early 1990s, even as he participated in ACT UP/LA actions, was extremely difficult for him and for others in the group:

In the early 1990s, I was feeling a lot of grief at the loss around and I felt like it wasn't okay to talk about that in ACT UP. ... We were supposed to be concentrating on the political work. It was like there wasn't time to cry about all these people, you were supposed to be out working. ... Another factor was the increase in fighting with each other ... which I thought ... looking back part of the reason we ended up fighting with each other so much then was sort of displaced grief ... because we were all very upset that Mark [Kostopoulos] and these other people had died, and instead of expressing that, we sort of took it out on each other and started fighting with each other.[6]

Walker came to attribute much of ACT UP/LA's slide to having leaders die of AIDS. He felt that

there got to be a bit of a leadership vacuum which is something that we never talked about in ACT UP ... we sort of had this pretense that we were leaderless, that we had no leaders, which I always thought was bullshit because ... being really involved in the organization like I was for a while then, I always knew who the leaders were ... at the same time like they were saying "oh we don't have leaders."[7]

Mark Kostopoulos died of AIDS on June 20, 1992; he was ACT UP/LA's co-founder and a leader of the leaderless ACT UP/LA. His death was a blow. For Ferd Eggan, Kostopoulos's death was an emotional turning point, a moment when the anger that fueled direct action turned into exhaustion:

[5] Email interview with author, 2012.
[6] Interview with author, 2011.
[7] Interview with author, 2011.

All of these ACT UP veterans got together, [Mark's] friends, people who had been in ACT UP for years, and we wanted to have a political funeral down the street. But at the same time, there was also a lot of discussion at that meeting. . . . A lot of us just wanted to feel sad. We didn't particularly want to have a political funeral. We just wanted to feel sad, to mourn. I mean, we had just sort of reached the end of righteous indignation. (Gould 1999: 435)

The memorials for Kostopoulos were politicized; activists grafted commemorations of Kostopoulos's death onto planned protest actions even while the death itself fueled new action. Locally, anti-AIDS activists were planning demonstrations in June 1992 to protest state and county budget cuts for the treatment of AIDS and to back California State Senator Milton Marks's plan to restore cuts in state AIDS spending.[8] ACT UP/LA scheduled a Day of Rage in Kostopoulos's memory on June 30, to take place at the LA County Hall of Administration where the Board of Supervisors met; they demanded "full funding for health care service to meet current and projected needs."[9] ACT UP/LA occupied the lobby of the nearby Ronald Reagan State Office Building as part of the same action, with several members chaining themselves to the building and vowing to disrupt "business as usual" until state funding for AIDS care was made current.[10] On the same day, ACT UP/LA members scattered Kostopoulos's ashes to protest cuts in funding at the county and state level that would result in the "political immolation" of the 5P21 AIDS outpatient clinic. The press release publicizing the action, referring to the Rodney King civil unrest less than two months earlier, read in part:

During the civil disturbances of May, ashes flew everywhere. They became the inescapable reminder of social injustice simmering to the flashpoint. The AIDS epidemic has produced a mountain of human ashes that are usually unseen. County government must take action to make health care a right for the people of Los Angeles.[11]

Helene Schpak, who was close to Kostopoulos, wrote a kind of eulogy for him for the ACT UP/LA *News* in the fall of 1992. She described his death as "a personal loss for me as well as a symbolic one, because in addition to losing a friend I also lost a guiding influence."[12] She wrote that "(i)t's strangely coincidental that Mark died at a time in ACT UP's evolution when many things organizationally were dying as well." Schpak linked Kostopoulos's death to the problems of burnout that the group had been experiencing and

---

[8] Unsigned. "ACT UP/LA Media Advisory: AIDS Budget Cuts Press Conference." June 9, 1992; ONE collection.

[9] ACT UP/LA. "Day of RAGE!" Flyer, dated June 29, 1992; ONE collection.

[10] ACT UP/LA. "Media Advisory: AIDS Budget Cuts Protest." June 30, 1992; ONE collection.

[11] Anonymous. "Scattering Activist Ashes to Save County Aids Clinic," p. 21, June 30, 1992; ONE collection. The "civil disturbances in May" is a reference to the unrest in the wake of the acquittal of the police officers who beat Rodney King.

[12] Helene Schpak, "Mark Kostopoulos October 26, 1954– June 20, 1991" ACT UP/LA News 5: 3 (Fall 92), p. 3.

counseled that the group needed to better plan actions in order to "(h)it as close to the source as possible." Significantly, Schpak also felt that the large demonstrations that had been the group's signature were no longer possible because its numbers had been dwindling. She urged ACT UP/LA to work more in coalition with other like-minded groups.

While it is difficult to measure the effects of Kostopoulos's death on ACT UP/LA in anything close to objective terms, we can look to the work of Bob and Nepstad (2007) who studied what the murder by the state of political leaders has meant for their movements. In the view of ACT UP/LA members, Kostopoulos's death and the deaths of other PWAs was the equivalent of state murder, a consequence of government neglect of the disease acting hand in hand with lethal society-wide homophobia. As such, the death of a visible and respected leader like Kostopoulos was at once confirmation of the righteousness of the anti-AIDS battle and of activists' sense that they were losing that battle. Bob and Nepstad (2007: 1376) also hypothesize that "(t)he murder of a movement leader is more likely to have a deleterious effect if the movement is weakly institutionalized," and, before them, Zald and Ash (1966: 338) predicted that, in the absence of efforts by a social movement organization to bureaucratize, the death of a charismatic leader would produce dwindling numbers. ACT UP/LA and the other ACT UPs existed in a decentralized network that actively resisted formalization, and all the ACT UPs were losing leadership to the disease. ACT UP/LA was proud of its informal structure and of the way that decisions about actions and agendas emerged from its members, but its very informality contributed to the leadership vacuum caused by Kostopoulos's death.

Kostopoulos's death was deeply mourned, and it was one of many. Because of his centrality to ACT UP/LA, Kostopoulos's passing was a reminder that even the most intense activism had not ended the AIDS crisis. Moreover, ACT UP/LA was still wrestling with local bureaucrats over public health provision for the AIDS-affected community. In early 1992, ACT UP/LA took action against USC/University Hospital (UUH), a new hospital privately owned by National Medical Enterprises (NME) and erected next to the publicly owned County/USC hospital. ACT UP/LA accused UUH of refusing to accept Medi-Cal patients and held a demonstration at the UUH site. Protestors were especially galled by the brand new state-of-the-art technology at UUH, which was dwarfed by County/USC, which activists described as "huge, understaffed, dilapidated ... jammed with the poorest people of the county."[13] The legal demonstration at UUH was accompanied by an affinity group action at NME corporate offices in Santa Monica (nearly twenty miles away), where six ACT UP/LA members chained themselves to an elevator in the lobby of the building

---

[13] ACT UP/LA. "NME University Hospital ... Is Breaking Our Hearts." Flyer. c. February 1992; ONE Collection; ACT UP/LA "Confrontation, Then Mediation: ACT UP/LA, NME, and Medical Apartheid." Anonymously (co?-) authored report, c. May 1992; ONE Collection.

while a seventh activist videotaped the action. All seven were arrested on charges of trespassing and failure to disperse by the city attorney of Santa Monica, who suggested mediation between ACT UP/LA and NME to resolve the conflict. The mediation took place in May 1992, but nothing concrete came out of it. ACT UP/LA members were not swayed by the argument that locating the new hospital next to County/USC would lead to "synergy" between the two institutions. Instead, the activists argued that UUH was clearly being added to be a money maker, specifically for USC. Mediation would do nothing to bridge the impasse between ACT UP/LA and NME/USC; ACT UP/LA was opposed in principle to the privatization that had led to the establishment of UUH, and NME/USC were not about to close UUH in order to satisfy activists' demands.[14]

As the confrontation with NME suggests, ACT UP/LA's 1992 agenda was in large part set by unresolved issues. LA County had established an AIDS ward and an outpatient clinic, but activists continued to see the County's responses as inadequate and underfunded.[15] Whereas in September 1988, ACT UP/LA could declare that "We've Won an AIDS Ward," in 1992, David Lacaillade, the ACT UP/LA member who reported to the GB about meetings with the County could only write about how staffing was still an issue at the 5P21 outpatient clinic and at "6700," as the dedicated AIDS ward at County Hospital had come to be known.[16] Lacaillade reported that physicians and physician assistants were leaving the clinic due to inadequate staffing. Non-HIV/AIDS patients were being admitted to 6700, lessening the number of beds available for PWAs. The County's overall budget for AIDS care, prevention, and education was considered by ACT UP/LA to still be far too low.

ACT UP/LA had some successes when dealing with the County. Its members helped physician assistants who wanted more money, and they persuaded the outpatient clinic to expand its walk-in hours. County officials whom ACT UP/LA had seen as obstacles to effective anti-AIDS strategizing were either transferred to other positions or announced their intentions to leave the County's employ. Nonetheless, Lacaillade's reporting on the County did not stress the positives, and it is easy to see why. Clinic patients were coming in sicker; more of the clinic's clients were homeless or mentally ill; the once pristine 6700 ward was starting to show wear. In June 1992, 5P21 actually stopped taking in new patients, a problem of short staffing that took months to clear up.[17] In late October 1992, Lacaillade and other activists were still meeting with Robert Gates, the director of health services

---

[14] "Confrontation, Then Mediation," ibid.

[15] Minutes, General Body Meeting, January 20, 1992; Flyer "What's Wrong with This Picture," about County/USC. c. February 1992. Author's collection.

[16] David Lacaillade, "While County Fiddles, People Die," ACT UP/LA *News*, 5: 3 (Fall 1992).

[17] ACT UP/LA, "County AIDS Fact Sheet." c. July 1992; ONE collection; David Lacaillade, "Small Bandages on Large Wounds: Reporting on the Second Gates Meeting Concerning AIDS Care at LA County/USC Medical Center." October 9 1992; ONE collection.

for the County of Los Angeles, seeking better oversight of both 5P21 and the 6700 ward.[18] The aforementioned salary raises granted for physicians' assistants had been "accidentally" deferred by the County for a year, a bureaucratic mistake that was corrected only with activist pressure. ACT UP/LA and other anti-AIDS groups demanded an audit of the clinic and criticized County bureaucrats for trying to pacify concerns about mismanagement by presenting activists with meaningless numbers that did nothing to actually illustrate how money at 5P21 was being (mis)spent.

Thus, in 1992, members of ACT UP/LA continued to face both the deaths of compatriots and the intransigence of local officials. The inevitability of death, coupled with the persistence of problems that activists faced in trying to end the AIDS crisis – and it has to be remembered that this was their goal – caused ACT UP/LA's numbers to dwindle. The narrative of despair leading to demobilization of the ACT UPs on the national level was complicated by events on the local level; despair came not just from (the denial) of grief in the face of loss, but from the intractability of the crisis itself.

SPIRALING DOWN IN 1992: THE PROBLEM
OF DWINDLING NUMBERS

ACT UP/LA members were demoralized by the shrinking of their group after the large numbers of new activists brought into the group by Governor Wilson's veto of AB 101, an anti-LGBT discrimination bill, began to fade away. Being composed of a small numbers of activists was not a problem in ACT UP/LA's earliest period, but to see the group's numbers dwindle after they had been large was demoralizing. Cat Walker remembered being particularly dispirited about the small numbers involved in ACT UP/LA's latter years:

One of the things I found hard then was that it seemed like it [ACT UP/LA] was just a shell of its former self ... because I had been there at the days when we had 200 people showing up at a meeting ... there was fifteen people, and they'd say "oh we have a really good turn out tonight."[19]

Wendell Jones, who had been particularly active in producing fundraising events for ACT UP/LA, started to pull away from ACT UP/LA in 1992 as well. Jones was burned out by the flurry of activity over AB 101 in late 1991 and, shortly thereafter, he began to care for fellow ACT UP/LA Treatment and Data Committee activist Wade Richards, nursing him through his final illness and death. Jones recalled taking time in 1994 to recover from Richards's death and then coming back to ACT UP/LA, which he described as "starting to unravel ... ACT UP was barely there. I didn't try to hold on ... " Another long-time ACT

---

[18] Lacaillade, ibid.
[19] Interview with author, 2011.

UP/LA activist, Larry Holmes, pointed to "exhaustion" as the reason he left the group.[20] Holmes explained that

(b)y mid-1990 I had been arrested +/– 100 times for some form of civil disobedience. I still worked full time at a job (managing a collection of artists) that required travel. My boss joked that lots of jobs had vacation time, but mine had jail time. Just living in LA seemed to take a lot of energy, and the work and activism and the omnipresent death all took a toll. We [Holmes lived with fellow activist John Fall] needed a break and headed to Seattle.

ACT UP/LA long-timers missed the joie de vivre of the earlier group, and yet leaving was still a difficult choice for many. Helene Schpak recalled that for her, "leaving ACT UP is not like anything clean. I remember being very conflicted about it for quite awhile, I remember being disappointed about the direction of the group but being torn, and it took awhile for me to kind of slip away on that."[21] And Brian Pomerantz stopped going to ACT UP/LA meetings in the winter of 1992, noting that the group seemed more factionalized by then and that he was also personally troubled by misguided suspicions some had about him being a government infiltrator.[22]

In summary, a lack of tangible successes coupled with the deaths of leaders combined to make ACT UP/LA a less attractive venue for battling AIDS. There were members of the group who recognized at the time that some troubling dynamics were starting to take place among members, and a committee called "Heart Politics" emerged to try to tackle the group's internal rifts.

HEART POLITICS: HEALING RIFTS AND MAKING CONNECTIONS

Some ACT UP/LA members were concerned about the group's internal dynamics even before the numbers of participants declined. A committee called "Heart Politics" had formed in 1990 in order to address questions of civility and solidarity among ACT UP/LA's members.[23] Some members felt that the way ACT UP/LA members expressed themselves to each other – the rawness of language used and people's pride in giving voice to their anger – was a liability, and thus Heart Politics took on the task of fixing the group emotionally. During the last months of 1990, Heart Politics planned a retreat for ACT UP/LA, which took place in February 1991. Cat Walker was cautiously hopeful about the retreat: "We may even find our way back to the feelings and solidarity we once had."[24]

---

[20] Email interview with author, 2012.

[21] Interview with author, 2011.

[22] Interview with author, 2012. Jeff Scheurholz also mentioned being mistakenly suspected of being a government infiltrator.

[23] Mickey Wheatley, Darren Goldstein, and Michael Albanese. "Finally, Health Care for ACT UP." Position paper dated August 27, 1990; ONE Collection.

[24] Funding for the February 1991 retreat was robustly debated in the General Body. (Field notes January 7, 1991; Minutes, General Body meeting, January 7, 1991; ACT UP/LA General Body meeting minutes January 21, 1991).

The 1991 retreat had good attendance by both men and women and seemed to do the group some good. A second retreat was held in March 1992 to discuss a characteristically ambitious range of issues about the group's internal workings and external face; as activist David Lacaillade quipped, "[w]hen the going gets tough, ACT UP/LA doesn't break up. It goes on retreat."[25] This second retreat was attended by forty or so people.[26] Attendees seemed particularly concerned about lack of communication among ACT UP/LA committees and therefore produced proposals for the GB to address these concerns. The retreat attendees asked that the Coordinating Committee, which helped to set the agenda for the GB meetings, help committees better coordinate actions; they also wanted a sound system and a chalk board set up at Plummer Park during GB meetings so that the action during the meetings would be easier to follow.[27]

The retreat attendees discussed how ACT UP/LA should relate to what they saw as the increasingly complex landscape of anti-AIDS and progressive grassroots organizing. ACT UP/LA conceived of itself as a coalition, and, since its inception, its members had participated in coalition work. Retreat participants wanted a clearer set of guidelines for participation in "true" coalitions, "where all member groups participate in setting the goals and strategies and share the burden of performance."[28] They recommended that ACT UP/LA take a more strategic view toward coalition work and reject coalitions that would not directly benefit ACT UP/LA. At the same time, they urged that ACT UP/LA's GB accept any differences it may have with the "style" of other groups – "whether it involves faerie dances in skirts or suits making windy speeches." The retreat attendees recommended that the Networking/Outreach committee "conduct an audit of the membership to identify ACT UP/LA members who are also members of other groups," so as to make those members liaisons with the responsibility of reporting to the GB about the actions of other groups.[29] While a complete record of discussions at the retreat does not seem to exist, the record as it stands does not show conversations about gender or racial/ethnic divides in the group. The challenges represented by the entrance of new members as a result of the AB 101 veto (see Chapter 4) or the growing centrality of Women's Caucus (WC) members' concerns do not appear to have been a major part of what members discussed.

It is difficult to gauge the effect of Heart Politics on ACT UP/LA. Interviewed many years later, Cat Walker referred to Heart Politics as a failure; he felt that

---

[25] David Lacaillade (for the Retreat Working Group). "Retreat." Packet including sign up sheets, c. late February/March 1992; ONE Collection.

[26] "ACT UP Camps!" Sign-in sheet, March 1992; ONE Collection.

[27] Minutes, General Body meeting, March 23, 1992; ONE Collection; Wade Richards and David Lacaillade, "ACT UP/LA Retreat." March 1992; ONE Collection. Richards and Lacaillade gave credit to retreat note-takers David Enos, Cat Walker, Neil Klasky, and Michael Albanese in writing their summary, which was five pages long, printed in small font and single-spaced.

[28] Richards and Lacaillade, ibid.

[29] Richards and Lacaillade, ibid.

the ideas of the committee/retreat never became integral to ACT UP/LA's process.[30] Indeed, there were members who felt that Heart Politics was a distraction and, alternatively, that Heart Politics members were trying to take over ACT UP/LA."[31] While Heart Politics aims were never universally supported, the retreats did give some in ACT UP/LA a safe space to think about the organization as such and about how they could better relate to each other. Walker believed that ACT UP/LA was beginning to lose its bearings; he described feeling that the energy at ACT UP/LA meetings was growing more "chaotic" as members' diverging interests split the group.[32] In retrospect, Heart Politics attempts to build time and space for members to connect – that is, to rebuild solidarity – may not have been enough to stop ACT UP's demobilization, but its efforts to recapture an earlier esprit de corps indicated that it had some sense that the early sense of commonality was crucial to maintaining the group.

"DISASTER": ACT UP/LA AT THE 1992 REPUBLICAN NATIONAL CONVENTION IN HOUSTON

Another crucial problem confrontinged the dwindling numbers of ACT UP/LA members was that the oscillation between local and national actions that had characterized ACT UP/LA's approach to anti-AIDS direct action was beginning to show diminishing returns for the local group. Events at the Republican Party National Convention in August 1992 illustrate how enervating poorly planned national actions could be for local activists. One hundred or so members of ACT UP/LA traveled to Houston to join ACT UPs and other anti-AIDS groups in protesting government inaction on AIDS at the Republican Party nominating convention, which took place August 17–20.[33] Cat Walker recalled that the relatively large ACT UP/LA contingent was made possible by Red, Hot + Blue money that had started to come into the group. The ACT UPs had also protested at the July 1992 Democratic National Convention in New York City; very few from ACT UP/LA joined in. Gregory Cooke, the co-facilitator of ACT UP/LA's Public Policy Committee, did go, and he reported that the protests were confrontational.[34] But the protests at the Republican Convention in Houston took confrontation to a different level, and the actions by the ACT UPs, allied affinity groups, and local community activist groups received a great deal of local and national media attention; on that level, the actions could be considered a success.

---

[30] Interview with author, 2011.
[31] Cat Walker, "Heart Politics," ibid.
[32] Interview with author, 2011.
[33] This is Cat Walker's estimate during his interview with author, 2011.
[34] Gregory Cook, "ACT UP LA at the National Democratic Convention." Report dated July 27, 1992, ONE collection.

The Houston actions nonetheless had a negative effect on the morale of ACT UP/LA. ACT UP/LA members who participated felt that the actions there were badly planned and badly supported, and they encountered a very aggressive Houston police who jailed protestors for days.[35] While many ACT UP/LA activists had been arrested in confrontational civil disobedience actions, they were not used to spending several days in jail under difficult circumstances; for those who were arrested, Houston represented the limit of what they were willing to endure. The recollections of ACT UP/LA participants in the Houston protests also suggest that the bad experiences had by activists who went to Houston created a split in the group afterward between those who had gone and those who had not. Pete Jimenez, who did go to Houston, felt that when those ACT UP/LA members returned to LA "you had this whole group of people who didn't go and wanted to pretend that Houston was no big deal and nothing happened."[36]

When I asked activist Terri Ford about the protests in Houston, Ford called the demonstrations there "a disaster" and became quiet.[37] I asked Ford what she meant by the term "disaster." She replied that since no one in ACT UP/LA had ever been to an action in Texas, they didn't understand that the police would be "out of control ... I mean they're bringing their horses in to trample us." Ford was part of a group that was able to sneak into the convention "in Republican drag" – conservative business attire – with the intention of interrupting Vice President Dan Quayle's speech. She noted that while she and other ACT UP protestors got in, the experience was "scary." Ford recalled that when her group revealed the "Silence = Death" shirts that they wore underneath their drag, they were "swarmed with I don't know what, Secret Service or I don't know what." Ford remembered that only the presence of a camera person kept the police from hauling the demonstrators off to a "back room."

ACT UP/LA's Brian Pomerantz also recalled police brutality in Houston.[38] Pomerantz described how one protest march at the beginning of the convention, headed toward the Astrodome, was led by police to a dead end where it became clear that the marchers were "going to get our asses kicked." Pomerantz described streetlights going out in the demonstration area and police "wailing on" demonstrators. Pomerantz echoed Ford as to the importance of enlisting the aid of media to stay safe; he recounted an incident in which an ABC television "Nightline" crew recorded one police officer instructing another not to hit a demonstrator while the lights were on. Pomerantz, along with several other

[35] Houston was given a heads-up in February 1992 about the planned demonstrations. The *Houston Chronicle* covered the arrival of an "advance guard for as many as 1,000 gays and lesbians intent on bringing chaos" to the Convention. The reporter's tone is alarmist, and one wonders why visiting organizers spoke with the press at all. (R. A. Dyer, "Dark Clouds Form for GOP Convention," *Houston Chronicle*, February 20, 1992, p. A17.)

[36] Interview with author, 2011.

[37] Interview with author, 2012.

[38] Interview with author, 2012.

activists, also recalled an ACT UP Women's Caucus "lie-in" at the end of the march were protestors were in danger of being trampled by mounted police. Standing protestors locked arms and stood between the police and the lie-in to protect those on the ground; everyone remained untrampled.

In his interview, Cat Walker vividly described how the Astrodome march was redirected by Houston police into the dead end "and we just found ourselves in this huge area ... and there was like hundreds of demonstrators ....and we were all just like milling around."[39] Walker recalled that some activists "started burning things, burning signs and burning effigies and creating these big bonfires." After the fires began,

all of a sudden it turned out that the Houston Police were hiding in the bushes that were surrounding this area and jumped out from behind the bushes and started hitting everybody with their batons. And started chasing, and everyone started running and it was just this mass chaos ... and of course they were doing this as a response to the anarchists and their fires.

While Walker blamed anarchists for the fires, he said that it was clear to him that the police wanted to chase all the demonstrators from the area, a task made difficult by the fact that there was no place to run. Walker, holding hands with two other demonstrators, ran as fast as he could to what looked like the way out; when they were close to exiting the scene, a police helicopter suddenly appeared above them, and police yelled at them to clear the area. Walker and the others were terrified because they did not know which way to go.

Houston was even scarier for those activists who ended up in jail. ACT UP/LA's. Richard "Doe" Racklin was one such activist. He was part of an affinity group of about seven protestors who entered the convention with fake press credentials, wearing his version of Republican drag: "I had like a white button down shirt and I think I was wearing a tie and a pair of kind of khaki pants."[40] Racklin waited for guests to arrive in an area reserved for the press, which was on a raised platform, and, when Bush took the podium to speak, they began their disruption:

A little bit after he started speaking that's when myself, and maybe one or two other people started yelling. "What about AIDS?" And things like that. Typical stuff. And I had a bunch of condoms in my pocket which I started throwing out into the audience, and I think a lot of the audience, a lot of the attendees were yelling to shut up and things like that, but we kept yelling "what are you doing about AIDS" and I think Bush was like putting his hand up to his ear. ... So I started throwing out the condoms in the wrappers ... he [Bush] couldn't understand what we were saying or was pretending not to, I figured I would just take out one of the condoms and unroll it and then maybe he would get the idea ... so I was yelling and waving it around in the air and there were all these flashes going off and because even though we were amongst all the media and the

---

[39] Interview with author, 2011.
[40] Interview with author, 2011

cameras they all turned around and started photographing us, and so that picture got around to *Time* magazine . . . with the condom in my hand. Then the security . . . the Secret Service was trying to get to us on the platform . . . we were yelling and carrying on for a little while before they could get to us on the platform . . . so then they finally grabbed me and whoever else was yelling and took us to a room.

Racklin's group was arrested; he was taken to jail and held there for days in poor conditions, separated from the other protestors by his inexperience. In order to stay together in arrest situations, ACT UP protestors would routinely answer "we are all living with AIDS" in response to questions about whether or not they were HIV-positive. In the tumult of his arrest, Racklin forgot about the strategy and simply answered "no" when asked if he had AIDS. He was put with, by his description, "some pedophiles and gay murderers and gay drug addicts." He was repeatedly harassed by the other inmates and he was humiliated by the guards. He managed to get his one phone call and called the ACT UP/LA office, crying into the phone. Racklin recalled that conditions were so poor that there were no mattresses provided for the first night he was in jail; mattresses showed up only after calls were made to the outside. Racklin's story of poor jail conditions was confirmed by other activists, including Jeff Schuerholz and Brian Pomerantz. A significant number of the Houston ACT UP protestors were held in custody until the end of the convention and possibly after its conclusion. Their supporters outside used the fact that phone calls were monitored to feed information to authorities. Brian Pomerantz recalled an instance of communicating to PWAs on the inside who were sick and having to sleep on bare concrete that a national news network was going to report about the lack of mattresses; after communicating this, the prisoners received mattresses. Pomerantz summed up the Houston experience very simply: "It was bad."

ACT UP/LA member Jeff Schuerholz was also jailed in Houston, arrested for disrupting a talk given at the convention by the Reverend Jerry Falwell.[41] Scheurholz remembered being dragged along the floor, and he felt a knee in his neck just before being thrown into a police wagon and jailed. Scheurholz described conditions in the jail as crowded, with lights on the entire time and "blaring" television coverage of the Republican convention; he recalled seeing himself on television being arrested over and over, until his cellmates took notice and assured him that "we hate that fucker [Falwell] too." Scheurholz also saw footage of Racklin and his affinity group interrupting President Bush's speech played over and over again. Scheurholz recounted being treated very badly in the Harris County jail. In contrast to Racklin, he described his incarceration was "an exciting time"; at the same time, from the standpoint of recalling Houston twenty years later, he dubbed the whole experience "a nightmare."[42] Scheurholz's partner, the late Pete Jimenez, stayed out of jail and tried to make trouble on the outside; angered by the police violence, he and others formed a group that

---

[41] Interview with author, 2011.
[42] Schuerholz and Tarley, p. 5, and interview with author 2011.

spontaneously tried to stop traffic on a freeway and then (thankfully) decided to leave the freeway and go back to the Astrodome, which had become a media circus.[43] Jimenez said that the events in Houston were traumatic, but it was also clear that he relished playing "cat and mouse" with the police as the police forced protestors to stay on the move, switching cars, and diving in and out of houses. Pete Jimenez and Jeff Scheurholz were able to integrate the violence of the Houston protests into their feelings about direct action; others, like Doe Racklin, couldn't. But they all recalled the actions in Houston as a drain on ACT UP/LA, using words like "disaster" to describe the events. The events generated media coverage; ACT UP/LA's Agitating/Legal Committee reported that, from a media standpoint, Houston had been "extremely successful with lots of local newspaper coverage."[44] The events surrounding the convention were also well covered in Houston, as one might expect. The *Houston Chronicle* reported that the Police Chief Sam Nuchia turned in a four-page report to the mayor and city council about two weeks after the march and police riot of August 17. Nuchia's report exonerated the Houston police of wrong-doing, claiming that activists had incited police by throwing bottles and lighting fires. Houston's mayor, Bob Lanier, supported the police chief's report of events, and the lesbian and gay community, members of the Houston civil rights community, and at least one city council member concluded that the report – which featured interviews with police officers only – was a "whitewash" of the events.[45]

For Cat Walker – who did not remember the Houston actions being well-covered in the media – the protests were dominated by "fairly new and young" activists from LA and elsewhere who

> just wanted to fight with the police ... and they would say things like "well we just got to get up in the police's faces" ... and it was kind of scaring the rest of us, because they didn't seem to have much political consciousness or understanding of what we were really trying to accomplish with the whole AIDS activism ... it was more like "oh this is fun, let's cause trouble."

Walker's comments about Houston suggest that something had shifted for ACT UP/LA members in their calculations about how worthwhile nationally coordinated actions were. As Walker recalled, "the actions in Houston were being orchestrated by activists from other ACT UPs, from other cities, because it seemed like they still had more of an intact leadership in a way than we did. But we didn't know those people."

After the Houston demonstrations in the summer of 1992, ACT UP/LA continued to slow down. Its leadership vacuum was manifested in its inability

---

[43] Interview with author, 2011.

[44] The minutes-taker cited coverage of the Houston events in the *New York Times* front page, *Time* magazine, radio stations in the region, local TV, CNN, and the ABC late-night news program *Nightline* (Minutes, General Body meeting, August 31 1992, ONE collection).

[45] John Williams, "Chief Lauds Police in GOP Row/Rights Groups, Gays Critical of Report on AIDS Protest Brawl." *Houston Chronicle*, September 2, 1992: 17.

to find a new treasurer after Rich Beecher, who had done the job for almost four years, stepped down.[46] Late in the year, the Coordinating Committee, which met on Sunday to set the Monday night GB meeting agenda, saw steep declines in its turnout, which led to less structure in GB meetings.[47] Members were tired. Successful actions were few, and rifts grew as energy dissipated. In a sense, Houston had been a revelation that national actions, which had previously been exhilarating, were not necessarily worth the effort. Attempts to refocus on the local were fraught with gendered and racial/ethnic tensions about what ACT UP/LA's purpose was regarding the many communities affected by the epidemic (see Chapter 4). In short, 1992 was a year of serious challenges to ACT UP/LA members' sense of effectiveness, although it would take years for the group to come to a dead stop.

SLOWING DOWN AFTER THE SLOW-DOWN: ACT UP/LA IN 1993 AND 1994

In 1993, ACT UP/LA continued to meet even with dwindling numbers of participants on a more or less weekly basis. The lack of numbers bothered those still coming; at one meeting in March, members expressed doubts about whether the few attending could even make decisions, ultimately deciding "that fourteen people can act as intelligently as a hundred fourteen."[48] The group still had no treasurer, and the Public Policy Committee had no facilitators.[49] The newsletter came out only occasionally. Still, ACT UP/LA continued to monitor LA County's public health AIDS provision, mostly through a few members' participation in a reorganized AIDS Community Advisory Council, where they sat with representatives from the County and the AIDS service sector. The County of Los Angeles did not appreciate ACT UP/LA's participation on the Community Advisory Council, and ACT UP/LA's David Lacaillade reported that the County made efforts to institutionalize the Council through the creation of bylaws, terms of representation, and the like. 5P21's chief administrator presented a proposal to Council members recommending a representative

---

[46] ACT UP/LA "*Ad Hoc* Financial Status Committee, 12, October, 1992; ONE collection. Beecher's resignation as treasurer apparently meant that taxes for 1991 on the merchandise ACT UP/LA sold had not been paid. Debts from Houston had not been entirely paid. Other monies seemed to have been squandered on poor planning; for example, the group paid for $6,000 worth of unused, nonrefundable airline tickets for members who did not go to Houston.

[47] Minutes, General Body meeting, December 7, 1922; ONE Collection. The minutes for the GB meeting of December 27, 1992, showed that no one actually went to the previous day's Coordinating Committee meeting, prompting attendees to eliminate the Coordinating Committee altogether.

[48] Minutes, General Body meeting, March 29, 1993; ONE collection.

[49] Minutes, General Body meeting, January 4, 1993, ONE collection. Minutes, General Body Meeting, February 15, 1993, ONE Collection. "ACT UP/LA May Be Bankrupt within Two Weeks," Unsigned, c. February 1993; ONE Collection.

structure that did not include activists. After Lacaillade and others objected, the clinic's chief administrator agreed to reconsider his proposal, and he eventually agreed to representation by those from the direct action AIDS protest sector and even unaffiliated individuals.[50] The fate of the 5P21 clinic was undetermined as the County made plans to replace the main buildings of the County/USC hospital complex; the hospital was built in 1932 and outdated to the point that many of its functions took place in trailers outside the huge edifice. ACT UP/LA was concerned about where the clinic would be moved to and what kinds of services would be available to PWAs in the interim.[51] The group's earlier jubilation at having once "won an AIDS ward" (see Chapter 2) drifted into consternation at the way that LA County's Department of Health kept dragging its feet.

ACT UP/LA also continued to deal with the deaths of its veterans. Richard Iosty, who had participated in ACT UP/LA during its heyday, died on December 29, 1992, and his last days exemplified the abysmal state of public hospital care for uninsured PWAs. Iosty had been in an NME hospital in Century City, in west Los Angeles, for almost two weeks toward the very end of his life. His care cost at least $93,000. Iosty lost his insurance, was kicked out of the NME hospital, and transferred to County/USC, where he was unable to find a bed in the 6700 AIDS ward that was housing leukemic patients. Outside the ward, Iosty was subjected to "homophobic interns and prayer meetings."[52] The GB voted to plan some sort of political funeral/memorial march for Iosty, with NME as a focus of protest.[53]

ACT UP/LA members tied Iosty's memorial to one for another member who had died, Jerry Mills, and put together a legal picket against the pharmaceutical company Amgen, located in Thousand Oaks, about thirty-five miles away from West Hollywood. ACT UP/LA targeted Amgen because members felt that the company charged excessive prices for two drugs – Epogen and Neupogen – that HIV/AIDS patients took to boost their production of red and white blood cells.[54] Planners hoped that a legal picket would be "the opening salvo" in a series of actions designed to pressure Amgen into lowering the costs of the drugs.[55] The legal picket took place on March 3, with ACT UP/LA providing the press

---

[50] David Lacaillade, "Two Meetings and a Third Postponed: Reorganizing the Council and Identifying New Principals in AIDS Care at LAC/USC Medical Center," February 1993 report to ACT UP/LA; ONE collection.

[51] Lacaillade, ibid.

[52] David Lacaillade reported to the General Body on Iosty's care. Minutes, General Body meeting, January 4, 1993; ONE collection.

[53] Minutes, General Body meeting, January 18, 1993; ONE collection.

[54] Neupogen cost approximately $1,350 per ten-day course, with an estimated 80 percent profit margin, which the LA times reported as "standard for prescription drugs produced by biotechnology firms." Stephanie Simon "AIDS Activists Decry Cost of Drug at Amgen Offices," the *Los Angeles Times*, March 4, 1993.

[55] Minutes, General Body meeting, February 15, 1993; ONE collection.

with information about how expensive Epogen and Neupogen were, and how Amgen had failed to adequately publicize their patient assistance program. ACT UP/LA also demanded that Amgen establish a community advisory board to guide further research and distribution of drugs, and it sought a promise that lowering the cost of the drugs in the US would not lead to cost rises in other countries.[56] According to the *Los Angeles Times*, "three dozen AIDS activists, blowing ear-piercing whistles and screaming bitter slogans" protested with chants like "Amgen, Amgen, you can't hide. We charge you with Amgenocide!"[57] The *Times* reporter felt compelled to minimize the protest as a "hullabaloo," but also quoted David Lacaillade on ACT UP/LA's demands.

Then, in late summer, David Lacaillade reported to the GB that he was no longer able to go to monthly meetings about 5P21 and the 6700 ward.[58] Lacaillade's swan song to the group contained this assessment of the state of AIDS care in LA County, after several years of protests and of meeting with County officials on AIDS care: "The state of AIDS care in Los Angeles County is abysmal ... 5P21 is bursting at the seams and treating sicker and sicker patients, and will soon be dislodged from its building." Lacaillade offered up his files to anyone from ACT UP//LA who wanted them, as "ammunition perhaps for whatever ACT UP/LA may decide to do about LA County health issues. Just let me know." Lacaillade's words betrayed his sense that ACT UP/LA did not in fact know what it wanted to do about the stalemate with the County.

In September 1993, the GB of ACT UP/LA saw another blow to their ranks as two participants apparently decided to organize their own ACT UP, "ACT UP County." ACT UP County went as far as submitting a prospectus about this reorganization to the GB itself, in essence inviting the GB to lop off a body part. The attendees at the GB meeting chiefly responded by assailing the breakaway activists for making their new group "invitation only" and for eschewing a focus on direct action. The GB response letter asked the ACT UP County group to find another name for their efforts since, without direct action, they appeared to be designing "another type of organization altogether." Nonetheless, the GB letter writers wished the break-off activists "the best of luck" in their efforts.[59]

ACT UP/LA's slide continued in 1994, a year that began inauspiciously for everyone living in the greater Los Angeles area. The Northridge quake occurred on January 17, 1994; it measured 6.7 on the Richter scale but had intense ground acceleration that caused it to be felt as far away as Las Vegas. The quake took at least seventy lives and was one of the costliest disasters in

[56] ACT UP/LA "ACT UP Visits Amgen: Because AIDS Is Big Business (But Who's Making a Killing?)." Press release/informational packet, c. March 1993; ONE collection.
[57] Simon, ibid.
[58] David Lacaillade, "They Still Lie," c. July 1993. Report to the General Body of ACT UP/LA; ONE collection.
[59] Letter signed by "The General Membership ACT UP/LA" to "Jeff and Gabriel," September 27, 1993; ONE collection.

US history up to that time.[60] Life for Angelenos was significantly disrupted for weeks, if not months. ACT UP/LA nonetheless continued to meet during all of 1994, albeit with very low attendance. Low attendance meant that the member-driven activist agenda, which always included a wide range of issues that were handled by committees, could not be maintained. Those attending the year's first GB meeting complained that the committee structure that had been in place could not be sustained, and it was recommended that participants drop the committee structure and meet together as one group.[61]

On the national level, the remaining ACT UPs worked on what came to be known as the "The AIDS Cure Project."[62] Activists wanted a "Manhattan Project" for curing AIDS; they wanted a reorganization and centralization of federal AIDS research with the aim of eliminating "extensive conflicts of interest endemic to medical research conducted within a market economy" (Cohen 2013: 65). But while the AIDS Cure Project interested local members, it did not generate enough local momentum to really sustain ACT UP/LA. ACT UP/LA's J. T. Anderson spoke about the AIDS Cure Project at an annual candlelight march sponsored by AIDS service organizations in May 1994, characterizing the Project as emerging from ACT UP/NY with input from other ACT UPs and community activists. Anderson told those assembled that the House bill would shake up the National Institutes of Health (NIH), which had become dominated by drug companies' agendas in its research, too stolid in its thinking about the disease, too tied to an "old boy network" when awarding grants to find a cure for AIDS.[63] The May march resulted in a "Candlelight Coalition" that sponsored a community forum on the AIDS Cure Project in September 1994.[64] Martin Delaney of Project Inform participated in the forum, as did representatives from the Treatment Activist Group (TAG), the group that had split off from ACT UP/NY. By then, the AIDS Cure Project (now HR 4370) had been endorsed by a number of Democratic politicians (like the once and future governor of California, Jerry Brown).

During most of 1994, ACT UP/LA meetings functioned more like a clearinghouse for information than a body working on its own actions. One exception was ACT UP/LA's actions in support of safer sex education in

---

[60] Kenneth Reich, "Study Raises Northridge Quake Death Toll to 72." *The Los Angeles Times*, December 20, 1995. http://articles.latimes.com/1995-12-20/news/mn-16032_1_quake-death-toll

[61] Minutes, General Body meeting, January 3, 1994; ONE Collection.

[62] Originally known as the "Barbara McClintock Project to Cure AIDS," named after a Nobel prize-winning scientist, the AIDS Cure Project started life as HR Bill 3310, introduced to the House of Representatives in October 1993; the bill went through different versions and name changes in the course of its life. See http://www.gpo.gov/fdsys/pkg/BILLS-103hr3310ih/pdf/BILLS-103hr3310ih.pdf.

[63] J. T. Anderson "ACT UP/LA Speaks at Candlelight March," ACT UP/LA newsletter, Winter 1995: p. 4. Anderson's May 1994 speech wasn't covered until ACT UP/LA's 1995 newsletter, which came out in early 1995, after a gap in publication of more than two years.

[64] ACT UP/LA "Demand a Cure for AIDS!" Unsigned press release dated September 26, 1992; ONE collection.

Glendale, a suburb north of downtown Los Angeles. Students at Glendale's Hoover High School contacted ACT UP/LA when the school board interfered with their plans to host a play entitled "Secrets," staged by Kaiser Permanente, the large non-profit HMO. The play contained information about safer sex; students were required to get permission slips from parents to attend. Despite the play's mainstream provenance and the permission slip safeguard, the Glendale school board cancelled the play. Some of the remaining members of ACT UP/LA had been working on questions of youth and safer sex education in the Los Angeles Unified School District (LAUSD) because LAUSD had begun publically debating whether to distribute condoms to high school students as part of safer sex education and AIDS prevention in schools.[65] In October 1991, ACT UP/LA members of the Treatment and Data committee had formed a working group called "Youth Action" to support "the passage of a comprehensive AIDS/HIV plan" within LAUSD; while the ACT UP/LA of 1994 had done away with the Youth Action committee, the remaining members were eager to help the students who had reached out.[66] On March 30, 1994, ACT UP/LA members brought "3,000 bright yellow condoms" to Glendale's Hoover High and handed out stickers in "neon yellow and green" that read "Safe Sex Is Hot Sex" to students to protest the cancellation of the play.[67] They were met with some "anti-condom" advocates of abstinence, but the action itself was peaceful. Several members continued to be involved in AIDS education in the Glendale schools.[68]

ACT UP/LA also demonstrated once again at the Westwood Federal Building on December 1, 1994, World AIDS Day, as part of a coalition of AIDS service organizations and students.[69] The demonstration was in part a memorial for recent losses in the AIDS activist community, and "mock coffins" were brought to the scene, which caught fire in the middle of the intersection of Wilshire Boulevard and Veteran Avenue, one of the busiest in the city. ACT UP/LA activist women, including Mary Lucey, Stephanie Boggs, Mary Nalic, Terri Ford, and She Welch "locked arms and refused to leave the street, risking arrest."[70] They were not arrested, although, according to Stephanie Boggs, it was not for lack of trying: "We . . . tried numerous formations, including sitting down in front of a police car, before we concluded that we were not going to be

[65] Berkley Hudson, "Shouting Unravels Press Conference," *The Los Angeles Times*, October 19, 1992, pp. B1, B3.
[66] "What Is Youth Action?" Unsigned report to the ACT UP/LA General Body, October 21, 1991. Collection of the author.
[67] Jennifer Oldham, "Condom Nation: Controversy Draws Safe-Sex Activists to High School," *The Los Angeles Times*, March 31, 1994. The *Times* reporter noted that the "Secrets" troupe had already staged the play for 700,000 students all over the state.
[68] Minutes, General Body meeting, April 11, 1994; ONE Collection.
[69] Stephanie Alana Boggs, "World AIDS Day Demonstration," ACT UP/LA newsletter, Winter 1995: pp. 1, 5; Minutes, General Body meeting, December 5, 1994; ONE Collection.
[70] Minutes, General Body meeting, December 5, 1994.

arrested, just beaten to death."[71] The GB minutes-taker who summed up the demonstration noted that group sentiment was that "ACT UP/LA should use the energy generated by the action to plan more actions."

The actions of a much smaller ACT UP/LA in 1993 and 1994 showed that there was still a small group of activists with a considerable amount of protest experience who were committed to ACT UP's brand of confrontational protest. At this point in the group's life, actions were focused on the local level only and followed, as they always had, members' concerns and initiatives. But the minutes-taker's note about using energy to plan new actions was poignant given the difficultly that a much smaller group of activists had in keeping their collective energy level high.

LAST GASPS: ACTIONS IN 1995 AND 1996

The last two years of ACT UP/LA's life showed how the much smaller group ultimately chose a politics of democratic principle over pragmatism. By 1995, members were meeting biweekly and working in an intermittent mode when it came to doing direct action. In April 1995, fourteen ACT UP/LA members demonstrated at St. Vibiana's Cathedral in Downtown LA during a visit by President Clinton and First Lady Hillary Clinton; they opposed Cardinal Mahony's stance on AIDS education as well as President Clinton's inaction on AIDS issues.[72] And the smaller ACT UP/LA protested an ad campaign by a long-time ally, the AIDS Healthcare Foundation (AHF), when members were disturbed by an AHF ad campaign in the local lesbian and gay press that stated "HIV is Treatable." These ads were meant to inform readers about protease inhibitors, a new class of anti-retroviral drugs that were giving many PWAs a new lease on life.[73] Jeff Scheurholz wrote letters to the press stating his objection to the campaign and to AHF's executive director, Michael Weinstein, who had been at the first meeting of ACT UP/LA and who was generally regarded as a friend. In GB meetings, Scheurholz suggested that ACT UP/LA run its own ad campaign with the slogan "HIV Is Treatable/ Then You Die." ACT UP/LA ran such an ad in *Frontiers*, a local gay community weekly, demanding that AHF "apologize to PWAs and their loved ones."[74] Taking on AHF meant eschewing coalitional ties that had once been important to ACT UP/LA, however difficult such coalitions could be in practice.

There was a return to form for the group when ACT UP/LA's last large-scale action took place – a February 1996 demonstration at Ronald Reagan's star-studded eighty-fifth birthday party held at Chasen's, a restaurant just outside

[71] Boggs, ibid., p. 5.
[72] Minutes, General Body meeting, April 17, 1995; ONE Collection.
[73] Minutes, General Body meeting, May, 16, 1995; ONE collection.
[74] Minutes, General Body meeting, June 5, 1995; ONE collection.

Beverly Hills.[75] The protestors wanted to remind the public of Reagan's inaction on AIDS during his presidency; the action was therefore largely symbolic as Reagan obviously had no executive powers. Jeff Scheurholz, who helped organize the demonstration, recalled getting a phone call from a friend tipping him off about the birthday party. In their joint interview in 2011, Pete Jimenez stated that he and Scheurholz did the bulk of the organizing for the action, which drew several hundred (according to the *Los Angeles Times*) or quite a few more (according to Scheurholz and Jimenez) to the site. Activists shouted at the party-goers, chanting "Shame" and "Over 300,000 AIDS deaths." Schuerholz described the demonstration as being a kind of reunion for ACT UP/LA, one that drew "people we hadn't seen for years came ... it was such a good demo because these limos would pull up ... and we would scream and scream [at the people getting out and] ... the police line would get charged."

But the Chasen's action did not permanently pull large numbers of old members back nor did it attract many new ones. The last few members of ACT UP/LA met bi-weekly through early 1997, chiefly to take positions on current AIDS issues; the group had gone from setting protest agendas to reacting to the stances taken by others. At about the same time, ACT UP/LA's last few members voted to reject, on matters of democratic principle, what might have been a lifeline for the group; they declined further funding from the Red Hot organization (see Chapter 2). ACT UP/LA's members objected to what they saw as the lack of democracy in the decision-making process about how to distribute funds.[76] In early 1996, ACT UP/New York had received $75,000 dollars from the Red Hot organization, and ACT UP/LA activists Terri Ford, Jeff Scheurholz, Stephanie Boggs, and J. T. Anderson participated in an ACT UP Network conference call in March to discuss how to disburse the monies. Anderson wrote in the April 1 meeting minutes about the call, stating that he and others in ACT UP/LA felt that the call had been a ruse and that decisions about how to disburse the monies had already been made by the time of the phone call. Accordingly, the ACT UP/LA representatives "requested a more democratic process," especially since their group had been so instrumental in making decisions five years earlier about how to distribute Red Hot + Blue (RHB) monies.

Another Network conference call was scheduled for the next week (i.e., early April), and, in the interim between the two conference calls, emails – a new medium of communication – began to fly back and forth between Los Angeles and New York. The point person for RHB in ACT UP/New York, Steven Shapiro, attempted to set an agenda for the April 7 conference call,

---

[75] *Los Angeles Times* Staff and Wire reports: "Luminaries Toast Ronald Reagan's 85th Birthday." February 7, 1996. http://articles.latimes.com/1996-02-07/local/me-33261_1_ronald-reagan, accessed July 16, 2012.

[76] Minutes, General Body meeting, April 1, 1996; ONE collection.

laying out the need for documentation of chapter ACT UP activities in each city and proposing different plans for distributing Red Hot money.[77] In each model, ACT UP/New York, the largest ACT UP, ended up with the lion's share of funds. Each model also included a scheme by which groups would receive Red Hot money in two disbursements, with the latter dependent on documenting how they had spent the former.[78] The April 7 conference call took place and apparently only ACT UP/LA objected to the distribution agreement. While ACT UP/LA stood to gain about $9,000 of Red Hot money, the six activists who attended the GB meeting the next day voted to refuse all Red Hot money, swayed by Jeff Scheurholz's report that "decisions made on the call were prearranged and that the call was a sham."[79]

In an email sent to ACT UP/NY and the other ACT UPs from J. T. Anderson's account, ACT UP/LA shared the news that it had unanimously voted to decline Red Hot money because it felt the process of deciding on distributions was "exclusionary, unfair and undemocratic."[80] It was clear that the remaining members of ACT UP/LA were aggrieved by what they saw as an attempt by the Network/ACT UP/New York to keep tabs on the existing ACT UPs in a play to become a kind of "ACT UP/Central," rather than remain a network. Shapiro immediately emailed back to ACT UP/LA, upset by what he saw as ACT UP/LA's intransigence. He argued that Red Hot monies had always come with the requirement of documentation. Shapiro claimed that the only change approved for the current round of disbursements was the request to have documentation given "mid-stream rather than at the end." He stressed that Red Hot money was the only real money coming to ACT UP/NY. Shapiro closed his message by expressing regret that ACT UP/LA had chosen "to divorce themselves from what must be necessary funds."[81]

It is impossible to know whether $9,000 worth of funding would have rejuvenated ACT UP/LA. Such a counterfactual assertion would have to take into account the growing complexity of the local and national landscape of anti-AIDS organizing and whether or not ACT UP's militant brand of organizing had a place in it. The success of the Chasen's action does give one pause; what if the six members of the group had acquiesced to requests for documentation? Would it have irreparably changed them? Would they have even had to follow-up in the manner that ACT UP/NY and the Red Hot organization wanted? It's impossible to know if the money could have helped; after all, in ACT UP/LA's history, just a few years prior, the Clean Needles Now controversy and many members' desire to keep ACT UP/LA's direct action character intact had led to intractable debates over what to do with new resources (see Chapter 4). The six

---

[77] Email, Steven Shapiro, April 7, 1996. "Re: Conference Call," ONE Collection.
[78] Email, Steven Shapiro, April 7, 1996. "Re: Report on the Conference Call"; ONE Collection.
[79] Minutes, General Body meeting, April 8, 1996; ONE collection
[80] Email, ACT UP/LA. April 10, 1996. "RED HOT MONEY"; ONE Collection.
[81] Email, Steven Shapiro, April 11, 1996, "Re: RED HOT MONEY (fwd)"; ONE Collection.

members who rejected the Red Hot money were, in this sense, following an organizational legacy of being unwilling to capitalize on opportunities for the mere sake of doing so.

In 1996, ACT UP/LA's last few members continued to attend and sometimes arrange protest actions. The last protest action seemed to be "zapping" President Clinton, who was running for re-election, at a fundraiser in order to protest his failure to support the most recent version of the AIDS Cure Act (now HR 761).[82] Protestors couldn't do much to confront the President except raise their signs higher as his motorcade went by and shout louder. Two ACT UP/LA members, J. T. Anderson and Peter Cashman, were able to speak to local broadcast media about Clinton's poor record at highlighting the AIDS epidemic and his failure to make good on his 1992 promise to appoint an "AIDS czar" tasked with coordinating the disparate and sometimes ineffective efforts at the federal level for fighting AIDS. Their actions were very much in line with ones that ACT UP/LA had always taken, but the actions themselves rested on very few individuals to carry out.

THE REAL END(S): THE DEATH OF ACT UP/LA

By early 1997, ACT UP/LA meeting attendance was never more than six members and was sometimes down to three. The group was dying. In contrast to its clean and coalitional start on December 4, 1987, ACT UP/LA's death sometime in 1997 or early 1998 was disputed in accounts by interviewees, and I uncovered two versions of the death of ACT UP/LA. According to Peter Cashman, J. T. Anderson, and the late Stephanie Boggs, jointly interviewed in July 1999, ACT UP/LA officially died at some point in 1998, when the three of them voted to end the group – or rather Cashman and Anderson voted to end it and Boggs voted "no." Arguably, ACT UP/LA still existed in 1999, since there was still a bank account open in the group's name with $206 in it. Thus, in this first version of ACT UP/LA's death, the group was ended by an orderly process in which activists committed to participatory democracy took a vote, and the majority will was followed. The two hundred or so dollars left in the account represented a die-hard hope of resurrection.

However, according to Jeff Scheurholz in his interview in 2011, ACT UP/LA was dead by the time of the 1996 Republican Convention in San Diego, when a few people from Los Angeles made the two-hour trip and held up signs in the protestors' pen. Scheurholz recalled that he was at the group's last meeting shortly after the convention – that is, in the fall of 1996, and that, furthermore, Cashman was not there. Scheurholz described Cashman as having actually "picked it [ACT UP/LA] up after it was over"; "all of sudden Peter Cashman had an email he sent out and he picked up being the contact. ... I remember

---

[82] ACT UP/LA. "ACT UP Zaps President Clinton at Hollywood Gala! AIDS Activists Charge: 'Four Years of Broken Promises.'" Press release dated September 13, 1996; ONE collection.

talking about it with a few other people, like, well that's a good thing because at least there was somebody to contact." Scheurholz remembered feeling relieved that *someone* had "picked up" the ACT UP/LA ball. In this second version, then, the group died a natural death when its energy just ran out. Of course, these two versions of ACT UP/LA's end are entirely reconcilable; the group likely fizzled out and Cashman, Boggs, and Anderson likely picked up the ball and carried it for a little while longer. At any rate, by 1998, ACT UP/LA was dead.

Ultimately, the story of the end(s) of ACT UP/LA is a story of activists' loyalty to a form of democratic decision-making *and* a style of direct action. At the very end, ACT UP/LA's last few members rejected money that came with strings attached and, in doing so, asserted their view of what the direct action anti-AIDS movement should look like: democratic, networked, with locally autonomous groups working on member-driven agendas. They didn't want to change to fit the times, and they didn't want to maintain coalitional links with those (like AHF) whom they saw as failing to keep up the level of outrage needed to defeat AIDS. The last few members of ACT UP/LA were solidaristic; they were not a coalition of diverse individuals. And, at a certain point, the making of coalitions took a back seat to the maintenance of a particular and valued identity.

In summary then, ACT UP/LA began a slow process of demobilization due to a variety of factors: the intersectional crises of gendered/raced and sexualized rifts among members (see Chapter 4), the deaths of key players leading to a leadership vacuum in the group, dismay over the intractability of local bureaucrats responsible for healthcare provision, and the evaporation of a local "pay-off" in the once generative oscillation between national and local action. While the timing of ACT UP/LA's demobilization fits the national trend, its demise is a local story that doesn't easily fit some general explanations for the end of the ACT UPs. Contrary to assertions that "success kills" social movements, lack of success very much affected ACT UP/LA. On the other hand, the case of ACT UP/LA gives some support for Gould's argument that emotions mattered in explaining why the ACT UPs fell apart because ACT UP/LA activists indeed were wrestling with burnout, grief, and exhaustion. But, even here, those feelings were affected by concrete local circumstances: exhaustion was exacerbated by the continued intransigence of LA County's public health bureaucracy, by the deaths of founders, and by the negative experiences of local actors at national actions. The refusal of the last few activists left in ACT UP/LA to give up their vision of how protest politics should be done needs to be seen in this context; they held on to something meaningful – and for them certain – as uncertainty about how to act settled in all around them.

6

From Streets to Suits: The Inside(r)s and Outside(r)s of ACT UP/LA

To me a successful political strategy is going to engage the full spectrum of political activity from grass roots on the streets all the way through to the collar and tie. We've [ACT UP] done it all ... and can do it all and have done it all and we've done it everywhere.

– Peter Cashman[1]

I must say I used ACT UP very well ... because when I went to the pharma [pharmaceutical companies] ... they knew I had contact with ACT UP. ... They were scared.

– Geneviève Clavreul[2]

INTRODUCTION: STYLES OF ACTIVISM AND ACTIVISTS IN ACT UP/LA

The two quotes juxtaposed above, taken from my interviews with former activists, reveal some barely audible but important aspects of disagreements within the AIDS Coalition to Unleash Power, Los Angeles (ACT UP/LA) about how to fight AIDS. Peter Cashman, one of ACT UP/LA's co-founders, suggests that members held common understandings about the differences between "grass roots on the streets" and "collar and tie" styles of activism; he links the two styles of activism to each other, implicitly placing them on a spectrum from radical to routine. In Geneviève Clavreul's statement, we can hear pride at what ACT UP/LA was able to accomplish through confrontation, but note how Clavreul describes her actions: she was personally comfortable with sitting

---

[1] Interview with the author, 1999. There is no real consensus on how to treat the term "grass roots" grammatically. "Grass roots" can also be spelled as one word – "grassroots" – and can be treated as either a singular or plural noun. Given the multiple constituencies that inhabit the space, I treat "grass roots" as a plural noun and hyphenate it as "grass-roots" when I use it as an adjective.

[2] Interview with the author, 2011.

down and speaking to authorities and confident that those in ACT UP/LA who were more committed to disruptive tactics would have her back. Her use of the first person voice acknowledges a separation between her individual actions as a negotiator and the group itself. Taken together, these two quotes hint at pervasive debates within ACT UP/LA about "insider" versus "outsider" strategies for ending AIDS, and they suggest that the lines between inside and outside activist spaces were blurry and easily crossed.

THE INSIDER–OUTSIDER DICHOTOMY IN SOCIAL MOVEMENT THEORY

In this chapter, I consider how members of ACT UP/LA managed issues raised by encounters with the "inside" – with institutions that were targets of anti-AIDS activism. The group debated the pros and cons of insider and outsider tactics even while insiders worked within ACT UP/LA, and ACT UP/LA members came from and entered insider spaces in order to further the battle against AIDS. Using a feminist intersectional perspective, I regender (Chappell 2006) the discussion of the role of inequalities in both outsider and insider activist space, and I argue that the experiences of activists who traversed these spaces complicates a vision of a hard line dividing them. I do this through reading the debates within the group about insider and outsider tactics and by listening to what former activists who were "straddling" (Newman 2012: 134) insider and outsider spaces thought about the contradictions involved in working in those spaces. In the 1980s and 1990s, the AIDS "establishment," as it was called by activists, was in fact newly established and porous, which gave rise to opportunities for activists to cross boundaries between institutional and grass-roots spaces. Access to resources, including positions of authority in government and social service organizations, was one of ACT UP/LA's demands. In Los Angeles, anti-AIDS organizations fought for the creation of government posts like that of the Los Angeles City AIDS coordinator, a position filled by former grass-roots activists throughout the 1980s and 1990s, including two from ACT UP/LA. Some activists wanted to be part of efforts to build the right kind of AIDS service organizations and programs; others wished to remain outsiders to institutional power.

In order to examine how ACT UP/LA participants related to – or didn't relate to – institutional power, I turn to the kind of debates that ACT UP/LA activists engaged in about dealing with institutional power, looking at a dispute that emerged in July 1990 among activists about whether the organization should "negotiate" with LA County officials or press those officials from the outside through disruptive protest. In looking at these debates, I consider what social movement scholars have said about the insider–outsider dichotomy in protest politics. I then consider the way in which some activists traversed the porous boundaries between outsider and insider activism by doing AIDS work (Brier

2009) in outsider and inside spaces; some activists came to ACT UP/LA from their work in institutional spaces, while others moved on to doing institutional activism as a result of their participation in direct action. I conclude that ACT UP/LA incorporated insider activists in doing disruptive protest, while institutional activists with experience in ACT UP/LA carried outsider attitudes about change into insider spaces. This suggests not just that the lines between outside and inside activist spaces were blurry in Los Angeles in the 1980s and 1990s, but also that those doing movement studies need to conceptualize the line between outsider and insider spaces as potentially porous and subject to degrees of erasure in the lives of activists themselves.

DEBATES ABOUT THE OUTSIDE AND THE INSIDE IN ACTIVISM

Former ACT UP/LA members recalled having different ideas about how to relate to instutionalized power. At one end of the continuum, Pete Jimenez referred to institutional activists as having gone over to "the dark side."[3] Jimenez relished being an outsider and enjoyed disruptive protest. And yet Jimenez and his partner Jeff Scheurholz actually met when Scheurholz was a volunteer for an AIDS service organization, Project Angel Food, which delivered food to homebound people with AIDS (PWAs). Jimenez was one such PWA. As Scheurholz recalled, in early 1991,

(a)ll my friends were dying. I had my store – my customers were dying. . . . I was already working for Project Angel Food – and that's how I met Pete. Pete was one of the clients and I would deliver food to him . . . and then I would try to get that route [we start laughing] because Pete was on the route, and I enjoyed seeing him. Then in October his name wasn't on the list – he was in Washington DC at the Universal Health Care Action and at the same time AB 101 happened here. So I was in the streets here every night for weeks and weeks and also immediately started going to the ACT UP meetings and the Queer Nation meetings where I found the coolest people ever around . . . a few weeks later Pete showed up at the meeting and everybody already knew him.[4]

Scheurholz and Jimenez were together for more than twenty years, until Jimenez passed away in May 2012. But they disagreed in their joint interview about whether or not institutional activists had indeed gone over to "the dark side" – a position of corruption and cooptation. Although Jimenez was adamant that working on the inside represented an inexcusable turn away from the street, Scheurholz felt that "a lot of people got hooked up with AIDS service organizations and took their ACT UP attitudes with them into those organizations." To further add to the complexity of attitudes about institutional work, both men agreed that they felt that there was something

---

[3] Interview with author, 2011.
[4] Interview with author, 2011. See Chapter 4 for discussion of the ramification of Governor Pete Wilson's veto of AB 101, an anti-discrimination bill focused on the rights of lesbians and gays, for ACT UP/LA.

unseemly about paid AIDS institutional activists who kept participating in direct action. Schuerholz described such people as "paid to be at the demo," while Jimenez, again the more adamant, stated that he was offended by professional AIDS workers who saw themselves as "big-time" activists.

Pete Jimenez was not the only one suspicious of institutional activists. James Rosen was a part of both ACT UP/LA and ACT UP/NY during the late 1980s and early 1990s as he and his partner Ty Geltmaker moved from coast to coast for work and family reasons. Rosen is HIV-positive and spent a considerable amount of his ACT UP/LA time working as part of the Treatment and Data committee. At one point, he acted as a liaison to Los Angeles County Supervisor Gloria Molina's office, which put him in touch with the Molina staff member in charge of AIDS and health issues. Molina had been elected to the Los Angeles County Board of Supervisors in 1991; she was the only female member on the Board when she was elected and the only person of color. Her election changed the balance of liberals and conservatives on the Board. Molina had a long background in Los Angeles and California politics, having been a community organizer and served as an LA City Council member and a California State Assemblyperson prior to being elected as Supervisor. In his interview in 2012, Rosen described Molina as having "had the potential to do great things" given her background. But he grew disenchanted with Molina, describing her as just another "worthless" Democrat who "just got sucked into the normal way of doing business."[5]

Rosen recalled that, because of his position as ACT UP/LA liaison to Molina's office, Molina and the County hospital expected him to "backchannel" information to Molina's office, which was painful because everyone in ACT UP/LA, including Rosen, thought that the group had some "genuine snitches that were there feeding information back to people at the County [hospital]." In August 1991, Rosen and Geltmaker co-signed a letter to the General Body (GB) excoriating a member of ACT UP/LA for taking a report intended for ACT UP/LA members and sharing it with the administration at the County's "5P21" outpatient AIDS clinic.[6] Rosen and Geltmaker had written the report about a meeting with LA County officials for the GB, and an ACT UP/LA member passed the report on to an administrator, who shared it with others; this action ultimately put the clinic personnel who had met with ACT UP/LA in danger of disciplinary action. The leaking of the report was ammunition for those who felt that meetings with anyone employed by the County was bad strategy for a direct action organization, and the action also bolstered arguments for greater secrecy within ACT UP/LA. Rosen and Geltmaker rejected these arguments even while they denounced the leak in no uncertain terms:

[5] Interview with author, 2012.

[6] Ty Geltmaker and James Rosen, "Scoundrel Time, or, The Silence of the Moles." Letter to the General Body of ACT UP/LA dated August 19, 1991; ONE collection. "5P21" referred to the number given to the clinic space in the County building in which it was housed.

We find this action reprehensible and a violation of the implicit trust necessary for us as a group to stay informed while elaborating policy. ...To those who would say we should not have made the report available to the general body, we respond: It is better to risk being duped by in-house fools and moles and visiting spies than to create an atmosphere of paranoid suspicion ruled over by a cadre of secretive leaders. ... We have every intention of continuing to meet with County employees and to keep ACT UP informed.[7]

Rosen also feared that meeting with County employees gave the County the opportunity to "lobby" ACT UP/LA members by using their face-to-face meetings with activists to communicate their own political agendas. Recalling a tour that he and other activists were given of the hard-won dedicated AIDS ward at County Hospital, Rosen remembered this scene:

I remember when we were given a tour of the [County USC] hospital by this nurse. We were in shock because she took us through the HIV ward and it was new, it was pristine, beautiful, everything was sunny and shiny and suddenly she opened these doors and she took us to the other end of the hospital and we were like, "oh my God." And she said "well this is what the rest of the hospital is like." And she said "you people have that, and this is what everyone else has." ... We had fought for those hundred beds and this new pristine unit, and the rest of the hospital was third world.

Like Jimenez, Rosen's take on the risks involved in institutional activism rested on an assessment of the potential for self-aggrandizement that institutional activism afforded. Without mincing words about ACT UP/LA's shortcomings, Rosen stated that he felt that ACT UP/LA itself "was so filled with Poo Bahs, *and* well-meaning people." Rosen seemed to use the expression "Poo Bah" to indicate a pompous individual rather than a bureaucrat – he situated the Poo Bahs in outsider space – but he was highly critical of the new insiders of the AIDS establishment:

(S)ome of the insiders [were there] for their own aggrandizement and their own power play and their own positions [and] would do certain things that were counterproductive to the greater good of what we were trying to achieve. And so there was a lot of that stuff going on and it was also people wanting to make their own position look good in the eyes of wherever they were working or in the eyes of the group as a whole or in the general ether of ACT UP itself.

At the very same time, Rosen explicitly stated that he didn't "disparage" anyone for working on the inside, and he acknowledged the need for an inside front against AIDS: "there's a limit to how much you can do outside the system." And, as an activist, he himself met with insiders despite his misgivings.

Brian Pomerantz, a former ACT UP/Philadelphia and ACT UP/LA activist, who at the time of his interview worked as a federal public defense attorney, stated that when he was an activist, he did not like hearing people inside the AIDS industry claim that they could do more from the inside: "I would have said

---

[7] Ibid.

that's 'bullshit' – you start taking money, you aren't an activist."[8] Pomerantz's solution to the quandary of the institutional activist was fairly simple: those working on the inside should not consider themselves to be activists. At the same time, Pomerantz stated that his mentor in ACT UP/Philadelphia, whom he regarded as an incredible activist, went on to work for the city of Philadelphia. Even while acknowledging these contradictions, Pomerantz was fairly adamant about what he felt were concerted efforts during the 1990s to calm down street protests by hiring AIDS activists for insider positions.

These recollections by activists in interviews selectively echo vigorous debates about "the inside" that took place in ACT UP/LA, and they reflect long-standing ideas that many other activists have about the reality of cooptation of protesters by outsiders. But, of course, the line between outsider versus insider activism is a blurry one; for example, Rosen was interfacing with authorities even as he walked the corridors of County Hospital. In the social movement literature, earlier ideas about the "non-routine" or "emergent" (Turner and Killian 1987) character of movements shifted in the 1970s to considerations of movements as politics by other means, where resources were mobilized in a rational manner by political actors who existed largely outside of institutions of power but who often supplemented confrontation with participation in routine politics (McCarthy and Zald 1977; McAdam 1988; McAdam and Paulsen 1993). By the 1990s, more recognition was given to "institutional activists"; that is, to people "who occupy formal statuses within the government … [and] pursue social movement goals through conventional bureaucratic channels" (Santoro and McGuire 1997: 503). Along the same lines, feminist scholars noted that American feminist activism in the 1960s and 1970s was aided by sympathetic women situated within institutions – in other words, institutional activists – who were pressing for the same kinds of changes as many of the outsiders engaged in protest (Banaszak 2011; Cobble 2004; Hartmann 1999; Katzenstein 1990, 1998a, 1998b; Roth 2003). Lastly, shifts toward thinking about protest politics as relational (see McAdam, Tarrow, and Tilly 2001) and global made it difficult to sustain the insider–outsider dichotomy as research revealed the existence of new kinds of political entities that straddled insider–outsider lines. For example, Keck and Sikkink's (1998) examination of transnational advocacy networks showed that these networks had within them traditional outsiders, traditional insiders, nongovernmental organizations and supranational organizations like the United Nations.

The reservations that some ACT UP/LA activists expressed about working with insiders echo debates in the literature stemming from the powerful work of Roberto Michels (1959), who argued that outsiders who attained institutional power were co-opted by institutions; these new insiders lost their radical edges and inevitably formed oligarchies that then lost touch with the mass base that brought them to power in the first place. Michels's argument was a powerful

[8] Interview with author, 2012.

one because the matters that he dealt with – of the vitiation, cooptation, and dismantling of radical grass-roots–driven agendas by encounters with institutionalized power – animated many social movement participants. While scholarly critics of Michels have argued that the positing of a unilinearity of outcomes for activists in institutions is belied by the variety of activists' experiences (Clemens 1993; Jenkins 1977; Katzenstein 1998a, 1998b; Meyer and Tarrow 1998; Staggenborg 1988; Zald and Ash 1966), the ideas that Michels put forward survive in the stock of "common sense" knowledge that many activists share.

One important critique of the Michels model comes from feminist scholars who argue that, far from being coopted, women and other structurally unequal actors are often marginalized within institutions. In her influential work, Patricia Hill Collins (1998) has called those marginalized within institutions due to their unequal social status "outsiders within." Outsiders within have socially disparaged statuses that limit their capabilities within institutions, and thus they find themselves "in marginal locations between groups of varying power" (1998: 5). As Hill Collins described it, the experiences of outsiders within institutions are a mass of contradictions; they are only begrudgingly, provisionally, partially, nominally accepted within institutions. Hill Collins argued that outsiders within bear the additional burden of being affected by their possession of oppositional knowledge: an understanding of non-mainstream, even hidden, cultural realities that others in the institution could easily ignore. Racial/ethnic minorities, women, and, LGBT institutional activists all easily fit into the outsider within category as members of socially marginalized communities (Taylor and Raeburn 1995). All are uncooptable in Michels's sense, both because of who they are *and* because of who they represent. And feminist intersectional movement scholars further criticized the romanticization of the grass roots as a space of inherent equality; the space of the grass roots is characterized by structural inequalities that exist in society at large, including but not limited to gender, race/ethnicity, and sexuality (Abu-Lughod 1990; Crenshaw 1989, 1991). Awareness of structural inequalities in grass-roots protest lies at the heart of "horizontalist" attempts by activists to do the hard and constant work of being attentive to inequalities that hamper activism.[9] As I have discussed in previous chapters, in lesbian and gay movement organizations, and in the specific case of ACT UP/LA, the shared status of sexual outsider did not eliminate the cross-cutting inequalities that existed in society at large nor did it eliminate different opinions about how much inequalities mattered in dealing with power.

---

[9] Horizontalism, or *horizontalidad*, refers to activism in which participants strive for democratic and anti-authoritarian relationships as a matter of political practice. See Sitrin (2006) on horizontalist practices among Argentinean activists and Juris (2008a) on horizontalist and, ultimately, contradictory efforts by US-based activists to ensure racial representation at the US Social Forum.

However, even if socially unequal activists are marginalized because of their structurally unequal status, does that mean that they could eschew insider activism? In the specific case of anti-AIDS activism in the 1980s and 1990s, activists were obliged – and sometimes eager – to deal with institutions and to go further into the institutional arena as they gained insider knowledge and scientific expertise (Epstein 1996). Anti-AIDS activists who entered institutional spaces engaged in what Newman (2012: 137), in her study of UK-based community activists called "border work"; their insider positions "required complex alliance-building between different struggles and movements; engagements between different scalar sites of governing in the constant search for funding; and difficult negotiations."

Activists who are in the midst of choosing among options constituted by the opportunities given by institutions as well as the resources they obtain or generate on the ground can feel obliged to come up with policies about how to approach those with authority. In ACT UP/LA, debates about how to approach insiders were a nearly constant and sometimes explicit concern. I next consider how ACT UP/LA members argued about the wisdom of working with those in power.

WHAT DOES IT MEAN TO "NEGOTIATE" WITH POWER?

One sustained and documented exchange about ACT UP/LA's approach to insiders took place during the summer of 1990. In July of that year, controversy erupted over the group's use of "negotiation" with insiders as a tactic. A number of ACT UP/LA members had been involved in ongoing talks with County public health officials and hospital employees over AIDS care provision. ACT UP/LA planned a "conditional" action against the County's Board of Supervisor for July 31, 1990, aimed at getting the Board to increase funding for AIDS care in the County budget; ACT UP/LA would call off the action only if officials increased the AIDS care budget and continued improving access to AIDS care through the County system. This local disagreement over negotiating with the public health establishment took place against a national backdrop that echoed the debate about cooperating with unjust authority. Most ACT UPs – ACT UP/NY was a significant exception – were boycotting the summer's Sixth International AIDS Conference in San Francisco. Activists were angry that the so-called Helms Amendment, passed by the US Congress in 1987, added HIV to the list of diseases that could bar an "alien" from the United States, thereby excluding HIV-positive people from attending the conference. The Immigration and Naturalization Service instituted a policy of granting waivers of the law's provisions for those HIV-positive visitors who passed a kind of balancing test as to whether the benefits of their visit outweighed risks to public welfare. Needless to say, the waiver policy did not appease activists, although it did satisfy the organizers of the San Francisco Sixth International AIDS conference who feared the disastrous public relations images of mass arrests of hundreds of visiting AIDS activists (see Wachter 1991).

In Los Angeles, four members of ACT UP/LA – Bill Rouse, Mickey Wheatley, Craig Carson, and Dwayne Turner – wrote and circulated a position paper entitled "Let's Not Negotiate Our Silence: Silence = Death" in mid-July. calling into question the group's ongoing negotiations with LA County over AIDS funding.[10] The authors stated that "negotiations are inappropriate for ACT UP/Los Angeles"; they were "uncomfortable" with the previous month's GB decision to participate in the Coalition for Compassion, an alliance of groups working directly with LA County officials, because they feared that ACT UP/LA would become bound by the Coalition's decisions. The position paper's authors argued that ACT UP/LA should participate in "dialogue" with officials but not negotiation as such. They envisioned dialogue as meeting "with interested parties to present and explain well-reasoned demands, answer questions relating to these demands and learn the other parties' perspectives." In contrast, they defined negotiations as "giving up something in exchange for receiving something." The position paper's authors felt negotiating with the County would damage ACT UP/LA's "integrity" for a number of reasons: (1) negotiations would make ACT UP/LA "a part of the secret 'backroom' dealings which have created many of the problems we face"; (2) negotiations would tie ACT UP/LA's hands for the future, trading potential voice for current promises; (3) negotiations would lead to ACT UP/LA agreeing to less than what had been demanded, which would make ACT UP/LA "party to exacerbating the funding problems of the health care systems; and (4) negotiations would undermine the skeptical stance that ACT UP/LA should take toward the Board of Supervisors because, the authors argued, the Board has "shown time and time again that their intentions are less than honorable."

Rouse, Wheatley, Carson, and Turner were also concerned that negotiating with the County would cause damage to solidarity within ACT UP/LA. They argued that it would be wrong if a small group of designated negotiators could make a decision about "whether or not an individual ACT UP member will risk arrest for something she feels is right." The position paper's authors decried the secrecy that negotiations might entail, worried that negotiating would redirect the group's energy into trying to justify their figures to government entities, and they warned that ACT UP/LA might try to retool demands to appease authorities rather than state its demands unequivocally to the County. Mincing no words, the writers' last line to other members was "(w)e call on you to renounce ACT UP's involvement in negotiation."

Mark Kostopoulos distributed a four-page position paper of his own to counter the anti-negotiation stance.[11] In his paper, Kostopoulos stated that

---

[10] Bill Rouse, Mickey Wheatley, Craig Carson, and Dwayne Turner "Let's Not Negotiate Our Silence: Silence = Death," Position paper dated July 16, 1990. The copy I have lacks Turner's signature; ONE collection.

[11] Mark Kostopoulos, "On Tactics: For ACT UP Members Only, Not to Be Reprinted." Position paper dated July 1990; ONE Collection. Although Kostopoulos's paper is dated "July 1990,"

the debate over negotiations was over tactics: whether ACT UP/LA should negotiate with County officials and whether they should use "conditional demonstrations." He recommended a course of pragmatism, with the only measurement of a tactic being whether it moved the group "closer to our goals of saving lives and ending AIDS." He argued that, given this standard, ACT UP/LA members needed to be "flexible and willing to adjust our assumption when faced with new information or arguments." Kostopoulos rejected the idea that negotiation with County officials blocked ACT UP/LA from future actions against the County, stating that "(a)s long as the Supervisors are standing in the way of AIDS care and prevention we will continue to raise our voices against them."[12] He also rejected the idea that ACT UP/LA working in coalition with other groups was in any way binding, noting that ACT UP/LA had always worked in coalition and that perhaps forming coalitions with other groups working on AIDS issues had always been difficult for some in the group. Kostopoulos was somewhat more generous toward the concerns of the anti-negotiation wing when it came to the question of cooptation: "I think there is a very real and realistic fear that ACT UP/LA will be co-opted by the political process. . . . But I do not think we avoid co-optation by refusing to wield our power in sophisticated ways." Kostopoulos was adamant that ACT UP/LA (and he personally) would only be coopted when and if "society as a whole adopts our goal, in which case I will gladly be coopted." He also stated that ACT UP/LA members had always and were currently members of committees and councils that were involved with planning AIDS services.

Beyond questioning whether the argument about negotiation was really "only" about tactics, Kostopoulos took the anti-negotiators to task for what he characterized as their emotionality. Arguing that fixation on expressing emotion through political action was a kind of "egotism," Kostopoulos wrote that

ACT UP/LA is not about giving people a place to express their anger, it is not about giving people a place to be involved in militant demonstrations or CD [civil disobedience]. We USE our anger and we USE demonstrations to save peoples [sic] lives. . . . People need to think about how we achieve our goals over the long haul.

Kostopoulos also rejected the anti-negotiators' stance about the tactic of negotiations as a threat to ACT UP/LA's "integrity":

It has also been argued that it is intrinsically immoral to sit down and talk to people or institutions which behave immorally. Claptrap. What would be immoral, is to avoid using every resources available to us to benefit people living with AIDS and HIV. And if that means sitting down and wrangling with the devil I'll do it.

a rebuttal to it on July 23 (the next General Body meeting) by two of the writers of the anti-negotiation position paper suggests that Kostopoulous's paper was distributed at the same July 16 meeting as the anti-negotiation position paper.
[12] "On Tactics," p. 3.

Kostopoulos wrote that "(s)ocial movements all over the world seek negotiations with the ruling powers," and these talks were not to be confused with friendship or acquiescence.

A week later, another position paper entitled "Let's Not Make a Pact with the Devil," this time signed by only Wheatley and Rouse, rebutted Mark Kostopoulos's pragmatism.[13] Wheatley and Rouse took aim at Kostopoulos alone in this second position paper, and their tone was quite specific and personal. Wheatley and Rouse argued that, on a philosophical level, ACT UP/LA "cannot be part of the system: the system is corrupt and unresponsive to the needs of our constituents." They further stated that "(o)ur gains should be made based on the merits of our claims, not because we are political insiders gaining from our connection with the Board. ... Unlike Mark, we are unwilling to make a pact with the devil." Wheatley and Rouse agreed in their papers that any increase in AIDS funding, even if it is not everything that ACT UP/LA wanted, was a victory, but Wheatley and Rouse disagreed that negotiations as such helped to get funding for PWAs, seeing only outsider agitation as a successful strategy. Wheatley and Rouse also attacked Kostopoulos personally for using "such a condescending tone toward us in his paper." They accused Kostopoulos of unfairly and dangerously framing the debate over negotiations as a

debate [of] the thinkers versus the feelers, insinuating that we have no good reasons for our positions. We cannot stand by and allow members to be divisive using such patriarchal tactics. Traditionally, men have silenced women by accusing them of being too emotional and not thinking. This false dichotomy has kept women oppressed, and we will not allow it to oppress us; we are not frivolous queens. ... Let's celebrate and develop our emotional faculties; let's listen to our queer's intuition.

It is impossible to know exactly how many ACT UP/LA members agreed with either side in the negotiation debates, but it is clear that some members of the group eschewed meetings with insiders and some members of the group continued to be involved for years in negotiations with the County over the public health budget for AIDS and over the quality of care provided. ACT UP/LA in theory was itself a coalition and in practice had room for activists to disagree about how to relate to institutionalized power. Still, as some members continued to talk with County officials, Kostopoulos's pragmatist stance on careful contact with the inside as part of an arsenal of tactics seemed to have won the day over principled non-negotiation. Others supported Kostopoulos's view that the only criterion for tactics was whether they worked. For example, in an undated piece that appears to have been distributed that same summer, ACT UP/LA member Bruce Mirken stated that ACT UP/LA had always used whatever "nonviolent

---

[13] Mickey Wheatley and Bill Rouse, "Let's Not Make a Pact with the Devil," position paper dated July 23, 1990; ONE Collection.

tactics work."[14] Mirken wrote that politics involved "compromise" and that "(l)ike it or not, negotiations will be held. . . . The question is not whether or not there will be negotiations about AIDS funding, services, and care. The questions is [sic]: Who will speak for us? Will we speak for ourselves or let others do it for us?" Mirken believed that ACT UP/LA members would not abandon "our broader principles" in negotiation with the County, adding, "(w)e are smart enough to keep from being co-opted."

In yet another position paper written in July 1990, apparently after the first back-and-forth about negotiations, Gunther Freehill, a central ACT UP/LA member and Kostopoulos's partner, stated that he found the discussion about whether to negotiate "offensive":

I don't like negotiating. I like dying less. I like feeling powerless while I die less still. I like even less than that the feeling that I am not doing everything possible to keep me and some of the people I love alive. I like least of all being told that my response is not valid because it is not emotional.[15]

Freehill noted that ACT UP/LA had, over a series of GB meetings, made the explicit decision to negotiate with LA County over questions of AIDS care provision; he allowed that it was possible that some members were not prepared for the group's decision to negotiate or had felt stifled. Freehill also suspected that some members did not trust those who were actually talking to the County. He reminded the group that ACT UP/LA empowered small groups of members to make decisions all the time:

There are a number of circumstances in which the body empowers a small group to make decisions. Affinity groups operate without the scrutiny of the body. Most demonstrations have empowered decision makers. Committee facilitators have discretion to get the work of their committees done. All of these things happen without rendering ACT UP/LA un-democratic because both the process of empowerment and the decisions made are open for contribution of opinions beforehand and review afterwards. . . . . The same principles apply to the negotiators designated to deal with the County.

Freehill saw negotiation as a mere tactic, in line with Kostopoulos's and Mirken's views, and stated that ACT UP/LA's major success – getting LA County to actually open a dedicated AIDS ward – was due to "combined tactics" of disruption and negotiation. But Freehill, who went on to have a long career in government working on AIDS issues (see later discussion), was more ambivalent about the question of "insiderness" than his July 1990 position paper let on. In ACT UP/LA's August/September 1990 newsletter, one dominated by articles about the Sixth International AIDS Congress in San Francisco, Freehill proclaimed his admiration for ACT UP/NY's work negotiating with insiders but had this to say about the situation in Los Angeles:

[14] Bruce Mirken, undated (c. July 1990) "Should ACT UP Negotiate?" Position paper, ONE collection.
[15] Gunther Freehill. "On Negotiation." Position paper dated July 30, 1990; ONE Collection.

I've seen how bureaucrats in Los Angeles County try to buy us off with a little flattery, and then try to distract us by asking us to do their work, leaving precious little time for us to pursue our own agenda and diminishing our ability to criticize effectively. I fear that enormous talent and finely honed anger in ACT UP/New York City may be diverted through similar ploys. How we know when we have crossed the line from working together to becoming part of the structure that tortures and oppresses us bedevils me. Being sure beyond a shadow of a doubt that you're right is usually a sign that you're wrong. The complementary danger is that by insisting on ideological purity and removing ourselves from the process entirely, we marginalize ourselves and our work. We make it impossible – rather than merely uncomfortable – for them to hear us. Righteousness can easily become ineffectiveness.[16]

Not quite two years later – and not quite two months before his own death – Kostopoulos had seemingly shifted his thinking about insider tactics. In a position paper dated April 6, 1992, he wrote about his fears that meetings with "a truly astounding number" of insiders – politicians, bureaucrats, various board members included – was causing ACT UP/LA to lose its action orientation: "I am very concerned that this 'inside' strategy has become almost completely disconnected from any 'outside' strategy."[17] Kostopoulos stated that

ACT UP's unique power and even moral authority come from our willingness to use direct action. There are a hundred AIDS groups which are willing to lobby their representatives or meet with pharmaceutical companies, but only ACT UP will surround their cars, occupy their offices, disrupt their public meetings and generally bring maximum public attention to their genocidal HIV policies.

Kostopoulos told his fellow activists that, in participating in meetings and hearings, "we don't have to play by the rules," and he expressed disdain for lobbying: "I would frankly like to excise the word lobbying from our lexicon. ... Lobbying implies petitioning our betters for some crumbs from their table."

In advocating disruptive action and rejecting lobbying, Kostopoulos seemed to be coming closer to the anti-negotiators in the group, and, not surprisingly, his statement angered others who believed that nondisruptive tactics worked. One week after Kostopoulos's statement, a rebuttal by Jim Bloor was distributed to the GB. Bloor wrote that there were "hundreds" of AIDS groups available to lobby and that there were few that ACT UP/LA could trust to really represent the community to insiders:

... (D)o we really trust the likes of APLA [AIDS Project Los Angeles], or the Ventura [County] Gay Community Services Center to meet face to face with politicians who ...

---

[16] Gunther Freehill, "After the Boycott." ACT UP/LA Newsletter, 3:4 (August/September 1990), p. 10. Author's collection.
[17] Mark Kostopoulos "How ACT UP/LA Is Losing Its Power." Position paper dated April 6, 1992; ONE Collection.

do indeed hold sway over our lives? . . . Shouldn't we seize each and every opportunity to educate these legislators?[18]

The debates about negotiating with power that occurred in ACT UP/LA in the summer of 1990 and afterward distilled the concerns that many in the organization had about the damaging effects of being too close to power. At the same time, some members of the group had already danced with the devil of institutions to the point where they were part of – or at least paid by – institutions. The work of some ACT UP/LA members with institutions informed discussions about the boundary between a grass-roots outside and an insider institutionalized sector and complicated depictions of the two spaces as distinct. I turn next to the stories of ACT UP/LA's institutional activists who, to various degrees and for various lengths of time, protested via direct action tactics *and* took positions as outsiders within government and social service agencies trying to address the AIDS crisis. These activists literally embody the way that outsider ACT UP/LA politics and insider institutionalist resources merged at times to allow activists to do AIDS work wherever they could. Their stories also show that while questions about the conflicts engendered by straddling insider–outsider lines come up for activists, at least some are able to feel like effective "outsiders within" through their AIDS work and that outsider spaces and organizations like ACT UP/LA can contain hidden insiders whose energy and knowledge aid protest politics.

PATHS ACROSS OUTSIDE AND INSIDE ACTIVIST SPACE

ACT UP/LA was a militant direct action anti-AIDS organization, but it was never a purely outsider space because insiders from the newly built AIDS establishment participated from the group's founding on. As evidenced by the various position papers on negotiating with power, members of ACT UP/LA certainly fought over the kinds of relationships the group should have with the inside, but many were willing to use insider tactics and thus engage the powerful in order to obtain results. Many members both relished disruptive protest and the opportunity for "ACT UP/LA representatives [to] sit on a number of County advisory committees as well as community AIDS and health care coalitions."[19]

As I consider the experiences of activists who worked in outside and inside spaces, I am influenced by Jennifer Brier's (2009: 4) critique of narratives of anti-AIDS activism that draw

a sharp distinction between "AIDS activism," defined as direct action targeted against the state and industry in hopes of producing dramatic change in AIDS policy, treatment

---

[18] Jim Bloor, "A Sort-of Rebuttal to Last Week's 'How ACT UP/LA Is Losing Its Power." Position paper dated April 13, 1992; ONE Collection.

[19] ACT UP/LA. Unsigned document, circa July 1990. "A Very Brief History of ACT UP/Los Angeles"; ONE Collection.

and prevention, and "AIDS service," defined as entities that developed to provide the actual "services" people with AIDS needed.

Brier's use of the phrases "AIDS work" and "AIDS workers" collapses the distinction between service and activism. I found that activists who straddled the insider–outsider divide started on both sides of the inside–outside divide; they inhabited both spaces for a time and saw their work in both spaces as connected. In the specific case of where the line was drawn between AIDS protest and AIDS service in Los Angeles, Kenney (2001) argued that there was a lesbian and gay tradition of blurring the boundary between direct action–protest activism and the provision of social services before the AIDS crisis hit. In the 1960s and 1970s, the radical Gay Liberation Front (GLF)'s Los Angeles incarnation quickly morphed into a social services network, and this "institutionalization of the GLF into a social services movement differentiated the Los Angeles experience from other cities, where the move toward social service provision occurred much later" (18). Thus, the provision of services to the community was seen as "an essential part of, rather than an alternative to, a radical political agenda" (83). Although none of the activists I interviewed directly referenced work in the GLF, each operated in a social movement culture where service was understood as a form of politics.

In the small sample of former activists I interviewed who straddled the insider–outsider line, two basic paths emerged. In the first path, taken by two interviewees, work in the newly created AIDS service sector led to involvement with ACT UP/LA; in the second, taken by five interviewees, participation with ACT UP/LA led to paid work fighting AIDS from government or service-sector positions. Each interviewee who straddled the line experienced periods (sometimes extensive ones) when he or she was participating in AIDS protest and paid anti-AIDS work at the same time. I turn to their stories next in order to illustrate how interconnected outsider and insider spaces could be for some ACT UP/LA AIDS workers.

PATH 1: AIDS SERVICE WORK TO DIRECT ACTION AND BACK TO ADVOCACY

The first path across the inside–outside line, taken by two of the former ACT UP/LA activists interviewed, was from AIDS service work to direct action with ACT UP/LA and back to advocacy. Phill Wilson was working for the Los Angeles Gay and Lesbian Services Center and for the Minority AIDS Project when Mark Kostopoulos approached him and asked him to help facilitate the December 4, 1987, town hall meeting that initiated ACT UP/LA. Kostopoulos was a member of the Lavender Left, a lesbian and gay socialist group, and very much committed to outsider activism, but he knew Wilson's partner, Chris Brownlie from the Lavender Left. Wilson agreed to help facilitate the town hall meeting. Wilson, who is African American, became an AIDS service worker in part because of Brownlie's illness and in part because of his own HIV-positive status. He recalled that, in 1987, he was regarded by leftists in the lesbian and gay community as a "moderate" primarily because of his position working in AIDS service organizations.

When I asked Wilson why he was asked to help facilitate ACT UP/LA's first meeting if he indeed had such moderate tendencies, Wilson replied that "by that time, I had a kind of street activist credentials but yet I was clearly someone who ... was kind of a moderate, so I brought to the table the whole notion of AIDS service providers." Wilson and Brownlie had both worked against the 1986 California Proposition 64, the Lyndon La Rouche–sponsored ballot measure that would have "returned" HIV to the list of communicable diseases in the state, and thus provided the grounds for mandatory HIV testing, the restriction of HIV-positive people from certain jobs (e.g., involving contact with children), possibly leading to quarantine (Faderman and Timmons 2006: 308–309). Wilson noted that he and Brownlie both worked with a group called the Stop AIDS Quarantine Campaign, which Wilson described as full of people with "genuine leftist credentials."

Wilson thought that his co-facilitation of the first ACT UP/LA meeting showed that Kostopoulos and other ACT UP/LA founders had the deliberate strategy of taking an "inside–outside" (Wilson's words) approach to fighting AIDS. He also thought he was asked to take a leadership position because he was Black and that there was a consciousness among ACT UP/LA founders that they would need to deal with LA's "multiculturalism." Wilson stated that, in 1987, those in nascent AIDS institutions and those who wanted to see grassroots direct action were acting in tandem: "we were the ones who urged the city to develop an AIDS coordinator's office, so that was the street activists saying you need to create an inside position ... it was certainly a part of our agenda to have inside and outside people."[20] Wilson soon became the second AIDS Policy Coordinator for the City of Los Angeles in October 1990, replacing Dave Johnson, an anti-AIDS activist and PWA who stepped down because of his ill health.[21] Wilson's history of institutional AIDS work and community activism, his personal links to those involved in direct action politics, and his willingness to openly support direct action meant that he was a sufficiently "complex" figure (Wilson's word) in the eyes of many anti-AIDS direct action activists so that he felt that he wasn't read as being a mere bureaucrat. And Wilson was probably right that he and some others in the new AIDS establishment who had "complex" backgrounds were treated differently by ACT UP/LA than those

---

[20] Interview with author, 1999.
[21] Patrick McGreevy, "Founder of Black Gay Group to Become City Coordinator," September 22, 1990, *The Daily News*, p. 3. (Jane Fritsch, "Activist Replaces Ailing City AIDS Coordinator," *The Los Angeles Times*, October 2, 1990, p. B7.) Johnson died in October 1994, at the age of 39. (*The Los Angeles Times*, "Dave Johnson, 39: LA's First AIDS Coordinator, Writer on Gay Issues." Unsigned obituary, October 29, 1994.)

whom ACT UP/LA did not know; Gunther Freehill noted in his 2000 interview that, as devoted as the ACT UP/LA was to militancy in dealing with the AIDS crisis, some lines were drawn and in general AIDS social service agencies were left alone.[22]

Ultimately, Wilson felt that his complex street politics plus moderate style was a bad fit for the AIDS policy coordinator position; he stated that "I didn't have the diplomacy [for the job], which is kind of shocking." As Wilson recalled, his job with LA City consisted of two distinct parts: (1) advising the mayor of Los Angeles directly regarding AIDS policy and (2) administering the budget for the provision of city funds for AIDS within the Community Development Authority. During the years that Wilson was policy coordinator, most of the city budget for PWAs involved housing, and his direct superior in the city bureaucracy was also a new employee with the Community Development Authority where his position was housed. His supervisor knew little about AIDS issues. Wilson felt stymied working in this environment because he had little patience with a bureaucracy that was slowly coping with a crisis that was quickly killing PWAs:

I didn't really want to do the bureaucratic part at all. . . . I was very interested in the policy part and where the city was going . . . but you know the kind of managing, budgets and programs and what have you, I wasn't particularly thrilled. . . . I did like fighting for more resources, I liked that part, I liked the fact that while I was there, you know, we found ways to like double the AIDS housing budget and what have you . . . so we were able to get a lot of housing money out there . . . but when you are dealing with housing programming, it's also not very rewarding, because you kind of fund someone in one year, and you don't see that product for five or six or seven years . . . in the AIDS arena then, that was like not . . . just not doing anything. . . . I mean *different* people would be around but the people that you are dealing with weren't going to be around.

Coupled with this frustration of the slow grind of bureaucracy was Wilson's admitted lack of "diplomacy." When he saw something he did not like, he would approach fellow bureaucrats as if they were in "ACT UP or someplace like that, [where] you would tell someone 'well you don't know what you are doing so no, we're not going to do it this way.'" As city coordinator, Wilson still thought of himself as part of an activist community where the rules of communication were decidedly different. He left city government, but he went on to found the Black AIDS Institute and is still the group's "president and CEO."[23]

For Terri Ford, work in AIDS services and activism in ACT UP/LA were two sides of the same coin. Ford was the director of global advocacy for the AIDS

---

[22] Interview with author, 2000. The informal policy of not going after service providers did not mean that activists didn't grumble about their displeasure with institutions or specific institutional activists. Freehill noted two instances where hostile graffiti was found directed at institutions. While the acts of vandalism were anonymous, Freehill suspected that someone from ACT UP/LA was responsible.

[23] www.blackaids.org.

Healthcare Foundation when I interviewed her in January 2012. The AIDS Healthcare Foundation was founded by AIDS activists, including its current president, Michael Weinstein, who former ACT UP/LA activist John Fall remembers as being among the actual organizers of the town hall meeting that led to ACT UP/LA.[24] Originally called the AIDS Hospice Foundation (AHF), its initial mission was to establish hospice care for dying AIDS patients. Phill Wilson described himself and his partner Chris Brownlie as co-founders of AHF, and the first hospice AHF established was named for Brownlie. AHF changed its name in 1990 as it broadened its mission from hospice care to other issues that those with HIV faced. Within ACT UP/LA, AHF was sometimes seen as a friend and sometimes seen as a member of the "AIDS establishment"; generally, AHF was better respected by ACT UP/LA than the other, larger local AIDS service organization, AIDS Project Los Angeles (APLA). One former ACT UP/LA activist, Richard "Doe" Racklin, described AHF as more "community-minded" than other service organizations;[25] another, Stephanie Boggs, described AHF as more "militant" than other AIDS service organizations.[26]

In the late 1980s, Ford was attending Santa Monica Community College and helping to revitalize what she described as a "pathetic" gay and lesbian student union there when a girlfriend recruited her to volunteer at the AHF-run Chris Brownlie Hospice. At about the same time, Ford heard about ACT UP/LA from her gay male student union co-president. She started attending ACT UP/LA meetings regularly in the fall of 1990; she described coming to those meetings as being "exciting," and she was immediately "roped in" to attending actions. At the hospice, Ford went from volunteering to working as a part-time paid cook. She then became director of the hospice's "dietary department" while participating actively in ACT UP/LA so that she was, in her words, "completely enmeshed" in AIDS work. In her interview in 2012, Ford emphasized that she made little distinction between paid AIDS work, volunteering, and the kind of activism she did with ACT UP/LA: "we were all so passionate about it, it didn't matter how many hours of the week [we worked]." Ford recalled that her position at the hospice even helped ACT UP/LA members who were sentenced to community service as a result of civil disobedience: "anybody who had community service from their arrests all did it with me in the kitchen," with one particular activist working at the hospice for "months doing dishes." Ford explicitly felt that participating in ACT UP/LA helped her in her paid AIDS work and vice versa, especially since it was work at a hospice:

I don't know if I would have been able to sustain in such a good way those four years at Brownlie without [ACT UP]. I had an outlet. I could go and kick the coffins in the middle of the intersections and burn them ... the other benefit to me was I also could tame that

[24] See http://www.aidshealth.org; Interview with author, 2012.
[25] Interview with author, 2011.
[26] Interview with author, 1999.

anger to be loving, because you had to be at Brownlie ... it didn't help the families and mothers to be angry activists.[27]

By the mid-1990s, Ford had risen to the job of head of hospice care for another AHF hospice. She stayed active in ACT UP/LA through much of this time, even as the group demobilized in the mid-1990s. She attributed her ability to manage paid AIDS work and AIDS activism to AHF's "ACT UP mentality"; she described the AHF ethos as being "advocacy-focused and we'll kick the door down if we have to, and sorry if we offend people ... we're not your normal AIDS service organization." Ford recounted that AHF's director Michael Weinstein showed support for her (and for ACT UP/LA) when he attended the Reality Ball fundraiser in June 1992; Ford, full of rage at the death of her mother and of yet another hospice patient to whom she had grown close, performed a monologue at the event about being arrested for civil disobedience. Ford stayed with ACT UP/LA for a long time – her name shows up on meeting minutes into 1996 – but, by 1997, she had become the director of a new AHF division for testing and prevention, and ACT UP/LA was functionally gone. At the time of her interview, Ford had been at AHF for twenty-one years, moving through a variety of positions; she described herself as generally having initially "no clue" about whatever was needed for each new position she started, but she also described herself as a "natural organizer."

Ford acknowledged that there were some in ACT UP/LA who were troubled by her becoming an increasingly powerful insider activist, and she recalled a number of people telling her so to her face. But she argued that, especially with her latest move into international AIDS advocacy, she had maintained a militant stance as an insider, stating that "I wish I could share with some of those people that I used to be on the front line with, that I'm on the front line now." Ford expressed fierce pride about the work AHF was doing around the world. It was her belief that looking at AIDS globally meant having a fairly sophisticated approach to thinking about grass-roots constituencies and governments: "first of all you can get a lot done on the inside. So I'm not against people working on the inside." Ford also believed that the global context defined relative insiders and outsiders differently in AIDS work, stating that, on a global level, AHF was often kept on the outside by fearful national governments.

As director of global advocacy, Ford described her work as coordinating on-the-ground teams that customized advocacy strategies for their local situations. She described these teams as essentially working from a modified ACT UP template: "You find out where these politicians are, you go to these meetings you publically confront ... but you have to do it in different ways. ... I can't act 'ACT UP' out of control in some of these countries, it doesn't work, you have to

---

[27] Interview with author, 2012.

adapt it." Ford used Uganda, the site of one of AHF's biggest projects, as an example of where AHF had to cultivate insiders who would help with AIDS prevention, testing, and treatment, despite the extreme anti-gay atmosphere that had developed in the country. Ford described having to work to influence Uganda's President Museveni through informal relationships, making contacts with high-level bureaucrats at cocktail parties and the like. When I noted in our interview that she was describing the kinds of insider network relationships that troubled some of ACT UP/LA's activists in the 1980s and 1990s, Ford responded that AHF as an organization was "not afraid to say what needs to be said . . . and I think a lot of that comes from ACT UP." For Ford, the lessons of her time with ACT UP/LA continued to reverberate in her paid AIDS work: "I mean ACT UP was a gift to me in my work with all the dying and AHF was a gift to me also as an AIDS activist . . . .it's still truly still that way."

PATH 2: OUTSIDER ACTIVIST TO OUTSIDER WITHIN

For five ACT UP/LA members I interviewed, direct action led them to find institutionally based AIDS service "day jobs" that helped them to continue participating in ACT UP/LA. Jan Speller was living in Orange County, south of Los Angeles, and had begun working with the Orange County Visibility League, a lesbian and gay rights organization. She was recruited to ACT UP/LA by another Orange County resident, Kevin Farrell, who had been going to meetings since late 1989. Speller was "very excited" by ACT UP/LA meetings and wanted to become more involved with the group, a difficult thing to accomplish given the distance and traffic involved in traveling between Orange County and West Hollywood. Speller moved to Los Angeles in order to be more easily involved in ACT UP/LA; at one point, she was living with Mark Kostopoulos and Gunther Freehill.

After making the move to LA, Speller continued working at a job at California State University, Long Beach, and she still faced a long commute. Kostopoulos encouraged her to find a new job. He had been volunteering with a group named Health Access, which was a coalition of organizations working on the issue of universal healthcare, and he wondered if she couldn't find some related work with the group. The organization that Speller went to work for, which she remembers as being called Los Angeles Homeless Health Care, was in the same building and on the same floor as Health Access. She became an administrative assistant in an AIDS education program that was

designed to do AIDS education for homeless service providers rather than with direct service to the homeless populations, because it was early on still, where many many homeless service providers . . . were, you know, slightly afraid of AIDS and afraid to work with people with AIDS, and didn't know how to help . . . didn't know about safe sex education and didn't really know how to deal with the health care needs of homeless people who were HIV-positive . . . so I began to work there . . .

When I responded to Speller's statement with the question "so then very quickly your professional life and activist life get pretty much enmeshed with each other?" Speller responded "exactly right."[28]

At the time of her 2000 interview, Speller was living in San Francisco with her partner and was involved in adult education, helping people get their GEDs. She no longer worked directly with issues involving HIV/AIDS. But she maintained that her experience in ACT UP/LA and in the nonprofit world of AIDS service prepared her well for dealing with her adult students:

Working with homeless and formerly homeless people in terms of education ... I think I have a deeper insight into, say, my students, in terms of the issues that have impacted their lives. In terms of racism and education and classism and access to health care and access to rehabilitation and drug services and ... many of my students are HIV-positive and mentally ill. ... And they've had learning disabilities that were never diagnosed or treated ... so you sort of see how the have-nots in this country have had assorted numbers of obstacles created [for them]. ... And probably prior to my work with ACT UP, I probably had sort of the typical working class/middle class kind of "well, you know, it's sad that people live that way, but if they'd get off drugs or just ....just get that high school diploma and go on and get that job and forget that felony arrest record you have. ..."

Although she did not define herself as a bureaucrat or an insider in the AIDS service sector, Speller was an example of an ACT UP/LA activist taking simultaneous tracks of insider work at an AIDS service–related day job and nights spent at ACT UP/LA meetings. She was mindful, however, of the contradictions that ensued from a militant, outsider group like ACT UP/LA having at least some members who worked on the inside or had long-term interactions with authorities. Speller felt that ACT UP/LA needed its insiders, people like Ferd Eggan and Gunther Freehill (both of whom are discussed later), who were willing to go "fight the fights at the Ryan White table and get on the committees."[29] At the same time, Speller acknowledged that some of the group felt "the internal conflict of the true leftist radicals who didn't want to be at the table." She characterized the internal conflict as being between the "true leftist radicals" and "pragmatists" who "said 'you know we fought so hard to get a voice ... why would we give it up?'" Speller understood the pragmatists, but also argued that insiders ran a real risk of being "absorbed" by institutions and that any given insider was always in danger of becoming an "AIDS fuck." Speller defined AIDS fucks as "people who were working in the system"; as

---

[28] Interview with author, 2000.

[29] "The Ryan White Comprehensive AIDS Resources Emergency (CARE) Act" was enacted in 1990 and began funding social service agencies in 1991. It was named after Ryan White, a hemophiliac, who was diagnosed with AIDS at the age of thirteen and died at age eighteen in April 1990, shortly before the act passed Congress. The CARE Act has been continuously reauthorized and refunded and has since been renamed "the Ryan White HIV/AIDS Program." See the federal Health Resources and Services administration website at http://hab.hrsa.gov /abouthab/ryanwhite.html.

one might imagine, she was quite clear in her interview that it was not a good thing to be an AIDS fuck. Despite her own experiences doing AIDS service work, Speller was ambivalent about the pluses and minuses of institutional activism.

Unlike Speller, who stayed employed in the social service sector but left AIDS work, other ACT UP/LA activists moved into institutionalized positions that allowed them to work on AIDS issues. Los Angeles City's third AIDS policy coordinator, Ferd Eggan, took over the job from Phill Wilson. Eggan had helped to found ACT UP/Chicago; when he came to Los Angeles in 1990, he participated in ACT UP/LA and was also executive director of Being Alive, a community-based self-help organization for PWAs. He was still in that position in October 1992, when he became city policy coordinator. Upon taking the policy coordinator job, Eggan immediately wrote to local "AIDS Service Organizations" – which apparently included ACT UP/LA – to introduce himself, to ask for continued good relations with the AIDS community, and to urge organizations "to utilize the resources available through this office. The AIDS coordinator and the AIDS Advisory Panel were created to help those who fight AIDS on a daily basis in their interaction with City government."[30] When I interviewed Eggan in 1999, he had been in the position for seven years; he served in it until 2001, at which point ill-health prevented him from continuing, and he died in 2007 at age sixty of liver cancer.[31]

Eggan came to his anti-AIDS direct action work after a long and mostly very radical background in left-wing politics. During his time with ACT UP/LA and Being Alive, Eggan was part of the network of AIDS workers actively combining service provision with attempts to pressure local government to provide more resources. When I asked Eggan why he decided to become a government bureaucrat – especially since his trajectory as an activist had started so far to the left – he told me where he thought his participation in government had been beneficial to the anti-AIDS movement:

What was mainly on my mind was that there were various things that the city probably should be doing ... and this position afforded some possibility for doing that. ... It was clear that the city should increase its funding of prevention activities. ... For a long time there's been an office in the City Attorney's office that handles HIV discrimination issues but there was no overall sort of thrust to what the city was doing in relationship to AIDS stuff. My predecessors struggled with that ... [they were] pretty disgusted with the inability of the city to respond to a number of issues, and I think I've been luckier than them, since I've gotten some good cooperation and support from this particular department ... from the City Council, the mayor's office in general, so that now, the

[30] Ferd Eggan, letter from Community Development Department to "AIDS Service Organizations," dated October 29, 1992; ONE Collection.
[31] Elaine Woo, "Ferd Eggan, 60; Ally for Those with HIV, AIDS." Obituary for *The Los Angeles Times*, July 12, 2007.

AIDS budget is significantly bigger ... and we play a role in a lot of national and local issues on AIDS because the council has been supportive.

In contrast to Wilson, Eggan described his government work as effective, and he stayed in the job for almost a decade. He also used his position to recruit another ACT UP/LA activist to the inside. Eggan hired Mary Lucey, an HIV-positive ACT UP/LA member who was a co-founder of ACT UP/LA's Women's Caucus and also a pivotal player in ACT UP/LA's prisoner rights committee because she had been incarcerated herself at one time. When I interviewed Lucey in 1999, her perspective on insider work was that former activists were the ones best positioned to propose innovative policy initiatives in city government. Lucey cited as an example of innovative policy a recently instituted program designed to check the spread of HIV in LA's huge pornography industry through education, the encouragement of safe sex practices, and regular testing. As an HIV-positive woman, Lucey felt that she had a spin on policy that emphasized the need to balance the rights of PWAs with prevention efforts, and she emphasized that the city's small prevention budget shouldn't be used for "boring, same old prevention programs." She felt that since HIV-positive people were overlooked in constructing prevention strategies, prevention programs often missed the mark in terms of getting PWAs to change behavior.

One of ACT UP/LA's early participants – he missed the first few meetings – was Gunther Freehill, a former academic/college administrator who had been active within the anti-AIDS community in Los Angeles before coming to ACT UP/LA.[32] Freehill started participating in ACT UP/LA in early 1988, after seeing ACT UP NY activists protest the Supreme Court's decision on *Bowers v. Hardwick* at the 1987 National March on Washington for Lesbian and Gay Rights. Freehill was impressed by ACT UP/NY's protestors and made some calls to see if anything was being organized in Los Angeles. At around the same time, Freehill started participating in the AIDS Regional Board, which he described as a "purportedly communitarian planning group for HIV services." The Board was composed of government and local social service agencies that cooperated regarding how to spend the money being released via the Ryan White CARE Act. As Freehill explained,

there was a lot of tension in the early years around how much involvement government was going to have, how much control government was going to have. And the AIDS Regional Board was an attempt to go to the polar opposite of a government-based model ... a combination of a sort of political organizing tool, a way of sort of assessing the need for services.[33]

Freehill was critical of the Board, which he said "floundered a lot" – but he was active in it for about a year and a half while he was active in ACT UP/LA. He saw no conflict between his participation with the Board and his activism with

---

[32] Interview with author, 2000.
[33] Interview with author, 2000.

ACT UP/LA because he saw the work with the latter as a complement to the former. Freehill went on to become the director of public affairs for the Los Angeles County Office of AIDS Programs and Policy, but even there he saw himself as doing the kind of anti-AIDS activity exemplified by ACT UP/LA.

In his interview, Freehill insisted that a commitment to the agenda laid out by ACT UP/LA was vital to effective insider work. But he was particularly concerned about the potential for "corruption" on the part of former street activists, reflecting the same kind of critiques of the inside from the inside that Jimenez and Rosen made from the outside. In contrast to Jimenez and Rosen though, and continuing the theme of activism being about effectiveness, Freehill equated corruption with incompetence and not personal enrichment:

You know, the things I struggle with are about the kinds of corruption I see in other people who used to be activists ... corruption in the sense that ... they are in jobs for which they are not qualified, or have really guilt tripped their way into it, they have arrogated to themselves an amount of personal authority that does not withstand scrutiny, they have confused the epidemic with themselves and. ... They continue to make AIDS services the planning for services around their own sort of social problems.[34]

In fairness, Freehill conceded that others might see him as similarly incompetent (and therefore corrupt). But his concerns about incompetence as corruption have little to do with the standard complaint, a la Michels, that former activists who move inside displace the goals of the movement for the goals of the institution. Freehill's definition of corruption does not even encompass the idea of using an office to get rich. Instead, he seemed concerned about former street activist/new insiders confusing the needs of PWAs and others with their own selfish needs. In essence, Freehill took the stand that the personal *should not* be the measure of the political; this stand was consistent with his earlier stance from outsider activist days about the importance of making unemotional assessments of needs in anti-AIDS work.

Nancy MacNeil, who was and is Mary Lucey's partner, was another example of an ACT UP/LA activist going from direct action to an insider AIDS service provision space. In MacNeil's case, the trajectory took her from work with ACT UP/LA into activist AIDS service work with HIV-positive women. While she was active in ACT UP/LA, MacNeil began working with Being Alive as the organization's office manager and, after a number of years, became the

---

[34] Interview with the author, 2000. In 2005, Freehill moved from working in LA County's Office of AIDS Program and Policy to Washington, DC, where he took a job as a grants and contracts manager for that city's HIV/AIDS administration. The LA County and DC offices were dogged by charges of corruption and incompetence, respectively. (Jack Leonard, "County Removes 7-Year Chief of AIDS Program," *The Los Angeles Times*, May 17, 2005; Elizabeth Weill-Greenberg, "AIDS Office Director Meets with Activists: Appleseed Promises Updated Report Card on HIV in DC," *The Washington Blade*, October 7, 2005; Debbie Cenziper, "Investigation: Earmarked AIDS Funds Lack Oversight," *The Washington Post*, October 19, 2009.")

executive director of Women Alive, a Being Alive offshoot. She was still in this position when I interviewed her in 1999. Reflecting the closeness that the two women shared as life and political partners, Mary Lucey first spoke to me about Women Alive's self-help orientation during her interview, noting that hundreds of women were involved with the group and that the standard of care for poor HIV-positive women was inferior, in part because of paternalism of social service providers who

drowned women in social services so that they won't pay attention to their treatment.... because "we'll handle it for them" ... "we'll give them child care, transportation, we'll send them to the doctors you want them to go to, we'll do food banks, we'll do the housing," like all this stuff, they drown them in social service, so they won't pay attention to what's really going on.[35]

Lucey argued that Women Alive, given its roots in the self-help group Being Alive, provided women with the information and support necessary for them to take charge of their disease. MacNeil explained that Women Alive wanted to serve women – especially women of color – beyond the boundaries of the lesbian and, especially, gay male communities. Here is her view as to why Women Alive needed to split from Being Alive:

Because we tried to make it work for so long with people in the AIDS community ... and it didn't work because of sexism on men's part ... the men didn't want, you know, kids ... they shouldn't have to put up with kids ... and the women didn't want to bring their kids to a place where men were wearing makeup ... and they shouldn't have to ... so in a nutshell, that's the reason ... those sort of reasons.

MacNeil described Women Alive's focus as being "treatment and education," with advocacy work undertaken when HIV-positive women needed help managing doctors, available services, and, especially, complicated medication regimens. When MacNeil headed it, the organization ran support groups and peer counseling, published a newsletter and informational pamphlets, and was funded by a mix of LA County, corporate, and foundation money.[36] In talking about her transition to institutionalized AIDS work, MacNeil described herself as increasingly unable to coordinate her AIDS worker "day jobs" and her unpaid activism with ACT UP/LA, although an actual break with ACT UP/LA was many years in the making. She described her paid AIDS service work as "doing AIDS stuff 24/7" and noted that working in the AIDS service sector was unlike having a normal job: "the demands of the job were ... far beyond like normal working hours ... so you know the time that you had off ... you wouldn't necessarily want to go to yet another meeting." MacNeil, alone among the institutional activists I interviewed, expressed the feeling that there was a general pull away from the street once one entered the inside:

[35] Interview with author, 1999.
[36] Women Alive is still in existence and still in located in the mid-Wilshire neighborhood of Los Angeles where I interviewed MacNeil; its website is http://www.women-alive.org/

You know I think it [paid AIDS work] kind of pulled a lot of us away ... that a lot of people in ACT UP became employed at the AIDS services organizations. It just consumed us ... to where, you know, okay so now [before working for Being Alive] I'm not focused on my job, I'm just being with ACT UP and bringing change that way, but now here I have this responsibility and this obligation to provide services, to reach out to women who are invisible.[37]

MacNeil's trajectory from outsider activist to incidental paid AIDS worker to executive director of an AIDS service organization was enabled by the fact that Women Alive was a "hybrid" (Whittier 2011) organization involving social service provision, self-help, and activist advocacy. As I have argued in Chapter 4, ACT UP/ LA did not want to become a hybrid organization itself and rejected having a role in service provision, but that did not stop ACT UP/LA activists from taking direct action style and attitudes with them as they moved inside. MacNeil noted that Women Alive produced stickers to raise visibility on AIDS issues, just as ACT UPs did, and that they as a group had protested at a conference on women and AIDS. One of the Women Alive's projects at the time that I interviewed MacNeil was forming a committee to convince the County of Los Angeles to keep its dedicated AIDS ward open at County Hospital, the very same ward for which ACT UP/LA had successfully agitated. Women Alive opposed County plans to close the ward, arguing that scattering AIDS patients throughout the hospital, where they could encounter opportunistic infections in multi-bed wards, was a mistake. MacNeil also noted that the committee wanted to publicize the very existence of the ward to poor HIV-positive women because many had no idea that it even existed. Through her work with Women Alive, MacNeil hoped that women's "angry" voices could help to, in her words, "resolve this on some level" and keep the ward open.

CONCLUSION: THE UNEASY SURVIVAL OF OUTSIDER PERSPECTIVES IN INSIDER SPACES

> I ask myself what it is that the AIDS movement taught me and how in the world do I apply the lessons? What sort of truths have I learned? How do I value communitarian work, you know ... grass roots politics?
>
> – Gunther Freehill[38]

Social theory has, with a lot of help from feminist and other theorists, dismantled the hard line once drawn theoretically between the outside and the inside in social protest and social change. Outsider spaces are not settings of perfect equality; insider spaces are not spaces of perfect acquiescence to power. Yet, as my discussion of debates within ACT UP/LA itself about negotiating with power shows, the group wrestled with the effects of working with power:

---

[37] Interview with author, 1999.
[38] Interview with the author, 2000.

some activists advocated the pragmatic use of whatever tactics would work, and others were leery of any routine engagement with institutional actors. While debates went on, ACT UP/LA, as an organization that worked according to the needs of its members, that saw itself as a coalition of impassioned participants, tended to accept a variety of tactics as legitimate, especially when the tactics appeared to get results. But unease about the potential for cooptation and vitiation of a radical anti-AIDS stance worried some members of the group even as other members worked across outsider and insider spaces.

As my small sample of ACT UP/LA members who straddled the line between outsider and insider spaces suggests, feminist intersectional scholars and others who have posited the survival of "outsider" thinking in insider spaces are right to insist that activist backgrounds and marginalized identities lead to resistance on the part of institutional activists (see Banaszak 2011; Newman 2012). The movement of these activists across boundaries of insider and outside show that the lines that scholars later draw between spaces are not necessarily clear to participants on the ground at the time; even when lines are drawn, some activists decide to cross them. At least in the case of ACT UP/LA, and contrary to what the "outsiders within" literature might predict, in the newly created institutional spaces for AIDS advocacy, potential outsiders within – in this case lesbian and gay activists – did not feel themselves to be inevitably marginalized. All the straddlers were able to make spaces for themselves for some period of time in the paid AIDS work sector, even while they experienced tensions brought by having an awareness of how little represented their communities were on the inside and how different their perspectives were from the typical bureaucrat. Activists shared an acute sense that the streets taught them something about what they should be doing to counter AIDS and help PWAs.

Thus, in this chapter I have shown that, within ACT UP/LA – a group that had insiders within it from its start and, simultaneously, a group that regarded itself and was regarded as practicing the most militant form of outsider activism – debates about how to interact with power were never really settled. ACT UP/LA's coalitional structure actually militated against settling the debates about interacting with power, and, while members disagreed about working inside institutions, institutional activists could remain under the ACT UP/LA umbrella as long as they wanted to with no real worry of being ejected from the group. The institutional activists who knowingly crossed the porous line between disruptive outsider activism and institutional activism were shaped by their outsider experiences and saw carrying oppositional knowledge and commitments into institutional spaces as an important part of what they had to give to their AIDS work. In the telling of their activist and insider histories, the former ACT UP/LA members who were institutional activists I spoke with saw their outsider and insider work as relatively seamless. But while the creation of such organic, even teleological, trajectories is partially an artifact of retrospectively recasting life events (and thus one of the hazards of interview research), the record supports the claims made that ACT UP/LA's institutional activists could blur the line between service provision, policy engagement, and disruptive activism by deciding to do work in these different arenas all at once. As institutional activists, however, they tended to judge their actions by outsider activist standards – it helped that ACT UP/LA was always concerned about the actual results of disruptive activism and not just expression – and they were willing to try to take institutions in new directions as to policy and advocacy. Certainly, we cannot tell from their stories if they were effective as such; that is a project that is beyond the scope of this chapter. But, given that anti-AIDS activists in the 1980s and 1990s struggled to access resources from established power (Epstein 1996) – given that for many activists the goal was institutionalizing a serious and thoroughgoing response by power to the AIDS crisis – we can understand the pull that institutional spaces had on even the most militant activists.

When I interviewed him in 1999, I asked Phill Wilson how he reconciled his activist history and orientation, not to mention his personal style, with his position as LA City's AIDS Policy Coordinator. Wilson replied that he developed "an ethical sleep test" that helped him reconcile insider status with outsider politics:

(I)t involves kind of asking yourself "did I do the best job that I could do today?" And when I evaluate the things that I did today, can I sleep given the fact that . . . . in my case, given the fact that tomorrow I may wake up and what I did today might be the last thing that I ever did. . . . And I've always tried to apply that test beforehand and the sleep part of it is that "Do you sleep at night?" And so far, I guess, the way I feel about it is that on most nights, I sleep.[39]

Wilson's ethical sleep test may not have satisfied all members of ACT UP/LA then or now, but it reflects a reality about the kind of challenges outsiders within faced when direct action resulted in some measure of institutional power; that is, when noisy protest *plus* more routine tactics actually worked.

CODA: NAMING ONESELF AN INSTITUTIONAL ACTIVIST

I interviewed former ACT UP/LA activist Richard "Doe" Racklin in 2011. Racklin's time in ACT UP/LA had seen him take part is some high-risk, high-profile activism and included a fairly traumatic incarceration for civil disobedience at the Republican National Convention in Houston in 1992 (see Chapter 5). Racklin was not someone who ever melded his paid work with AIDS activism. He worked at Northrup Grumman, an aerospace company, for fifteen years subsequent to his ACT UP/LA involvement; he had been given a lay-off notice from the company shortly before our interview. Racklin was like the probable majority of ACT UP/LA members: an activist who came to the

---

[39] Interview with the author, 1999.

group without trying to make his life one seamless blend of paid and unpaid activism.

Racklin emailed me shortly after our interview:

Benita,

I've read your project description and wanted to add some things I am doing for the community. It wasn't as obviously activism and certainly not the street activism that we have done and that I miss a little bit. In the 15+ years that I have worked at Northrup Grumman, using my position in the Diversity & Inclusion, EEO, Contributions and Community Relations department, I was able to influence the company to provide grants and funding to many HIV and GLBT organizations ... because I brought my whole self to work in 1995 ... to a very conservative defense/aerospace company. So in 16 years about $750,000 has been donated to these organizations. On the Diversity side, I was also instrumental in helping the company to attain a 100% rating on the Human Rights Campaign Corporate Equality Index. With the help of my manager (and nudging her!), I've attained DP [domestic partner] benefits for over 125,000 employees. We also have added sexual orientation and gender identity to the company's non-discrimination clause.[40]

I wrote Racklin back, suggesting that he was a corporate LGBT activist and telling him about work on the movement for LGBT equality in corporate America (see Raeburn 2004). He responded: "YES! That's what I am, a corporate activist ... I never thought of it that way."[41]

Of course, Racklin's work at Northrup was not made any more real by having a name given to it, but our exchange and his eagerness to claim the name "corporate activist" seems important to me for at least two reasons. First, our interview about his ACT UP/LA days clearly catalyzed him into thinking about how to characterize his corporate activism, which, if viewed strictly from the standpoint that only disruptive protest from the outside is real protest, might not have seemed like "real" activism at all. Second, it is clear that Racklin's corporate activism was in part a result of his learning how to take risks in ACT UP/LA, of his willingness to "bring his whole self" to his paid work. Certainly, research on the biographical consequences of activism suggests that activists tend to remain committed to their politics and seek alternative ways to be political when street activism evaporates (McAdam 1988, 1989; Whalen and Flacks 1989). Racklin's awakening to his status as a corporate activist suggests that even those former members of ACT UP/LA who did not continue with institutionalized AIDS work integrated their time in direct action directly into their lives.

---

[40] Email sent to author, May 22, 2011.
[41] Email sent to author, May 24, 2011.

7

Looking Back on the Life and Death of ACT UP/LA

> ACT UP pushed the envelope. We did things that had not been done before in ways that people had not imagined doing them before. But it was for a purpose . . . And it was the time and we were the people who did the pushing. I think it was hugely successful in that way.
>
> – Helene Schpak[1]

RECAPTURING THE DIRECT-ACTION STRUGGLE AGAINST AIDS

In writing about the AIDS Coalition to Unleash Power, Los Angeles (ACT UP/LA) more than twenty-five years after the organization's birth, I have been made continuously aware of how far we are removed, as a political culture, from the acute and deadly homophobic fear that greeted AIDS in the 1980s. I teach courses about social protest at SUNY Binghamton, and I include the history of anti-AIDS activism in my teaching. My students there – mostly middle-class, mostly white, mostly heterosexual, and mostly born in the 1990s – by and large accept their LGBT peers. They live in a world where there has always been AIDS. They have always known about the need to practice, or at least pay lip service to, safe sex. They have grown up seeing prominent lesbian, gay, and transgender personalities in media, and they see more every day. Magic Johnson, whose announcement of his HIV-positive status was seen as such a momentous event in November 1991, is a name students might recognize because they have read about his openly gay son E. J., maybe even on the same sports sites that covered his father's NBA games.[2] While it is an overstatement to say that HIV/AIDS has become only one disease among many, my students understand HIV infection as preventable

[1] Interview with author, 2011.
[2] http://espn.go.com/los-angeles/nba/story/_/id/9177551/ej-johnson-son-magic-johnson-talks-being-gay

if one takes personal responsibility and treatable so long as one is covered by insurance. For them, the absence of information about HIV/AIDS is emphatically not a problem; they can read what they like about HIV and any other health issues that worry them by looking at one of their many screens. For their generation, the consequences of HIV infection have been minimized. Avoiding HIV is more or less like avoiding anything that is bad for one's health.[3]

In the second decade of the twenty-first century, my students – and the rest of us – are also very far removed from the militant direct action response to AIDS exemplified by ACT UP/LA and the other ACT UPs. When my students learn about the history of anti-AIDS activism, they immediately understand the vitriol and ignorance directed at HIV-positive people in the years after the epidemic broke as egregious responses. What is new for them, and what shouldn't be, is knowledge of the hard battles fought by anti-AIDS activists against government neglect, medical establishment prejudices, pharmaceutical company misbehavior, and society-wide heterosexism and homophobia. It is that history that I want to help to partially restore through the admittedly selective lens of analyzing the rise and fall of ACT UP/LA.

In Chapter 1, I introduced the case of ACT UP/LA as an anti-AIDS direct action social movement organization, and I argued that it was an important case to look at for several reasons. First, I argued that the conflation of ACT UP with ACT UP/NY minimized the broad appeal of anti-AIDS direct action politics and minimized the coalitional nature of that social movement in the 1980s and 1990s. Second, I made the case for the importance of the politics of place for understanding social movement organizing, employing the concept of Ray's (1999) social movement "field" to argue that there were factors specific to Los Angeles as a metropolitan region that influenced ACT UP/LA. The features of the Los Angeles metroscape that influenced the formation and trajectory of ACT UP/LA was LA's "segregated diversity" (Pulido 2006: 52), the County of Los Angeles' role in healthcare provision, and the local history of LGBT politics. Third, I argued that ACT UP/LA was, like other ACT UPs, an exemplar of progressive, multi-issue, anti-corporate, confrontational movements of the late twentieth century. Last, I stated that I would use a feminist intersectional theoretical lens in order to understand the dynamics around inequalities in ACT UP/LA, showing how members grappled with the challenges that inequalities posed to their desires to engage in democratic and coalitional politics.

I started examining ACT UP/LA's birth and mobilization in Chapter 2. Beginning in December 1987, ACT UP/LA's founders sought a direct action

---

[3] The idea of HIV as avoidable has seemingly taken root among young gay men who reportedly have been having more unprotected sex based on a strategy of "sero-sorting" – choosing one's partners based on the perception or test results that show that they are HIV-negative or have undetectable viral loads. (Donald G. McNeil Jr., "H.I.V. Concern Rises Along with Unprotected Sex," *The New York Times*, September 29, 2013, p. A4.)

response to the AIDS crisis modeled on the participatory democratic example of ACT UP/NY. ACT UP/LA's initial organizers brought together a coalition of groups and individuals committed to activism that was officially leaderless and open to agendas set by participants. They structured their organization along the lines of ACT UP/NY's "General Body plus committees" model in order to capture energy and maximize members' participation. ACT UP/LA members oscillated between actions that addressed local concerns and those that were nationally coordinated with other ACT UPs; during the group's heyday, the oscillation between the local and the national infused the group with regular bursts of energy. National campaigns against the US Food and Drug Administration (FDA) and the Centers for Disease Control (CDC) dovetailed with local and intense battles to force the County of Los Angeles to devote resources to care for public health–dependent people with AIDS (PWAs). Once the County opened a dedicated AIDS ward at County/USC hospital, members of ACT UP/LA kept pressure on a sluggish bureaucracy that failed to keep promises about the delivery of care in its hospitals and outpatient clinics. ACT UP/LA members' efforts ranged from theatrical actions designed to capture a national audience, like stopping the Rose Parade or invading the Academy Awards ceremony, to locally based sit-ins, vigils, and phone and fax "zaps." The group began to turn its attention to women's AIDS issues as a Women's Caucus (WC) formed within its ranks.

I examined the opportunities and challenges that feminist ACT UP/LA women in the WC faced in interactions with the wider group in Chapter 3. Feminist women in ACT UP/LA used the organization's "feminist-friendliness" to organize, and they had some real successes in the group despite continuous efforts to keep members' attention on women's AIDS issues. Drawing an internal boundary between themselves and ACT UP/LA's men allowed feminist women to draw on, and draw out, the support of actively feminist ACT UP/LA men. Being in the WC also allowed feminist women to become legitimated within the group as ACT UP/LA's "official women," a development that had beneficial and unintended effects; while the WC could expect male deference from others in respect to its political agenda, being official women led to the compartmentalization of women's AIDS issues as feminist women took up a larger share of the burden of representation of and activism on behalf of women. Ultimately, the WC, as dependent as it was on the help of ACT UP/LA's men in order to accomplish its agenda, also reshaped the trajectory of ACT UP/LA, such that members of the wider group could not ignore gendered politics.

In Chapter 4, I looked at the "intersectional crises" that enervated ACT UP/LA. I looked at three such crises: (1) the influx of participants into ACT UP/LA in late 1991 as a result of California Governor Pete Wilson's veto of Assembly Bill 101 (AB 101), a lesbian and gay rights bill that challenged ACT UP/LA to accept new members not versed in the gender and racial/ethnic stances of the group; (2) disputes about the gendered and raced boundaries of ACT

UP/LA beginning in early to mid-1992 that focused on resources used for the needle exchange project, about the wisdom of using ACT UP/LA to deliver a social service, and about efforts to move the Monday night General Body (GB) meetings to different sites around LA in order to reach more people of color; and (3) local and negative reverberations about "competing" gendered national protest actions that took place in April 1993 during the March on Washington for Lesbian, Gay, and Bisexual Rights and Liberation. Gendered, racial/ethnic, and sexual difference were all at play in these debates, although the salience of forms of inequality shifted in each case. Ultimately, intersectional crises help to fracture solidarity and demobilize the group.

I explored ACT UP/LA's demobilization and death in Chapter 5. ACT UP/LA's demobilization took place over a period of five years, from the latter half of 1992 until late 1997. After reviewing the general consensus in movement studies about why the ACT UPs demobilized, I discuss the local issues that led to ACT UP/LA's demobilization. In addition to the enervating effects of intersectional conflict in the group, I argued that ACT UP/LA lost leadership to death, and, at the same time, members experienced a sense that they were becoming less effective as a group. I also discuss how the oscillation between the local and the national, once a generative process for the local group, became hurtful to local esprit de corps after badly planned, highly confrontational actions at the 1992 Republican Party Convention in Houston. I chronicle the last few years of the group, when a very small group of activists resisted national plans for the distribution of funds to ACT UPs and thus rejected money that might have helped ACT UP/LA hang on. Last, I explored the meaning of the fact that ACT UP/LA's last few members disagreed about how the group ended; that is, whether the death of the group was a natural, unheralded petering out or a democratically made decision by its last few die-hards.

In Chapter 6, I considered how ACT UP/LA's participants managed issues raised by encounters with the "inside" – with institutions that were targets of anti-AIDS activism – by reading through debates that took place within the group about the wisdom of using insider and outsider tactics. I also use interviews with former activists whose lives straddled insider and outsider spaces to show how porous the newly established AIDS "establishment" was in the 1980s and 1990s. I argue that ACT UP/LA was never truly "outsider" space and that former ACT UP/LA activists who moved into insider spaces often kept one foot in outsider protest politics and were influenced deeply by their experiences in ACT UP/LA. The evidence in this chapter supports views of social movement activists as having a variety of relationships with institutionalized power, relationships shaped by life experience but also by structural inequalities of gender and sexuality. I therefore suggest that those researching movements conceptualize the line between outsider and insider spaces as potentially porous, subject to degrees of erasure in the lives of activists themselves and, in any case, a matter for empirical investigation.

THEORETICAL LESSONS FROM THE CASE: INTERSECTIONAL PERSPECTIVE, INESCAPABLE INEQUALITIES, POLITICS OF PLACE, AND THE BLURRING OF OUTSIDER–INSIDER SPACES

There have been several interlinked theoretical threads running through the account of the life and death of ACT UP/LA: namely, (1) the importance of a feminist intersectional perspective for explaining the trajectory of social movements, (2) the role of inequalities in movements, (3) the significance of local politics for movement action, and (4) the variable relationship of insider and outsider spaces in social movement activism.

First, I looked at the case of ACT UP/LA through a feminist intersectional lens, arguing that more studies of movements should incorporate an intersectional perspective in order to understand how gender inequalities dovetail with other social structural inequalities. Gendered analysis of social phenomena needs to incorporate awareness of other relevant social divides. Gendered politics in ACT UP/LA were played out among activists who were themselves members of a community marginalized on the basis of sexual orientation. The bonds that were created between lesbians and gay men in ACT UP/LA were real ones, albeit impacted by the unequal status that men and women occupy in society at large and influenced by men's "epidemiological pre-eminence" (Altman 1994: 72) in the AIDS epidemic. Race and, to a lesser extent, class and sexuality were implicated in the decisions members made about where to meet as a group, what kinds of links to make with other groups, and what actions to take. It is easy to think about why gendered or racial politics matters when feminist women come together to form a women's caucus or people of color come together to form a people of color caucus; it is more difficult to think through what intersectional politics means when matters of gender, race, or sexuality are not the explicit subject of discussion. As I argued in Chapter 4, the intersectional crises that, along with other organization factors considered in Chapter 5, enervated the group are not intelligible without an intersectional lens looking for where and how complex inequalities mattered for social movement organizing. In looking at ACT UP/LA's trajectory, then, feminist intersectional analysis shows how the burdens of social inequalities shaped activists' interactions with each other in complex and contextualized ways.

A second theoretical contribution that follows from taking a feminist intersectional perspective to examining the case of ACT UP/LA shows how both grass-roots and institutional spaces were crosscut by inequalities that shaped how activists were able to be activists. Exploring the internal dynamics of ACT UP/LA contributes to a welcome deromanticization of the grass roots as a pure space of action by equals. Such deromanticization is quite advanced in activist practice, as the hard work done by activists concerned with creating "horizontal" spaces (Sitrin 2006) shows. In ACT UP/LA, members' radically democratic and egalitarian intentions were nonetheless continuously challenged by the interactional burdens placed on the group of large-scale, long-standing relationships of unequal social locations. Even while activists decried the societal discrimination that made the AIDS pandemic more deadly to the marginalized, efforts to call attention to inequality were met with ambivalence. The formation of the ACT UP/LA WC was both heralded and met with suspicion; efforts to make ACT UP/LA more racially inclusive were fraught; and the interactional burdens of inequalities dovetailed with other less than conducive elements – stalemate with authorities, death, and burnout – in leading to ACT UP/LA's eventual demise. In short, the interactional burdens that intersectional inequalities conferred in grass-roots spaces create challenges for the creation of unity – or, if one prefers, solidarity – in social movement organizations because it through interaction that movement members create collective identities (Diani and Bison 2004).

In suggesting that the grass-roots space of politics was one of crosscutting inequalities, I do not mean to suggest that we do away with the idea of a "grass roots." Rather, I suggest that we complicate our understanding of how power and inequality operate in *all* social spaces, even oppositional ones. Kimberlé Crenshaw's (1989, 1991) original formulations of intersectionality included an awareness that oppositional groups were themselves coalitions. In practice and in theory, coalition members cope with varying access to power. I thus took a "process-centered" (Choo and Ferree 2010) intersectional approach, noting circumstances of relative privilege and relative disadvantage within ACT UP/LA. Privilege and disadvantage adhere to individuals and groups located in the matrix of social structural inequalities whether or not members make claims on behalf of redressing the injuries caused by inequalities. Inequalities complicate the construction of collective identity because identity categories exist prior to group mobilization and thus construct (and are reconstructed through) activism. And if gender and other significant markers of social inequality are always elements of interaction, it is likely that they will create lines of social cleavage that challenge the ability to construct solidarity.

A third theoretical thread that moves through my account of ACT UP/LA is taking seriously the politics of place for understanding social movement organizations' trajectories and for understanding what faces organizations situated in different social movement fields. Studying ACT UP/LA contributes to our knowledge of how local histories and relationships condition social movement activism. The case of ACT UP/LA shows that, as much as the ACT UP model or brand of activism was attractive to activists in various locales and as important as nationally coordinated campaigns were, each of the ACT UPs was situated in different social movement fields (Ray 1999). What mattered in LA – the segregated diversity of the metroscape, the distances involved in getting from community to community, LA County's responsibility for public healthcare, and the LGBT tradition of meshing political action and service provision – might matter for other ACT UPs, but that is a question that needs local answers. Some ACT UPs had, as Los Angeles did, a history of activist lesbian and gay organizing in place by the 1980s (Faderman and Timmons 2009; Kenney 2001);

others didn't. Some ACT UPs organized within gay and lesbian enclaves; in Los Angles, both the Silverlake neighborhood of LA and the recently incorporated city of West Hollywood provided crucial spaces in which to organize and populations to draw from in what was otherwise a diverse and spread-out urban landscape. Some ACT UPs had to, as ACT UP/LA did, struggle with their local governments for public health provision; in Los Angeles, the years-long struggle with LA County mobilized ACT UP/LA and led to its earliest successes, while continuous engagement with the County also proved frustrating and demoralizing. In short, even when a group is part of a national network, the local matters for understanding what activists actually can do.

Last, my study of ACT UP/LA contributes to studies that problematize the hard line once drawn between the outside and the inside in social protest. We know that insiders can bring outsider mindsets to insider spaces and that outside spaces are not settings of perfect equality. This study showed that AIDS insiders in the newly established AIDS establishment brought inside with them a perspective drawn from the streets and that some were drawn to the streets while doing AIDS work. This suggests not only that insiders can hold on to outsider values, but that social movement organizations can accommodate relative insiders and still be very militant in their tactics and aims. It is true that, within ACT UP/LA, debates raged about the kinds of relationships with power that made sense and whether routinized tactics – like lobbying or even more confrontational face-to-face negotiations – would get results. Some members were worried about how contact with authorities could vitiate ACT UP/LA's radical anti-AIDS stance, but most were willing – following the group's ethos of promiscuity in issues and tactics – to let members try what they thought might work to fight AIDS. What the case of ACT UP/LA shows is that it is possible, given an organization's structural commitment to coalition, to allow for a variety of approaches to exist under *one* organizational roof – not just in one movement, and not just in one collection of organizations that have formed around an issue. ACT UP/LA's coalitional structure may have militated against the group ever settling debates about strategy and tactics when facing power, but that very unsettledness allowed institutional activists to stay under the ACT UP/LA umbrella with no real fear of being purged. Coalitions of individuals with different ideas about how to do protest politics can coexist in one organization, particularly if the issue is new and emergent and the lines between outside and insider have not yet been established.

THE ACT UPS' LEGACY AND THE ONGOING AIDS CRISIS

> Organizations either serve their purpose or they do not. When they do not, they
> should cease to exist. I don't believe in making mummies out of corpses.
>
> – John Fall (Larry Holmes's partner)[4]

---

[4] John Fall, email to author, August 20, 2012.

Another ACT/UP? Well, you push a bunch of sick and dying people with nothing
to lose up against a wall – you're gonna get what you deserve.

– Larry Holmes (John Fall's partner)[5]

While I was conducting interviews for this book in May 2011, a friend, Tom
Carter, introduced me to Brigitte Tweddel, the executive director of Project
New Hope; Carter was doing some bookkeeping work for the organization.[6]
Project New Hope, founded in 1990, grew out of grass-roots efforts to provide
affordable housing to people with AIDS and their families. Tweddel's time was
limited, and, as such, our conversation – about the Project's efforts, the limits of
government resources, and the ongoing nature of the HIV/AIDS epidemic –
lasted perhaps forty minutes. Brief as it was, two moments occurred during our
talk that I think hold significance for assessing the legacy of ACT UP/LA, the
other ACT UPs, and the direct action anti-AIDS movement.

The first moment actually occurred at the end of my visit to Project New
Hope. Tweddel handed me five different glossy magazines to peruse. Four were
aimed at HIV-positive people, and one, *Real Health*, was aimed at the Black
community, but featured a prominent story about how marriage *increased*
Black women's risk of contracting HIV.[7] All five of the magazines included
stories accompanied by glamorous portraits of attractive individuals. For
example, the May/June 2011 issue of *HIV Plus* featured singer Annie Lennox,
wearing a shirt from the AIDS Treatment Action Campaign reading "HIV
POSITIVE." All of the magazines had articles about HIV drugs, about drug
trials, and about ways to stay healthy; all of them had full-page or two-page
advertisements for AIDS medications. Although the sociologist in me knew not
to read too much into an extremely convenient sample of five magazines,
I couldn't help but be struck by the magazines' slick production values and
their messages about HIV disease as treatable, chronic, almost glamorous.[8]
I was also struck by how the magazines represented – indeed, were doing
the work of – the incorporation of HIV illness into the everyday world of the
mediascape. I asked myself if the glossy, attractive world of the HIV-positive
depicted in the magazines was a victory for anti-AIDS activists. Or were the
magazines, with their shiny ads accompanied by pages of very small print about
medications' side effects – a kind of collective, mainstreamed lie?

---

[5] Larry Holmes, email to author, August 10, 2012.

[6] www.projectnewhope.org.

[7] Cristina Gonzalez, "In Sickness and in Health: Love, Marriage, a Baby Carriage and . . . HIV?"
Real Health 25 (Spring 2011), p. 9.

[8] In his recent book, *Body Counts: A Memoir of Politics, Sex, AIDS, and Survival*, Sean Strub
writes about the 1994 founding of *POZ*, the first, in his own words, "glossy lifestyle magazine for
people with AIDS" (2014: 285). *POZ* is still published (see http://www.poz.com/). Strub, who
sold the magazine after about a decade, details the political and financial struggles involved in
getting the magazine out; chief among these political/financial struggles was whether and when to
take advertising money from pharmaceutical companies.

A second moment of significance for thinking about the legacy of direct action anti-AIDS protest took place while Tweddel and I were talking. Tweddel noted that thousands of new HIV cases were still being diagnosed in Los Angeles County each year. According to the 2010 Annual HIV Surveillance Report conducted by the LA County Department of Public Health, reports of new HIV infections have been rising in the County, although the report's authors hedged their bets by speculating that the rise might be an artifact of changing reporting requirements.[9] The report gave a figure of 2,036 new diagnoses of HIV infection in 2009 for LA County, including 1,312 cases of AIDS; overall, in 2009, more than 40,000 PWAs lived in LA County. New infections were concentrated in West Hollywood, in the district that contained the County Men's Central Jail, and in downtown Los Angeles, with its large homeless population. Black women were disproportionately represented among women with new HIV infections. While death rates from AIDS were down, the County's institutions and nonprofit service agencies were still faced with a considerable public health challenge.

Beyond LA County, the picture of HIV/AIDS in the United States is a steady-state grim one, punctuated by cautious good news. While great strides have been made in treating HIV disease, new infections of the virus in the United States have held at 50,000 per year for nearly a decade.[10] The rate of new infections has come down since the peak numbers of the 1980s, but prevention programs have been less successful at making inroads into at-risk communities, and infection rates have risen for young Black gay men and for Black women. In the United States, HIV disease is still centered among men who have sex with men, but HIV disease disproportionately affects the poor, young men of color, and women of color, with nearly a third of new infections being contracted through heterosexual sex. According to the *Washington Post*, the HIV rate of sero-prevalence in Washington, DC, in 2008 was 3 percent, a rate higher than that of West Africa and "on par with Uganda and some parts of Kenya," with all modes of transmission on the rise.[11] In the Navajo nation, a recent report found that new HIV cases had increased fivefold since 1999, defying the national trend of holding steady.[12]

The costs of treating HIV disease remain high. While the difficult regime of taking dozens of pills to control the virus has morphed into a few or even one pill a day, the new drugs are not cheap. The FDA recently approved a once-a-day pill from Gilead Sciences, named Stribild, which will cost patients/insurance

[9] http://publichealth.lacounty.gov/hiv/

[10] Donald G. McNeil Jr. "New HIV Cases Remain Steady Over a Decade." *The New York Times*, August 4, 2011, p. A16.

[11] Jose Antonia Vargas and Darryl Fears. "HIV/AIDS Rate in D.C. Hits 3%," *The Washington Post*. March 15, 2009, p. A1.

[12] Dan Frosch, "Navajo Confront an Increase in New H.I.V. Infections," *The New York Times*, May 20, 2013, p. A12.

companies $28,500 dollars for a year's course.[13] AIDS drug regimens – the so-called cocktail or combination of the thirty or so antiretroviral drugs that now exist – have helped millions of PWAs live with a chronic illness, but the drugs have side effects that induce inflammatory diseases and lead to premature aging in some users.[14] In the United States, big "pharma" is targeting non-infected gay and bisexual men with Truvada, a drug aimed at "pre-exposure prophylaxis" (known as "PrEP"). In May 2014, the FDA approved the anti-viral drug made by Gilead Sciences, as the first PrEP drug for "high-risk" HIV-negative populations – i.e., younger gay men. The cost of a year of Truvada is roughly $13,000, which would be covered by insurance – if one has insurance. The populations at highest risk for HIV infections in the United States are gay Black and Hispanic men, and they are the least likely to have health insurance.[15] The AIDS Healthcare Foundation (AHF)'s president and founder Michael Weinstein remains one of the few leaders in the anti-AIDS service community who has questioned the wisdom of PrEP. AHF's objections to PrEP rest on whether HIV-negative men would take a drug they don't need daily and if the ability to take a daily pill would erode "condom culture" among men who have sex with men. AHF fears that Truvada will erode safer-sex culture, but others in the health establishment argue that "PrEP's effectiveness in preventing transmission outweighs the risk that people will not take their pills, or will stop using condoms."[16]

The drug regimens to prevent or treat HIV disease cost thousands of dollars a month and thus anti-retrovirals are beyond the means of most PWAs worldwide. Globally, HIV disease is a major cause of death, dislocation, and social misery. UNAIDS estimates that, in 2012, there were 35.3 million people living with HIV/AIDS, with perhaps 2.3 million newly infected per year. While the latter number of new infections represents a falling rate of new transmission from its height in the mid-1990s, hopes for ending transmission of the virus rest on overcoming a difficult constellation of obstacles. Ending AIDS rests not just on remedying access to and the cost of antiretrovirals, but on implementing testing regimes, ending poverty, stopping gender violence, rescinding punitive anti-gay laws, and on combating what the UN terms a "(l)ow political commitment to reducing new infections among people who

[13] Andrew Pollack, "F.D.A. Approves Once-a-Day Pill for H.I.V." *The New York Times*, August 28, 2012, p. B4.

[14] Jerome Groopman, 2014 "Can AIDS be Cured?" *The New Yorker*, December 22 and 29, pp. 78–96.

[15] Donald G. McNeil, Jr. "Are We Ready for H.I.V.'s Sexual Revolution." *The New York Times*, May 25, 2014 pp. SR 6–7.

[16] Weinstein's anti-Truvada stance has caused many in the AIDS prevention community to condemn him; see Josh Barro, "Drug to Lower H.I.V. Risk Has Lone Public Naysayer," *The New York Times*, Monday November 17, 2014 p. a16. But Weinstein's public willingness to question the wisdom of PrEP may represent the opinion of public health professionals who cannot speak out.

inject drugs."[17] The stark inequalities between Global North and Global South are strongly implicated in the abilities of countries like South Africa to control HIV disease; while aspects of the epidemic are under better control in that country, the public healthcare system for HIV/AIDS care was heavily dependent on the United States' President's Emergency Plan for AIDS Relief (PEPFAR), which poured billions of dollars into the country beginning in 2003.[18] As PEPFAR funds dry up, the overburdened local healthcare institutions struggle to keep up with what is still considerable demand for their services. In short, the HIV/AIDS crisis is far from over either here or abroad. Our having learned to live with HIV disease in the United States has not eliminated the ability of AIDS to shorten and immiserate lives.

The AIDS crisis is not over, and the ACT UPs collectively have had a major impact on how grass-roots groups around the world continue to address the HIV/AIDS crisis *as a* crisis. Nguyen (2010) has noted that an anti-AIDS group in Abidjan, Ivory Coast, renamed itself "ACT UP Abidjan" to link itself to the style of activism that the ACT UP name represented. In the United States, there are currently at least two ACT UPs with roots in the 1980s still alive. ACT UP/NY continues to stage protests aimed at raising awareness about the ongoing HIV/AIDS crisis; in 2014, they staged a "die-in" at New York City Mayor Bill de Blasio's inauguration.[19] ACT UP/Philadelphia also continues to be active. ACT UP/Philadelphia staged a protest by seven naked activists with slogans painted on their bodies in House Speaker John Boehner's office in November 2012; three women protestors (out of a mixed-gender group of seven) were arrested for "lewd and indecent acts."[20] While there is no longer an ACT UP in Los Angeles, ex-ACT UP/LA activists have used social media to keep in touch. In 2004, an online newsletter announced the formation of "ACT UP Southern California," so named, according to the release's anonymous author because some members of ACT UP/LA still wanted to keep their name.[21] In early 2011, a Facebook page entitled "ACT UP/LA" counted three hundred friends; by early 2012, the page was apparently gone. In early 2012, the Facebook page "ACT UP Southern California" had one member who had last signed in during December 2009, promising "re-organization."

---

[17] See http://www.unaids.org/en/media/unaids/contentassets/documents/unaidspublication/2013/ JC2571_AIDS_by_the_numbers_en.pdf

[18] See Donald G. McNeil, Jr. "AIDS Progress in Peril," *The New York Times*, Tuesday August 26, 2014 p. D1.

[19] See http://actupny.com/actions/.

[20] ACT UP/Philadelphia's website is http://www.actupphilly.org/. On the Boehner protest, see Trudy Ring, "Naked AIDS Activists Protest at Boehner's Office," *The Advocate*, November 27, 2012 (accessed January 14, 2013 at http://www.advocate.com/politics/2012/11/ 27/naked-aids-activists-protest-boehner-office).

[21] "Action Newsletter Volume One August 2004"; see http://www.actupny.org/indexfolder/ AUsocal.html

The ACT UPs – direct action anti-AIDS activists responding on local, national, and international levels to what became a global health threat – were one of the first of the batch of globalized, decentralized, multi-issue, multi-constituency movements that characterized late twentieth-century protest. The ACT UPs were an early embodiment of the loosely bound, networked (Juris 2009) coalitions of autonomous direct action activists that are perhaps the modal form of activism in a globalizing world. ACT UP members made use of what was then only an emerging new set of communication technologies, coordinating actions through teleconferencing, cell phones, and, toward the end, email and the Internet. Anti-AIDS activists asked questions about political exclusion, about the realities of social inequalities and the potential for social rights, and about the meaning of democracy. Their concerns animate many movement organizations and networks today. Even given conflict and fracturing, the ACT UP network and individual ACT UPs helped to bring about large-scale changes in the way we provide for those with HIV/AIDS disease, in what scientists do research on, and how we think about LGBT communities.

I have written about ACT UP/LA's internal struggles, but these struggles should not lead us to downplay or dismiss the group's successes or the accomplishments of other groups like it. As HIV/AIDS disease continues to threaten the lives and well-being of so many, it should not be forgotten that the model of activism that anti-AIDS protestors fashioned in the 1980s and 1990s produced results. In January 2009, cable news network MSNBC analyst Rachel Maddow memorialized Martin Delaney, the founder of Project Inform, the AIDS activist treatment organization, on her television show. In the course of doing so, Maddow called the anti-AIDS movement a "hidden huge success story about people power changing the world." She was right about the movement's success and right about its being hidden from the public. It is my hope that this book about ACT UP/LA contributes to keeping alive the history of how social change is made by people who desperately need change to survive.

APPENDIX

Multiple Methods and Multiple Perspectives

DATA: DRAWING FROM THE ARCHIVES, PARTICIPANT OBSERVATION, AND INTERVIEWS

In writing this book, I have taken a historical and sociological approach to understanding the life and death of the AIDS Coalition to Unleash Power, Los Angeles (ACT UP/LA). A historical sociological approach has as its fundamental premise that events could have occurred differently and thus require explanation as to why they occurred as they did.[1] Typically, historians work from archival records; less typically, they compile oral histories or interviews. But I have gone beyond the archival in assembling the sources of data I used in this book. I used archival material, interviews, and my participant observation with ACT UP/LA from late 1990 to mid 1992; the latter method especially is not normally part of the historical studies arsenal.

My use of multiple sources of data meant that I needed to consider questions that historians normally do not; specifically questions of identity and confidentiality. Guenther (2009: 412) has pointed out that "the act of naming is an act of power" and lamented the lack of discussion by social scientists about how they decided to identify organizations and individuals that they researched. Guenther argues that "the business of naming is not simple, often involving on-going dialogue between a researcher and her/his respondents, research goals, analytic strategies, and personal and professional ethics" (12). Guenther makes a distinction between the maintenance of confidentiality for individuals and the maintenance of confidentiality for organizations, noting that even the American Sociological Association's Code of Ethics gives researchers no guidance as to how and when to make research sites, as opposed to personal identities, public.

Guenther questioned the ethnographic convention of giving the German feminist organizations she studied pseudonyms and decided against doing so

[1] I am indebted to Karen O'Neill for reminding me of this simple but key insight.

for two main reasons. The first was that the effort to maintain an organization's anonymity in the era of the easy Internet search was fruitless. The second reason, and the one that I resonate with, was that giving organizations pseudonyms could

result in lost meanings as the names of these organizations represent specific histories, goals, and ideologies which even the cleverest pseudonyms would be unlikely to capture. Hiding these names would both devalue the strategic work of women's organizations and reduce the strength of my analysis. (2009: 419)

For the reasons that Guenther gives, and because I was committed to writing a history of ACT UP/LA, I never thought of giving the group a pseudonym or otherwise disguising it. Additionally, I had already published ethnographic work on ACT UP/LA and had not used a pseudonym in that article because of my desire to let readers know about the group's very existence (see Roth 1998).

My decisions about how and when to identify individual activists were more complex. Usually, historians make straightforward use of the names appearing in documents. In interview-based research, the names of interviewees may or may not be revealed depending on the purpose of the study and the agreement between interviewer and interviewee. My research was complicated by the fact that I had done participant observation on ACT UP/LA and had published work on the group; in that work, I employed the ethnographic convention of using pseudonyms in the place of real names. I decided to keep to this convention in this book when using the material drawn from participant observation. There was a practical and ethical reason for doing so; since I used pseudonyms instead of real names in my field notes, I would have to rely on my memory to reinsert real names. That seemed to me to be presumptuous, especially in the light of the fact that no human subjects research committee at UCLA had ever approved the ethnographic research, which I had originally done as graduate coursework. I could not recall our professors ever asking us to submit our research to such a committee; that may have been the result of the laxer standards in the 1990s, or it might have been a principled stand that one should not have to ask a committee in order to write about what one experienced. In any case, the safest course seemed to be leaving field notes as they were. I should note, however, that the decision to keep pseudonyms in place has elicited comments by two former ACT UP members. One ACT UP/LA member who I interviewed and who had read the previously published article based on my participant observation with the group was frustrated by the use of pseudonyms because he could not figure out who was who in the article. Another former ACT UP/NY activist who I encountered in presenting work from this book felt that the use of pseudonyms had the effect of erasing LGBT history; she urged me to reinsert the real names.

As for interviews, these were conducted in two "batches"; in both cases, they were done after I had my research project reviewed by Binghamton University's Human Subjects Research Review Committee (HSRRC). I submitted a consent form and a schedule of interview questions to the HSRRC and received the go-ahead to start after reviewing a required online module of relatively useless information about conducting human subjects research. As I was conducting open-ended interviews, the interview schedule was useful in keeping me on track, and the actual questions I asked during an interview deviated significantly from the approved list. The consent form that interviewees signed asked for permission to record the interview (only one person refused this); asked whether or not interviewees were okay with being identified by name (all were); and stated that interviewees could ask to see any part of the book that contained quotes or other material attributed to them (again, only one person explicitly wished to do this). Given the wonders of digital technology, the second batch of interviewees received digital recordings of the interviews themselves.

Thus, in this book, the reader will find that, in the majority of instances, I refer to people by their real names. Because of my participant observation, there are a few instances where a person given a pseudonym in my field notes also appears in the text with their actual name. I note where pseudonyms are used by enclosing a name in quotation marks when it is a pseudonym, and I did not "match up" the pseudonyms and real names in telling ACT UP/LA's story. In the spirit of Guenther's call for social scientists to acknowledge the power of naming, I will just say that I have taken the tack of letting the field notes stand as is in order to make the following methodological point: the convention of using pseudonyms in the field note excerpts serves to emphasize that notes are *my* filtering of events and personages, while interview excerpts, even though drawn from co-constructed conversations with me, nonetheless feature activists' interpretations, recall, and opinions of events and actions.

Like having multiple cameras filming one event, using multiple methods to explore ACT UP/LA provides some "coverage" in terms of getting at the internal dynamics of the group. Each method has also exposed the limitations of the others. Archival records are indispensable to reconstructing an organization's history for several reasons. First, they fill in the "before and after" for me as a participant and allow me to actually tell a story about ACT UP/LA from beginning to end. Second – and this became very clear to me as I conducted two rounds of interviews – my immersion in the archival material made it possible for me to ask different questions of the interviewees than I would have had I not been in the archives. Counterintuitively, it led me to ask *fewer* questions about specifics and thus changed the tone of the latter set of interviews considerably. Third, researching ACT UP/LA's archival record and conducting interviews showed me that, however vivid and rich my participant observation data was, my observation was inescapably partial in terms of capturing the dynamics of ACT UP/LA as a whole. The archival work especially illustrated to me how sheer experience, even in the self-reflexive mode of participant observation, is by its very nature incomplete.[2] Fourth, my

---

[2] On the question of the role of experience in historical exploration, see Joan Scott (1991).

participant observations answered questions – and in interviews, forestalled questions – about practices in ACT UP/LA. While I may not have been everywhere at once, I was there enough to understand what some of the core interactions might have been like among activists. Last, the interviews allowed me to "test" some of my inductive hypotheses about events and outcomes, and they provided data about activists' motives, about their emotions, and about their interpretation of the groups' decisions and, thus, ultimately, its legacy. This testing could only occur through the structured conversation of the interview; one cannot ask documents questions, and testing ideas during participant observation is a tall, and perhaps impossible order because the participant observer's goal is to attempt to record the world around her.

In the next section, I consider the specifics and the process of gathering archival research, using participant observation data, and interviewing in turn.

ARCHIVAL RESEARCH/PRIMARY SOURCES

During my time with ACT UP/LA, I collected documents and "ephemera," as any other member would. That collection constitutes a small part of the archival record that I relied on in writing this book. The other archival collections I used are located at the ONE National Gay and Lesbian Archives in Los Angeles. The ONE archive has two major collections of materials on anti-AIDS efforts: the ACT UP/LA Collection and the AIDS History Project Collection. The ACT UP/LA Collection consists of unprocessed, uncatalogued material that covers roughly the entire life of the group, with various degrees of completeness from year to year. Going through the papers required anti-allergy medications on my part and a great deal of patience from the archivists at the ONE as we tried to figure out what might be in each box and what I had already looked at.[3]

The ACT UP/LA collection consists of newsletters, minutes, agendas, position papers, flyers, and the like, and it includes documents gathered from other organizations and media sources. The AIDS History Project Collection was created by merging documents gathered by two LA gay community activists, Jim Kepner and Phill Wilson. Wilson, whom I interviewed in 1999, was present at the first meeting of ACT UP/LA, and he became LA City's second AIDS Policy Coordinator. He gathered materials for a collection he entitled "The Southern California AIDS Social Policy Archive," and which was deposited at the ONE. Kepner put together a collection about the history of the AIDS epidemic, focusing on Southern California, for what he called the "International Gay and Lesbian Archives"; these papers became part of ONE as well. In contrast to the ACT UP/LA papers, the AIDS History Project Collection is processed and contains a fair amount of material about the AIDS crisis in general. Chronologically, the two collections more or less overlap and cover the

---

[3] It is my understanding that the archive has since received funding that will allow it to begin processing the ACT UP/LA Collection.

period from the mid-1980s to the late 1990s. While the documents produced by and about ACT UP/LA are invaluable in aspects of the group's self-understandings, the documentary evidence for the group's history is thinner after 1992. My well-founded assumption is that many boxes of significant ACT UP/LA's papers lie in ex-participants' homes.

Other important sets of primary sources that I used were not necessarily archival in the same way as the collections just noted. In order to inform myself about ACT UP/NY and its national role in the ACT UPs, I read through the available interviews of the ACT UP Oral History Project (http://www.actuporalhistory.org/), a collection of nearly 130 videotaped and, in most cases, transcribed interviews with ACT UP/NY activists. Since the ACT UP Oral History Project focuses on interviews with activists with ACT UP/NY, I used the interviews to give me a sense of how ACT UP/LA might have differed from the ACT UP/NY. Another set of primary sources I looked at was the writing done by AIDS activists in the 1980s and 1990s, which I deemed "primary sources" because they were written as salvos from the battle lines. Last, news articles from local and national media formed a last set of primary sources; these included, but were not limited to, material from *The Los Angeles Times, The Los Angeles Herald Examiner, The Daily News,* the *LA Weekly,* the *LA Reader,* and, in the lesbian and gay press, from *Frontiers, The Advocate,* and *LN (Lesbian News).*

PARTICIPANT OBSERVATION

Feminist ethnographers have written about how important it is for the field researcher to self-reflect on her status with regards to the group that she writes about (see McCorkel and Myers 2003; Moore 2011). In writing this book, I have drawn on the field notes that I took during participant observation that I conducted within ACT UP/LA, and thus I will give the reader some more detailed background about the participant observation itself.

In November 1990, I came to ACT UP/LA through a desire to study the Women's Caucus (WC) of the group, and I began going to WC meetings with the intention of doing an ethnographic study of ACT UP women. I was in graduate school at the time and taking a course on ethnography. I had been using archival material to study 1960s and 1970s feminist organizations, and I was interested in studying political activism through my own engagement, influenced especially by "new social movement" scholars of engagement like Melucci (1989) and Touraine (1981).

My participation in the WC quickly escalated into participation in the larger group since, in practice, the WC and the General Body (GB) of ACT UP/LA were not discrete entities, as I discuss in Chapter 4. I discovered that the WC was truly a caucus, a bounded part of a larger whole, but that it operated with the help of that larger whole. After a few months, I was chosen to represent the WC at the upcoming AIDS Clinical Trials Group (ACTG) meeting in

Washington, DC, in March 1991, so I was sent to Treatment and Data Committee meetings to familiarize myself with those issues. Thus, my involvement in the WC and GB grew from one WC meeting every second Sunday attended mostly as a course requirement to those Sunday meetings, plus a weekly Monday night meeting of the GB, plus bimonthly Treatment meetings, plus attendance at demonstrations and fundraisers, some in town, and of course, that trip to DC. The only conscious decision I made about my escalating ACT UP/LA involvement was not joining affinity groups or being arrested for civil disobedience.

My situation as a researcher/activist in ACT UP/LA felt complicated, although perhaps the tugs and pulls I felt were the same ones ethnographers feel no matter where they are. I did see that escalating involvement in the group was a common experience and not one that befell me because of my research interests as such. Because of ethical concerns, I sought the explicit approval for my research from the WC members after two weeks. When I did so, one of the WC members mentioned that she had been taking notes on the previous WC meeting for her sociology class. Obviously, I was not the first one to think that ACT UP/LA was an interesting object of study.

Significantly, I never similarly "came out" as a researcher to the larger ACT UP GB, nor did I ask for the GB's approval. I also never asked for the approval of members of ACT UP/LA's Treatment and Data Committee to take notes, even when I was sent as a WC representative to the ACTG meetings. Given that the WC claimed to represent women in ACT UP/LA, I took an "insider" stance on the question of permission to observe; since it was the WC's view that the WC had the authority to represent women, I concluded that they could sanction my role as researcher vis à vis ACT UP/LA as a whole. This stance was, of course, convenient for me, but it is important to note that no WC member ever suggested that I ask the GB for permission to study the group. Moreover, no one in ACT UP/LA really seemed to care if a few of us were engaged in research. While I participated in ACT UP/LA, I knew of at least two other UCLA graduate students (both male) who were doing research on the group, and their status seemed to be generally known and accepted. I have no idea and never asked them if they were conducting research with the group's permission.

Some readers may shudder at this story and see it as an example of my taking an old-fashioned and methodologically "covert" approach to research. However, I did ask an organized part of ACT UP/LA, the WC, for permission, so I was "out" to those with whom I most frequently interacted. If I had to do it over again, given my current set of concerns and my current store of knowledge, I probably would have asked the GB for permission to record events as I saw them. I have no way of knowing if that permission would have been granted, but I suspect my request would have been met with an "okay" and a general shrug of indifference.

INTERVIEWS

I started interviewing ACT UP/LA activists in 1999, after I had left Los Angeles for a tenure track job at the State University of New York, Binghamton. In 1998, I published an article based primarily on my participant observation with the group (Roth 1998). At the same time, I was working on what would become a book on racial/ethnic dynamics in US post-war feminist movements (Roth 2004). But I never stopped thinking about my experience in ACT UP/LA, and, since by 1998, ACT UP/LA was no longer active as an organization, I decided to interview former activists about what life was like after street activism had subsided. Interviews provide invaluable understandings of the experience of activism, particularly so when combined with archival research designed to inform the interviewer and counter partial and partisan memories (Morris 1984; Blee and Taylor 2002). I conducted twenty open-ended interview sessions, with twenty-three total participants, and three more "email interviews" for a total of twenty-six participants; all but two of the interview sessions were one-on-one. Eleven activists were interviewed in 1999 and 2000, and twelve were interviewed in 2011 and 2012. The email interviews were conducted in 2012, chiefly to see if previous interviews had covered enough ground; these email interviews were not conducted in real time and were thus much shorter and less textured than the face-to-face conversations I had. I nonetheless found them valuable.

In order to find interviewees, I used a snowball sample based on my participation with ACT UP/LA. I asked interviewees via letter (for the first round) and via email (for the second round) if they were willing to be interviewed. With one exception, all interviews were taped or digitally recorded with the express written permission of the interviewee, and, as discussed earlier, real names were given and are used in this book. The interviews lasted from approximately one hour to more than three hours.

I had several theoretical questions in mind in conducting the earlier round of interviews, and these initial interests both remained and shifted over the years. Initially, I wanted to know how former militant street activists had adapted to the institutionalization of their social movement concerns; that is, how they had gone from "streets to suits." However, not all the activists I interviewed fit the pattern of transitioning into government or social service work, and yet it was clear that former activists' time with ACT UP/LA had been hugely transformative regardless of their career paths. I also wanted to know how the lesbian and gay activists from ACT UP/LA compared to other activists who had engaged in high-intensity activism (McAdam, 1989; Whalen and Flacks 1989), and I was particularly curious as to whether lesbian and gay activists paid high prices for their identities within institutions (Taylor and Raeburn 1995).

I coded the first round of interviews using a "grounded theory" approach that yielded thirty-five codes, and, in grounded theory style, I constructed "theoretical memos" for each code. As one might gather, many of the codes were not useful for this project, but the process helped me think through the material, and many codes – for example, "borders of community," "complacency/cooptation," "feminism," "race," "resources and money" – were significant in helping me decide what would go into the book.

After I interviewed twelve more ex-ACT UP/LA participants in 2011 and 2012, I took these digitally recorded interviews, semi-transcribed them, and coded them using the initial thirty-five codes. These codes' boundaries expanded somewhat to accommodate the new material, but, in the main, the initial coding seemed pretty robust. At the same time, there were significant differences in the interview process from the first round to the second. From a technological standpoint, there is no question that the development of easy, portable, digital recording technology made interviewing easier and less formal. I had conducted the first round of interviews with a large black audiocassette recorder that whirred a bit while it recorded and a large black conventional microphone set up between me and the interviewees. The quality of the sounds captured by an audiocassette recorder and mike was, to be blunt, frustrating. In contrast, the second round of interviews was conducted using a finger-length, completely silent, silver digital recorder placed discreetly by my side; the lapel microphone I used was miniscule but powerful, and I was able to persuade most interviewees to wear it. Because of the ease of digital duplication, the second set of interviewees were all sent copies of their interviews for their own personal use and for comment and correction (although, to date, none of the interviewees has chosen to comment or correct his or her interviews as a result of listening to them). The impact of digitization on conducting interviews – how or if it changes the collection of data, and especially, who owns what data in the age of digitization – is a complex question far beyond the scope of this appendix. My sense, though, is that digitization potentially opens up the interview process to more egalitarianism. For example, in 2011, one of my interviewees set up a small video camera to tape us as the interview proceeded, turning the tables on me as to whose purposes were being served by the interview. Unfortunately, the camera malfunctioned and kept turning itself off.

A second difference between the rounds of interviews had to do with their timing. Simply put, the interviews conducted in 1999 and 2000 yielded more detailed data about events: times, names, and places. Ten years later, during the second round of interviews, the emotional tenor of interviewees was distinctly different. It was as if ACT UP/LA had receded far enough into the past that it had become incorporated as part of life stories and memories that were part of the activists' bodies. Some activists' recall of details was certainly missing, but since I had spent extensive time with archival records, I was far less worried than I might have been about getting names and dates. The elegiac tone of most of the interviews was something I did not expect.

A third difference between the two rounds of interviewing, and one that I encouraged, was that the 2011–2012 interviews were also much more like conversations, more informal than the first set, although my open-ended interview schedule had barely changed. I was much more inclined during the 2011 and 2012 interviews to disclose aspects about my experiences in the group and my recall of events. This was not always a good thing. At one point, an interviewee told me "you are putting words in my mouth." That was a useful cautionary experience, and I went on to actually use the phrase as a question – "Am I putting words in your mouth?" – during subsequent interviews. But, at the same time, and much more so than in the first round, people wanted to know what I thought about things. Since I had better recall of some names and dates by virtue of my archival work, I might have appeared to be more "expert" about ACT UP/LA than the first time, and perhaps that prompted interviewees' questions.

That perceived expertise affected my "positionality" as a researcher in the interviews (McCorkel and Myers 2003), and it was in conducting interviews that I most strongly felt the influence of my intersectionally constructed social location, although not necessarily in the ways that the literature on identity politics might predict. A feminist intersectional approach to research would emphasize the interplay of, at least, race, gender, class, and sexuality in the co-construction of the interview. Some aspects of these identities were salient in the interview process, but added to the mix was my position as an academic and as a former ACT UP/LA participant. In other words, a key part of my positionality was that of "knowledgeable ex-activist"; I believe I was seen as an expert on ACT UP/LA.

The idea of the interviewer as expert necessarily implies a power differential between the interviewer and interviewee. At the same time, in ACT UP/LA, everyone was an expert on something; that was how the group functioned. Nonetheless, my standing as an academic seemed important to others during the interview process. When I began conducting interviews for this book, I was already a tenure track academic at a good public university, one whose "start up" money was funding my visits back to Los Angeles for interviews and archival work. Although, as noted earlier, my knowledge of ACT UP/LA gained through participation was necessarily partial, my archival work was giving me an overall sense of the scope of the organization's activities. Not all of the interviewees had that kind of comprehensive knowledge of the group. I believe that my institutional standing was especially significant for those activists who had gone into insider positions in government and social service; we could all relate to being part of institutions. But the "knowledge rapport" as I've come to think of it was also based on the fact that I had participated in the group; my face was recognized by some of the interviewees, my name was familiar to others, and I had my own memories of certain events.

I do not wish to argue that "knowledge rapport," or my standing as an academic, or as an ex-activist somehow trumped the inevitable effects of master statuses such as race, gender, class, and sexuality on the interview process. I do wish to argue that we think in even more concrete terms about the kinds of identities that are salient in constructing positionalities as researchers. As to those master statuses, their salience in the interview process was variable. I believe that I was read as white by the interviewees, although my race did not come up; since most of the interviewees were white, and since I am white, in most of the interviews, our racial statuses faded into the background. This did not mean that interviewees were not sensitive to the racial politics of ACT UP/LA; rather, those politics and controversies were not recapitulated in the interviews themselves. One aspect of ethnic identity that did emerge during interviews was Jewish identity; since one of the interview questions focused on how the interviewee identified in racial/ethnic terms, Jewish interviewees named themselves as Jewish, prompting a "me, too" response on my part. I cannot say that the "me, too" response was a result of my thinking through the ethics of positionality in research; rather, it's more or less what Jewish people do in social situations where one's Jewish ethnicity is not immediately apparent. As to class, although class background was also part of the interview schedule, my own class background seemed irrelevant to the interviewees. It is possible that my position as an academic stood in for whatever class background I might have come from.

Interestingly, considering how central questions of sexuality were to ACT UP/LA, my sexuality was not much of an issue for most of the interviewees. There were exceptions. One male interviewee asked me flat out how I identified, to which I answered "bisexual"; sexual experiences with women were part of my personal history, but the label "bisexual" was not one I would claim in everyday life. Two other interviewees, both women, made passing references to my sexual life, but these were fleeting enough so that they seemed unremarkable. The rest of the activists answered the question about how they identified sexually in a forthright manner and seemed unconcerned about my sexual identity as such. As I interviewed another female activist, I remembered having a conversation with her back in the 1990s about my status as a more or less straight woman in ACT UP/LA, but I did not bring the memory up to her, and thus I have no way of knowing if she remembered that conversation. My "gender presentation," to use sociologist Mignon Moore's (2011; see Chapter 2) term for how we choose to style ourselves in public, is basically "femme"; that is, someone whose presentation corresponds to mainstream ideals of feminine display. Except as noted earlier, I cannot say how my mainstream display of my gender/sexuality affected the interviews.

WEAVING TOGETHER PERSPECTIVES: FEMINIST INTERSECTIONALITY, GROUNDED THEORY, AND EXTENDED CASE METHOD AS COMPLEMENTARY RESEARCH STRATEGIES

In writing *The Life and Death of ACT UP/LA*, I have drawn from three distinct theoretical orientations: feminist intersectionality; grounded theory, first promulgated by Glaser and Strauss (2012 [1967]); and Burawoy's (1991a, 1991b) extended case method. Feminist intersectionality is discussed in some detail in Chapter 1. Therefore, in the next section, I argue for the way that feminist intersectionality can dovetail with grounded theory and extended case method. The latter two approaches to qualitative data are often counterposed to each other, chiefly because of Burawoy's critique of grounded theory; however, I found elements of each to be useful to me in conducting my research, and I found both to be compatible with a feminist intersectional approach to research.

A feminist intersectional perspective/sensibility sensitizes the researcher to the workings of power, sameness, and difference structurally and in specific social situations and guides the researcher toward taking a critical stance to constructed activist identities and political solidarities. An intersectional perspective can initiate a "process of discovery" (Davis 2008: 77) about what activists face as they act within a nested set of social milieus shaped by large-scale, long-term inequalities. That process of discovery is precisely what is appealing about Glaser and Strauss's (2012 [1967]) "grounded theory" method, and, as mentioned earlier, I took a grounded theory approach to coding my interview data.

Glaser and Strauss wrote *The Discovery of Grounded Theory* as a reaction to what they saw as the preeminence of stultifying deductive approaches to theory in the sociology of the 1960s. They argued that sociologists should do more than test received theories: "some theories of our predecessors, because of their lack of grounding in data, do not fit, or do not work, or are not sufficiently understandable to be used and are therefore useless in research" (2012[1967]: 11). Stating that "it does not take a 'genius' to generate a useful grounded theory," Glaser and Strauss argued that qualitative research could generate new theories about social phenomena that had been previously badly theorized or ignored (2012 [1967]:11). They advocated taking an inductive approach to theory generation through the close and continuous examination of data that the researcher was in the process of gathering; that is, they argued for an approach to theory that regarded "theory as process" (2012[1967]: 43). Ongoing close work would allow researchers to further refine categories of observed phenomena and would allay the critique of qualitative research as ungeneralizable beyond a specific context and unverifiable (see discussion on Glaser and Strauss, pp. 15–18).

Grounded theory had great appeal to ethnographers in sociology who were looking for ways to apply methodological rigor to their data because Glaser and Strauss gave ethnographers techniques for organizing data in a systematic way. As all data analysis involves the reduction of the data to make theoretically meaningful statements, grounded theory techniques helped qualitative researchers make sense of their data because their methods of participant observations and interviewing generated "too much" data. Above all, Glaser and Strauss insisted that grounded theory could, to use a current phrase, help sociologists "think outside the box." They give an instructive example of the problem of thinking inside the box, taking to task a study on women's prisons that only seeks to "verify" Erving Goffman's theory of the total institution:

An instructive example [on the limits of verification] is *Women's Prison*; the authors have simplistically assumed that since the theory about prisons is based on men's institutions, a study of a women's prison will both qualify the theory – by pointing up differences between men's and women's prisons – and support the theory by underlining similarities between the prisons. They do not, however, understand that such a comparison limits them to generating theory within the framework of existing theory, nor do they recognize that more effective comparative analysis would permit them to transcend it. (2012 [1967]: 255–256)

I see a strong similarity between Glaser and Strauss's cautionary words about "generating theory within the framework of existing theory" and the challenges to existing theories about inequalities issued by feminist intersectional analysts. Collectively, those in intersectionality studies are critical of received wisdom about the social construction of inequalities and advocate new thinking about interaction among structured inequalities. Thus, performing intersectional analysis via grounded theory techniques is viable research strategy for the feminist intersectional researcher.

By the 1990s, some social scientists worried that grounded theory itself had limitations, chief among them Michael Burawoy. Burawoy's work focused chiefly on questions of class and interactions in industrial workspaces. In his ethnographic work, he argued for using what he called "extended case method" to understand ethnographic data. While Burawoy welcomed grounded theory's engagement in the making of new theory based on empirical cases, he critiqued it as simultaneously too "micro" and too abstract in its approach to ethnographic research. In Burawoy's view, it was possible for the ethnographer to keep a focus on a single micro site in all its complexity while, at the same time, using the site to learn about "a larger set of structural dynamics and relationships" (1991a: 5). For Burawoy, the researcher should not lose sight of how any specific social situation is shaped by external forces; she or he should use a sociological imagination, a la C. Wright Mills, in order to connect "'the personal troubles of the milieu' to 'the public issues of social structure'" (1991a: 6). And, in contrast to grounded theory's emphasis on the generation of new theory, Burawoy was specifically interested in using ethnography to reconstruct existing theory (1991b: 279). As Burawoy explained, "(t)he importance of a single case lies in what it tells us about society as a whole rather than about the population of similar cases" (1991b: 281). In a similar way, feminist intersectional theorists advocated for the theoretical reconstruction of received categories explaining macro-level inequalities, with particular attention paid to the co-construction of categories (McCall 2005).

In addition to the reconstruction of extant theories, Burawoy asserted that extended case method could construct what he called "genetic" explanations for social phenomena; that is, "explanations of particular outcomes" – he saw this as a different aim than grounded theory's expressed goal of providing new "generic" explanations of invariant laws of interaction that obtain in a similar set of social situations (1991b: 280). Obviously, to a historically minded researcher, this emphasis on the genetic explanation of outcomes over the generic delineation of social laws is attractive. I would argue that, in intersectionality studies, researchers tend to reject new explanations of generic laws of social interaction in favor of looking for genetic explanations of particular and contingent outcomes that result from actors' continuously re-enacted relationships of co-constructed unequal power.

Without homogenizing the differences between grounded theory and extended case method, and without arguing that they are both subsumed under feminist intersectional analysis, I will simply note that, in conducting my research on ACT UP/LA, I found both grounded theory and extended case method to be valuable in the research process and valuable for looking at archival and interview data as well as ethnographic material. The "generic" and "genetic" oscillated in considering what happened in ACT UP/LA. As for the generic, it was clear to me that intersectionally constituted structures of inequality predated the formation of ACT UP/LA – indeed, necessitated the formation of ACT UP/LA – and that these same inequalities manifested themselves within the group, sometimes generating explicit efforts to fight inequality and sometimes going unmarked. Grounded theory guided me through the surfeit of information that I had from participant observation, archival work, and interviews with former ACT UP/LA activists. Glaser and Strauss's powerful idea of "theory in process" helped me focus on the question of the dynamics of interaction within ACT UP/LA even as every new piece of data shifted the picture of the group that I had to that point; grounded theory techniques helped me to refocus earlier emphases in this iterated project as I shifted from concerns with transitions from militant street activism to institutional activism, to a desire to understand the role of inequalities in social movement activism. Additionally, the emphasis in grounded theory on the "new" helped me to continuously think about countering received wisdom about the ACT UPs as a social movement.

Extended case method helped make sense of the "genetic" possibilities for explanation in exploring the trajectory of ACT UP/LA as a social movement organization. Extended case method's focus on explaining outcomes over time made the method congruent with historical study and the use of archival material. My view of interactions in ACT UP/LA having been impacted by large-scale social forces of gender and other intersecting inequalities is squarely in line with Burawoy's argument that exploring a micro-site in rich detail can uncover information about the macro, about how large-scale social forces operate. Much of what I attempt in this book is exactly an explanation of ACT UP/LA's trajectory as a social movement organization as a result of endemic and, to some extent, intractable pressures generated by social inequalities.

To summarize, in writing about ACT UP/LA, I have used multiple sources of data – archival research, participant observation, and interviews – that I believe complement each other. I have also drawn from critical methodological traditions – feminist intersectionality, ground theory, and extended case method – that, while remaining distinct, have points of overlap that have helped guide me as a researcher. It is my hope that in drawing on multiple methods and multiple critical traditions, I have managed to tell a coherent and consequential story about ACT UP/LA's life and death.

References

PRIMARY SOURCES

Interviews by author with former ACT UP/LA activists, listed in chronological order.

1999–2000

Jan Speller, July 13, 2000, San Francisco, CA.
J. T. Anderson, Stephanie Boggs,[a] and Peter Cashman, July 23, 1999, West Hollywood, CA.
Jeri Deitrick, July 26, 2000, Los Angeles, CA.
Phill Wilson, July 26, 1999, Los Feliz, CA.
Mary Lucey, July 29, 1999, Los Angeles, CA.
Nancy MacNeil, July 29, 1999, Los Angeles, CA.
Ferd Eggan,[b] July 30, 1999, Los Angeles, CA.
Judy Sisneros, August 1, 2000, Los Angeles, CA.
Gunther Freehill,[c] August 4, 2000, Los Angeles, CA.

[a] Stephanie Boggs died in April of 2010 of metastasized breast cancer.
[b] Ferd Eggan died in 2007 of liver cancer.
[c] Gunther Freehill died in 2013 of heart failure.

2011–2012

Walter "Cat" Walker, May 12, 2011, West Hollywood, CA.
Genevieve Clavreul, May 15, 2011, Pasadena, CA.
Richard "Doe" Racklin, May, 17, 2011, West Hollywood, CA.
Jeff Scheurholz and Peter Jimenez,[d] May 18, 2011, Los Angeles, CA.
Doug Sadownick, May 18, 2011, Culver City, CA.

Helene Schpak, May 18, 2011, Glassell Park, CA.
Ty Geltmaker, May 21, 2011, Silverlake, CA.
Wendell Jones, May 23, 2011, West Hollywood, CA.
James Rosen, January 14, 2012, Los Angeles, CA
Terri Ford, January 17, 2012, Los Angeles, CA.
Brian Pomerantz, January 17, 2012, Los Angeles, CA (not recorded).

d Pete Jimenez died of AIDS in May 2012.

August 2012
Interviews conducted via email, with date indicating individuals' responses to emailed questions.

Jake Epstine, August 4, 2012, from Los Angeles CA.
Larry Holmes, August 10, 2012, from Portland, OR.
John Fall, August 20, 2012, from Portland, OR.

Field notes
I took field notes on meetings (General Body, Women's Caucus, Treatment and Data), events, and actions from November 1990 to mid-1992. The following notes are cited in the text:

Women's Caucus meeting, November 11, 1990; "Women and AIDS" Teach-in, November 17, 1990; Women's Caucus meeting, November 25, 1990; Women's Caucus meeting, November 30, 1990; Women's Caucus meeting, December 1, 1990; General Body meeting, December 10, 1990; Women's Caucus meeting, December 23, 1990; General Body meeting, January 7, 1991; General Body meeting, January 14, 1991; Women's Caucus meeting, January 27, 1991.

BROADCAST

January 30, 2009. "Martin Delaney 1945–2009." "The Rachel Maddow Show," MSNBC. Available online at http://www.bing.com/videos/watch/video/martin-delaney-1945–2009/687ciy8.

Archival Collections
I used documents from my own collection (1990–1992) and from the ONE National Gay & Lesbian Archives at the USC Libraries (see http://one.usc.edu or www.onearchives.org). Documents from the ONE Archive came from either of two collections: the ACT UP/LA Collection, which was uncatalogued at the time that I looked through it, and the AIDS History Project Collection, which was a broader, catalogued collection of documents relevant to the history of AIDS. Documents listed here are from the ONE collections unless noted.

ACT UP/LA Minutes
Between my collection and the material at the ONE Archive, I was able to review approximately 90 percent of ACT UP/LA's General Body meeting

minutes. Minutes from those and other committee meetings on the following dates were used in the text:

From the "General Body meetings": January 25, 1988; March 14, 1988; March 28, 1988; June 13, 1988; July 11, 1988; September 12, 1988; September 26, 1988; January 7, 1991; January 21, 1991; February 25, 1991 (Author's collection); April 4, 1991 (Author's collection); June 3, 1991 (Author's collection); January 20, 1992; February 17, 1992; March 8, 1992; March 23, 1992; April 6, 1992; April 13, 1992; April 20, 1992; June 15, 1992; July 13, 1992; July 20, 1992; July 27, 1992; August 24, 1992; August 31, 1992; September 21, 1992; October 19, 1992; October 26, 1992; December 7, 1992; January 4, 1993; January 18, 1993; February 8, 1993; February 15, 1993; March 8, 1993; March 29, 1993; May 3, 1993; January 3, 1994; April 11, 1994; August 1, 1994; August 8, 1994; August 15, 1994; December 5, 1994; April 17, 1995; May, 16, 1995; June 5, 1995; April 1, 1996; April 8, 1996.

From Women's Caucus meetings: October 28, 1990 (Author's collection). From the Coordinating Committee: July 5, 1992.

ACT UP/LA Position Papers/Reports
Position papers and reports were given/handed out at ACT UP/LA meetings. Some were signed by authors. Where there is no author listed, authorship is attributed to "ACT UP/LA."

ACT UP/LA. 1988. "The New INS vs. Lady Liberty," c. January.
ACT UP/LA. 1988. "Appendix Bathhouse Background in the Context of the AIDS Epidemic." Three-page unsigned document, c. February.
ACT UP/LA. 1990. "Sexism in ACT UP/LA," c. late January 1990.
ACT UP/LA. 1990. Report on "Minutes – ACT-Now General Membership Meeting in Chicago – April 22, 1990."
ACT UP/LA. 1991. "Needle Exchange Program," c. March. Author's collection.
ACT UP/LA. 1991. "What Is Youth Action?" October 21. Author's collection.
ACT UP/LA. 1992. "CNN/ Clean Needles Now" statement, c. April.
ACT UP/LA.1992. "Confrontation, Then Mediation: ACT UP/LA, NME, and Medical Apartheid." Anonymously (co?-) authored report, c. May.
ACT UP/LA.1992. "Scattering Activist Ashes to Save County AIDS Clinic 5p21," June 30.
ACT UP/LA Treatment and Data Committee. 1991. "Current Scope of Need," January 4. Author's collection.
ACT UP/LA Treatment and Data Committee. 1991. "ACT UP/LA Treatment & Data Committee Treatment Issues Report." Number 8, August 19.
ACT UP/LA Treatment and Data Committee. 1990. "ACT UP/Los Angeles Treatment and Data Committee Treatment Primer" table of contents, c. December. Author's collection.

Alternative Budget Coalition. 1990. "The "A,B,C'S" of the LA County Budget," c. June.

Bloor, Jim. 1992. "A Sort-of Rebuttal to Last Week's 'How ACT UP/LA Is Losing Its Power,'" position paper dated April 13.

Burke, Jim. 1998. "An Open Letter to the Community," c. February.

Chang, Henry. 1992. "Let the Needles Do the Talking!" CNN/Clean Needles Now position paper, April 20, 1992.

CNN/Clean Needles Now. 1992. "Policy Statement on Needle Exchange, Harm Reduction, and Treatment on Demand," April.

Cook, Gregory. 1992. "ACT UP LA at the National Democratic Convention," Report, July 27.

Day, Larry, Ed Williams, and Brad Confer (Education Committee of ACT UP/LA). 1988. "ACT UP/LA Position Paper: Los Angeles County Bathhouse Closure," February 29.

Freehill, Gunther. 1990. "On Negotiation," July 30.

Fuller, Doug, and Tay Ashton. 1991. "Coalitioning," c. November 1991.

Geltmaker, Ty. 1991. "Hospital Update," June 10. Author's collection.

Kimball, John. 1992. "The Trouble with ACT UP/Los Angeles," c. June.

Kostopoulos, Mark. 1990. "Sexism Discussion," February 5.

    1990. "On Tactics: For ACT UP Members Only, Not To Be Reprinted," July.

    1991. "Red Hot and Blue," February 11. Author's collection.

    1992. "How ACT UP/LA Is Losing Its Power," April 6.

Lacaillade, David (for the Retreat Working Group). 1992. "Retreat." Packet including sign up sheets, c. late February/March 1992.

    1992. "Small Bandages on Large Wounds: Reporting on the Second Gates Meeting Concerning AIDS Care at LA County/USC Medical Center," October 9.

    1993. "Two Meetings and a Third Postponed: Reorganizing the Council and Identifying New Principals in AIDS Care at LAC/USC Medical Center," February.

    c. July 1993. "They Still Lie." Report to the General Body of ACT UP/LA.

Meyer, Amy. 1991. Report on "ACT UP Action Network Conference Call," July 10.

Mirken, Bruce. 1990. "Should ACT UP Negotiate?" c. July.

Richards, Wade. 1990. "Girl! Where in the World Did You Get That White Sheet? Or What Did Wade Really Say at the ACT UP/LA Retreat?" December.

Richards, Wade, and David Lacaillade. 1992. "ACT UP/LA Retreat." March.

Rouse, Bill, and Mickey Wheatley, Craig Carson, and Dwayne Turner. 1990. "Let's Not Negotiate Our Silence: Silence = Death," July 16.

Simmons, Mark, and David Brown. 1991. "ACT-UP/Los Angeles' Network & Outreach Six Months Goal Setting Strategy," July 1. Author's collection.

Simmons, Mark, and Members of ACT UP's People of Color Caucus. 1991. "Report from Seattle," c. December.

Wheatley, Mickey, and Bill Rouse. 1990. "Let's Not Make a Pact with the Devil," July 23.

Wheatley, Mickey, Darren Goldstein, and Michael Albanese. 1990. "Finally, Health Care for ACT UP." Position paper dated August 27, 1990.

Wildes, Lee, and Steven Corbin. 1992. "ACT UP – Get Moving!" June 23.

ACT UP/LA Newsletter Articles
Listed by author; if unsigned, author is listed as "ACT UP/LA."

ACT UP/LA. 1988. "Emergency Community Meeting." *ACT UP/LA* 1: 9, November/December, pp. 5–6.

ACT UP/LA. 1988. "Condensation of Demands to be Presented to the County as Formulated by Being Alive." *ACT UP/LA* 1:9, November/December, pp. 3–4.

ACT UP/LA. 1989. "Vigil Support." *ACT UP/LA* 2:1, February/March, p. 3.

ACT UP/LA. 1989. "Times Is Up!" *ACT UP/LA* 2:2, April/May.

ACT UP/LA. 1992. "CNN/Clean Needles Now (ACT UP/LA) Policy Statement on Needle Exchange, Harm Reduction and Treatment on Demand." *ACT UP/LA News* 5:1, March/April, p. 9.

Anderson, J. T. 1995. "ACT UP/LA Speaks at Candlelight March." ACT UP/LA Newsletter, Winter, p. 4.

Beecher, Richard. 1989. "ACT UP Throws a Piece of the Rock!" *ACT UP/LA* 2:6, December 1989/January 1990, pp. 1–2, 12.

Bledsoe, Joe. 1990. "From the Inside Looking Out." *ACT UP/LA News* 2:6, December 1989/January 1990, p. 8.

Boggs, Stephanie Alana. 1995. "World AIDS Day Demonstration." ACT UP/LA *Newsletter*, Winter, pp. 1, 5.

Cashman, Peter. 1988. "ACT UP Fights Lying Down." *ACT UP/LA* 1:6, August, p. 3.

Day, Larry. 1988. "What a Week It Was!" *ACT UP/LA* 1:4, June, p. 3.

1989. "ACT UP/LA Attends LAC/USC AIDS Community Advisory Council Meeting." *ACT UP/LA* 2:3, July.

1990. "Campaign Continues." *ACT UP/LA* 3:4, August/September, p. 2.

Eggan, Ferd. 1990. "ACT NOW to Network." *ACT UP/LA* 3:5, October/November, p. 9.

Fall, John. 1988. "A Brief Personal View of the Happenings in Washington October 8–11." *ACT UP/LA* 1:8, October, p. 4.

Farrell, Kevin. 1990. "Why Stop the Rose Parade?" *ACT UP/LA* 3:1, February/March, p. 3.

Ford, Terri, and Judy Sisneros. 1991. "Lights! Camera! AIDS Action Now! ACT UP Hits the Oscars." *ACT UP/LA News* 4: 2, April/May, p. 1.

Freehill, Gunther. 1990. "After the Boycott." *ACT UP/LA News* 3:4, August/September, p. 10.

Iosty, Richard. 1992. "Magic Johnson and the Spectacle of Male Heterosexual Sentimentality." *ACT UP/LA News* 4:5, December 1991/January 1992, p. 4.

Kostopoulos, Mark. 1988. "People with AIDS: Care and Uncaring." *ACT UP LA* 1:3, April/May, p. 4.

———. 1988. "ACT UP/LA's January Action." *ACT UP/LA* 1:9, November/December, p. 3.

———. 1989. "Montreal AIDS Conference." *ACT UP/LA* 2:3 Newsletter, July, p. 10.

McDaniel, Jim. 1991. "Interview with three founding members of ACT UP/LA." *ACT UP/LA News* 4:5, December 1991/January 1992, pp. 6–7.

Morello, Enric. 1988. "We've Won an AIDS Ward." *ACT UP/LA* 1:7, September, pp. 1–2.

———. 1989. "From the Editor." *ACT UP/LA* 2:1, February/March, p. 2.

Lacaillade, David. 1991. "Back to the Rose Parade: American Are Still Dying for Health Care." *ACT UP/LA News* 4:1, January/February, p. 6.

———. 1991. "Shrine Tours Interrupts Oscars, ACT UP/LA Member Arrested." *ACT UP News* 4:2, April/May, p. 6.

———. 1992. "While County Fiddles, People Die." *ACT UP/LA News* 5:3, Fall.

Merkin, Bruce. 1991. " 'AIDS Is a Disaster! Prisoners Die Faster!'" *ACT UP/LA News* 4:3, June/July, p. 1.

Norman, Connie. 1990. "LA County Board of Stupes." *ACT UP/LA* 3:5, October/November, p. 5.

Podolsky, Robin, 1989. "Shutting Down the Feds." *ACT UP/LA* 2:6, December 1989/January 1990.

Puente, Michael. 1988. "AIDS in the Latino Community." *ACT UP/LA Newsletter* 1:3, April/May, pp. 5–6.

Reece, Ray. 1990. "Déjà vu: Back to the Baths." *ACT UP/LA* 3:5, October/November, p. 14.

Roy, Chris. 1989. "Health Services Action." *ACT UP/LA* 2:2, April/May.

Satterlees, Mark. 1991. "Inter/Views You." *ACT UP/LA News* 4:2, April/May p. 3

Schuerholz, Jeff, and Philip Tarley. 1992. "Jailtime in Houston." *ACT UP/LA News* 5:3, Fall, pp. 4–5.

Schpak, Helene. 1992. "Mark Kostopoulos October 26, 1954–June 20, 1992." *ACT UP/LA News* 5:3, p. 3.

Schultz, Randy. 1988. "AIDS and People of Color." *ACT UP/LA Newsletter* 1:3, April/May, p. 5.

Simmons, Mark. 1991. "People of Color AIDS Activist Conference." *ACT UP/LA News* 4:3, June/July, p. 8.

———. 1991. "AB 101, Race and AIDS." *ACT UP/LA News* 4:5, December 1990/January 1991, p. 3.

Sisneros, Judy 1990. "Women's Caucus Report." *ACT UP/LA Newsletter* 3:4, August/September, p. 15.

speller, jan [sic]. 1990. "Women Demand Action." *ACT UP/LA* 3:4, August/ September, p. 8.

Tausner, Mauri. 1991. "93 Arrested in National CDC Action." *ACT UP/LA News* 4:1, January/February, p. 3.

Yellowbird, Ellen. 1991. "Frontera: The Struggle for Humane Conditions Continues." *ACT UP/LA News* 4:1, January/February, pp. 1, 8.

ACT UP/LA Ephemera: Almost of all these documents are unsigned and thus authorship is attributed to "ACT UP/LA." They are listed chronologically.

ACT UP California. 1991. " Prisoners & AIDS: Some Facts." handout c. May. Author's collection.

    1991. "ACT UP Demands." Flyer c. May. Author's collection.

ACT UP/LA. 1987. "Bring the Spirit of Washington Home!" Flyer, December.

ACT UP LA. 1987. "Agenda for 12/4/85" [sic].

ACT UP/LA. 1988. "Demonstration Against AIDS Hysteria and for Lesbian and Gay Rights." Unsigned press release c. January.

ACT UP/LA. 1989. Agenda, July 31.

ACT UP/LA. 1989. "Proposal for Fall Action." August 7.

ACT UP/LA. 1989. "ACT UP Attacks Archbishop's Reversal on Safe Sex Education." Press release dated December 8.

ACT UP/LA. 1990. "ACT UP/LA Structure." March.

ACT UP/LA. 1990. "National AIDS Actions for Healthcare." Flyer/schedule regarding Chicago events, April 20–23.

ACT UP/LA. c. 1990. "A Very Brief History of ACT UP/Los Angeles." July. Author's collection.

ACT UP/LA. 1990. "Week of Outrage/ November 26–December 3, 1990." Author's collection.

ACT UP/LA. 1991. "Proposal for National Action." c. February. Author's collection.

ACT UP/LA. 1991. "Proposed Response to RHB Letter." c. February.

ACT UP/LA. 1991. "Attention New Members." March, Author's collection.

ACT UP/LA. 1991. Flyer announcing May 6 Sacramento protest. Author's collection.

ACT UP/LA. 1991. "This Clinic Is Built on a Fault." Leaflet, June 3.

ACT UP/LA. 1991. "Rally A.B. 101." Flyer, June. Author's collection.

ACT UP/LA. 1991. "AB 101 Letter Writing Guide." c. June. Author's collection.

ACT UP/LA. 1991. "What Does It Take to Make You Angry?" Flyer, c. August.

ACT UP/LA. 1991. "ACT UP/LA Condemns Cardinal Roger Mahony's Censorship." Press release, c. August.

ACT UP/LA. 1992. "Dateline: 21–27 January 1989." Reprint of article from the AIDS Project LA Newsletter, as part of the *From the Archives* series.

ACT UP/LA. 1992. "Public Policy Survey." January.

ACT UP/LA. 1992. General Body Meeting Agenda, March 2. Author's collection.

ACT UP/LA. 1992. "CNN Needle Exchange Budget Expenditures – 1 Year of Distribution: May 1, 1992–May 1, 1993." c. April.

ACT UP/LA. 1992. "ACT UP/LA's 1992 Reality Ball." May 20.

ACT UP/LA. 1992. "ACT UP/LA Media Advisory: AIDS Budget Cuts – Press Conference." June 9.

ACT UP/LA. 1992. "Day of RAGE!" Flyer, dated June 29.

ACT UP/LA.1992. "Media Advisory: AIDS Budget Cuts Protest." June 30.

ACT UP/LA. 1992. "What's Wrong with This Picture." Flyer about County/USC Hospital. c. February. Author's collection.

ACT UP/LA. 1992. "NME University Hospital … Is Breaking Our Hearts." Flyer. c. February.

ACT UP/LA. 1992. "ACT UP Camps!" Sign-in sheet, March.

ACT UP/LA. 1992. CNN [Clean Needles Now]. Press Release, March 23.

ACT UP/LA, c. 1992. "County AIDS Fact Sheet." July.

ACT UP/LA. 1992. "Demand a Cure for AIDS!" Press Release, September 26.

ACT UP/LA. 1992. "Ad Hoc Financial Status Committee." October 12.

ACT UP/LA. 1993. "ACT UP/LA May Be Bankrupt within Two Weeks." February.

ACT UP/LA. c. 1993. "ACT UP Visits Amgen: Because AIDS Is Big Business But Who's Making a Killing? Press release/informational packet. March.

ACT UP/LA. 1993. "ACT UP Goes to Washington." April.

ACT UP/LA. 1993. "ACT UP Itinerary in DC." April.

ACT UP/LA. c. 1993. "ACT UP Itinerary in DC." c. April.

ACT UP/LA. c. 1993. "ACT UP Marches on Washington." Press Release, c. April.

ACT UP/LA. 1993. "Support Lesbians with AIDS." Multi-page publicity/information packet, April 23.

ACT UP/LA. 1993. "ACT UP/Los Angeles to Demand Lesbians with AIDS Research at Health and Human Services." Press Release, dated April 19.

ACT UP/LA. 1993. Letter signed by "The General Membership ACT UP/LA." to "Jeff and Gabriel." September 27.

ACT UP/LA 1996. Email "RED HOT MONEY." April 10.

ACT UP/LA. 1996. "ACT UP Zaps President Clinton at Hollywood Gala! AIDS Activists Charge: "Four Years of Broken Promises." Press Release, dated September 13.

ACT UP/LA People of Color Committee. 1992. People of Color Committee Working Document, April 6.

Beeker, Richard L., and Joshua Wells, 1991. "Dear Friend." Letter, September.

Geltmaker, Ty, and James Rosen. 1991. "Scoundrel Time, or, The Silence of the Moles." Letter dated August 19.

Kostopoulos, Mark et al. 1991. "Creation of a 'Red Hot and Blue' Committee." Letter dated July 12.

1991. "Letter to ACT UP/Network Members." July 13.

Perkins, David Lee. 1990. "Press Release for Frontera." November 30. Author's collection.

Non-ACT UP/LA Documents
Listed by author.
ACT UP/DC. 1991. "Time to Become an AIDS Activist." Flyer, September.
ACT UP Network. 1991. "Universal Health Care: A Handbook for Activists."
    October. Author's collection.
ACT UP/NY. 1991. "The 2nd ATAC 72 Hrs of AIDS Treatment Activism."
    Flyer, c. September.
ACT UP National Women's Network. 1993. Letter, "Dear Friends." March 29.
ACT UP National Women's Network. 1993. "Support Lesbians with AIDS."
    Packet, April.
Arias, Yolanda. 1991. Letter to ACT UP/LA, September 13.
ATAC 2. 1991. "About the Strategy Sessions." Flyer, c. September.
Eggan, Ferd. 1992. Letter from Community Development Department to
    "AIDS Service Organizations." October 29.
Fowler, Brad. 1989. "Los Angeles County Health Care: A Fashion Victim." Set
    of ten postcards/color photos in art paper envelope credited to "Stiffsheets:
    Brad Fowler."
Gates, Robert C. 1988. Memorandum dated September 23 from Director of
    Health Services, Los Angeles County to Los Angeles County Supervisors.
Nowlin, Eric and Ann Northrup. 1991. "Red, Hot and Blue Letter to all ACT
    UPs." April 14. Author's collection.
Queer Nation. 1991. "Do You Care Enough About Your Rights to Make a Few
    Simple Phone Calls?" Flyer c., May. Author's collection.
S.A.N.O.E. 1990. "AIDS Activists to Stop Rose Parade." Press Release,
    January 1.,
Shapiro, Steven, 1996. Emails,. "Re: RED HOT MONEY." April 7, April 11.

PUBLISHED PRIMARY SOURCES: BOOKS, COLLECTIONS, AND
ARTICLES BY ACTIVISTS

The ACT UP/NY Women & AIDS Book Group. 1990. *Women, AIDS and
    Activism*. Boston: South End Press.
Cox, Cece, Lisa Means, and Lisa Pope. 1993. *One Million Strong: The 1993
    March on Washington for Lesbian, Gay, and Bi Equal Rights*. Boston:
    Alyson Press.
Crimp, Douglas with Adam Rolston. 1990. *AIDS Demographics*. Seattle: Bay
    Press.
Geltmaker, Ty. 1992. "The Queer Nation Acts Up: Health Care, Politics, and
    Sexual Diversity in the County of Angels." *Society and Space* 10, pp.
    609–650.
Leonard, Z. 1990. Lesbians in the AIDS crisis. Pp. 27–30 in *Women, AIDS and
    Activism*, edited by The ACT UP/NY Women and AIDS Book Group.
    Boston: South End Press.

Lurie, R. 1990. Translating issues into actions: Introduction. Pp. 135–138 in *Women, AIDS and Activism*, edited by The ACT UP/NY Women and AIDS Book Group. Boston: South End Press.

NEWSPAPER AND PERIODICAL ARTICLES

Listed by author.

Altman, Lawrence K. 1993. "Widened Definition of AIDS Leads to More Reports of It." *The New York Times*, April 30.

Askari, Emilia. 1989. "Officers in Gloves Jail 80 at AIDS Protest: Activists Angry with Inaction by Federal Officials." *Herald Examiner*, October 7.

Barker, Karlyn. 1991., "Taking AIDS Battle to Capitol Hill." *The Washington Post*, September 29.

Barro, Josh. 2014. "Drug to Lower H.I.V. Risk Has Lone Public Naysayer." *The New York Times*, Monday November 17, p. a16.

Behrens, Steve. 1991. "Cardinal Blasts Airing of Documentary: Like Some Viewers, He's No Fan of Point-of-View Shows." *Current*, September 9, accessed online March 3, 2013, at http://www.current.org/wp-content/themes/current/archive-site.

Berke, Richard L. 1991. "AIDS Battle Reverting to 'Us Against Them.'" *The New York Times*, October 6.

Bernstein, Sharon. 1991. "'Stop the Church' to Be Part of KCET Special." *Los Angeles Times*, August 21.

    1991. "KCET Pays Price in Flap with Church." *Los Angeles Times*, October 10, pp. F1, F10

Cenziper, Debbie. 2009. "Investigation: Earmarked AIDS Funds Lack Oversight." *The Washington Post*, October 19.

Cimons, Marlene. 1990. "Activists Call for Expanded Definition of AIDS in Women." *Los Angeles Times*, December 27, p. A5.

Clark, Jeff. 1991. "LA Streets Still Sizzle." *Vanguard*, 2:16 October 18, p. 1.

Clark, Keith. 1991. "Near Riot in San Francisco." *Vanguard News and Reviews*, 11:15 October 4, p. 1.

Coady, Elizabeth. 1990. "300 Protest Definition of AIDS: ACT UP Group Claims CDC Is 'Killing Women.'" *Atlanta Journal and Constitution*. December 4, p. D-2.

Cockburn, Alexander. 1991. "Unchallenged, the Censors Will Prevail." *Los Angeles Times* September 20.

Dawes, Amy, and Claudia Elle. 1991. "Security Tight, Skies Clear, Traffic Smooth at Shrine." *Daily Variety*, March 3.

Dawsey, Darrell. 1989. "80 Arrested as AIDS Protest Is Broken Up." *Los Angeles Times*, October 7.

Dyer, R. A. 1992. "Dark Clouds Form for GOP Convention." *The Houston Chronicle*, February 20, p. A17.

Ford, Terri. 1991."'Stop the Church' Stop the Censorship." *Frontiers*, September 13, p. 27.

Fox, David J. 1990. "Star Studded AIDS Fundraiser." *Los Angeles Times*, September 7. Accessed July 10, 2012, at http://articles.latimes.com/1990–09-07/entertainment/ca-778_1_aids-research.

Freehill, Gunther, and Eliseo Acevedo Martinez. 1991. "Blasphemy, Lies, Videotape: The Encounter Over AIDS: Public TV." *Los Angeles Times*, September 13.

Fritsch, Jane. 1990. "Activist Replaces Ailing City AIDS Coordinator." *Los Angeles Times*, October 2, p. B7.

Frosch, Dan. 2013. "Navajo Confront an Increase in New H.I.V. Infections." *The New York Times*, May 20, p. A12.

Furillo, Andy, Robert Davilla, and Patrick Hoge. 1991. "Downtown Engulfed by Gay Protest." *The Sacramento Bee*, October 11, p. 1.

Gonzalez, Cristina. 2011. "In Sickness and in Health: Love, Marriage, a Baby Carriage and ... HIV?" *Real Health* 25 Spring p. 9.

Grimaldi, James V., and Donna Wares. 1990. "Frontera Wants Doctor Charged." *Orange County Register*, December 6, pp. 1, 26.

Groopman, Jerome. 2014. "Can AIDS be Cured?" *The New Yorker*, December 22 and 29, pp. 78–96.

Gunnison, Robert B. 1991. "Gay Rights Protest at State Capitol." *The San Francisco Chronicle*, October 12, p. 1.

Harris, Scott. 1991. "Gay Protests Spreads to LA Airport." *Los Angeles Times*, October 10, pp. B1, B3.

1992. "Freed AIDS Patient Seeks Prison Reform." *Los Angeles Times*, April 2, p. B2

Hudson, Berkley. 1992. "Shouting Unravels Press Conference." *Los Angeles Times*, October 19, pp. B1, B3.

Lacey, Marc. 1992. "Riot Death Toll Lowered to 51 After Coroner's Review." *Los Angeles Times*, August 12.

Leonard, Jack. 2005. "County Removes 7-Year Chief of AIDS Program." *The Los Angeles Times*, May 17.

Los Angeles Times. 1989. "Edelman Backs Bigger AIDS Ward in Speech at Vigil Site." January 29.

Los Angeles Times. 1991. "Letters to the Times: Controversy over ACT UP Film." *Los Angeles Times*, September 13.

Los Angeles Times. 1991. "Commentary: Catholic Policy on AIDS Programs: Acts of War or Love?" October 5, p. F14.

Los Angeles Times. 1994. "Dave Johnson, 39: LA's First AIDS Coordinator, Writer on Gay Issues." Unsigned obituary, October 29.

Los Angeles Times. 1996. Staff and Wire Reports: "Luminaries Toast Ronald Reagan's 85th Birthday." February 7. http://articles.latimes.com/1996–02-07/local/me-33261_1_ronald-reagan. Accessed July 16, 2012.

Martinez, Al. 1989. "Peter and the Dilletante." *Los Angeles Times*, June 3.

McGreevy, Patrick. 1990. "Founder of Black Gay Group to Become City Coordinator." *The Daily News*, September 22, p. 3.

McNeil Jr., Donald G. 2011. "New HIV Cases Remain Steady Over a Decade." *The New York Times*, August 4, p. A16.

2013. "H.I.V. Concern Rises Along with Unprotected Sex." *The New York Times*, September 29, p. A4.

2014. "Are We Ready for H.I.V.'s Sexual Revolution." *New York Times*, May 25, pp. SR 6–7.

2014. "AIDS Progress in Peril." *The New York Times*, Tuesday August 26, p. D1.

Merina, Victor. 1989. "15 Seized in AIDS Sit-In at Board Meeting. *The Los Angeles Times*, May 17.

Mirken, Bruce. 1991. "Needles as an A.I.D.S. Tack." *Los Angeles Reader*, March 22: 8.

1991. "Needle Vote Nettles Antonovich." *Los Angeles Reader*, March 29: 5.

1991. "Best ACT UP Award at the Oscars Show." *Los Angeles Reader*, March 29.

Muir, Frederick, and Charisse Jones. 1991. "Police on Horseback Break Up Gay Protest." *The Los Angeles Times*, October 24, p. B1.

Newton, Edmund. 1990. "'Supervisors' Rip Priorities of Real Board." *Los Angeles Times*, June 10. Accessed June 18, 2012, http://articles.latimes.com/1990–06-10/local/me-415_1_board-meeting.

Ohland, Gloria. 1992. "The Eye of the Needle." *LA Weekly*, September 4–September 10, pp. 14–15.

Oldham, Jennifer. 1994. "Condom Nation: Controversy Draws Safe-Sex Activists to High School." *Los Angeles Times*, March 31.

Pollack, Andrew. 2012. "F.D.A. Approves Once-a-Day Pill for H.I.V." *The New York Times*, August 28, p. B4.

Pyle, Amy. "Clean Needles Put Into War on AIDS." *The Los Angeles Times*, September 9, 1992, pp. B1, B4

Reich, Kenneth. 1995. "Study Raises Northridge Quake Death Toll to 72." *Los Angeles Times*, December 20. http://articles.latimes.com/1995–12-20/news/mn-16032_1_quake-death-toll

Rourke, Anne C. 1990. "Research Office for Women's Health Answers Complaint of Bias in Research." *Los Angeles Times*, November 11, pp. A1, 40.

Sadownick, Doug. 1989. "ACT UP and the Politics of AIDS." *LA Weekly* October 6–October 12, pp. 20–25.

1990. "ACTing UP Against the Health-Care System: National AIDS activists' Conference Debates Tactics." *LA Weekly*, May 4–10, p. 12.

1990. "AIDS Treatment, Steerage Class: AIDS Programs for Women in and out of Prison, Say Critics, Are Nonexistent or Worse." *LA Weekly*, November 30–December 6.

Simon, Richard. 1990. "27 Arrested in Protest to County Over AIDS Budget." The *Los Angeles Times*, May 23.

Simon, Stephanie. 1993. "AIDS Activists Decry Cost of Drug at Amgen Offices." *Los Angeles Times*, March 4.

Solis-Marich, Mario. 1991. "The New Movement Must Empower People of Color." *Vanguard* 2:16 October 18, pp. 6–7.

Stein, Jeanine. 1990. "Stars Turn Out to Support AIDS Benefit." *Los Angeles Times*, September 10. Accessed July 10, 2012, at http://articles.latimes .com/1990–09-10/news/vw-76_1_aids-benefit.

Tobar, Hector. 1990. "Protest by AIDS Activists Halts Procession for a Short Time." *The Los Angeles Times*, January 2.

Vargas, Jose Antonio, and Darryl Fears. 2009. "HIV/AIDS Rate in D.C. Hits 3%." *The Washington Post*, March 15, p. A1.

Wares, Donna, and James V. Grimaldi. 1990. "Secret Frontera Pact Confirmed: State Officials to Sign Deal with Suspended Medical Chief." *Orange County Register*, November 15, pp. 1, 26.

"Inspectors Assail Frontera Infirmary." *Orange County Register*, November 16, pp. 1, 4.

Warren, Jennifer. 1990. "Protestors Decry Segregation of HIV Inmates." *Los Angeles Times*, December 1, p. A30.

Weill-Greenberg, Elizabeth. 2005. "AIDS Office Director Meets with Activists: Appleseed Promises Updated Report Card on HIV in DC." *The Washington Blade*, October 7.

Weigel, George. 1991. "KCET's Action: The Antithesis of Freedom." *Los Angeles Times*, September 20.

Wilkinson,Tracy. 1991. "Gay Republicans Say Wilson's Veto Betrayed Them." *Los Angeles Times*, October 3, http://articles.latimes.com/1991-10-03/ news/mn-4417_1_gay-republicans.

Williams, John. 1992. "Chief Lauds Police in GOP Row/Rights Groups, Gays Critical of Report on AIDS Protest Brawl." *Houston Chronicle*, September 2, p. 17.

Woo, Elaine. 2007. "Ferd Eggan, 60; Ally for Those with HIV, AIDS." *Los Angeles Times*, July 12.

SECONDARY SOURCES

Abu-Lughod, Lila. 1990. "The Romance of Resistance: Tracing Transformations of Power Through Bedouin Women." *American Ethnologist* 17:1 February, pp. 41–55.

Adam, Barry D. 1987. *The Rise of a Gay and Lesbian Movement*. Boston: Twayne Publishers.

Agustin, L. R., and S. Roth 2011. Minority inclusion, self-representation and coalition-building: The participation of minority women in European women's networks. Pp. 231–247 in *Transforming Gendered Well-Being in Europe. The Impact of Social Movements*, edited by A. E. Woodward, J. -M. Bonvin, and M. Renom. Farnham, Ashgate.

Alexander, Priscilla. 1994. Sex workers fight against AIDS: An international perspective. Pp. 99–123 in *Women Resisting AIDS: Strategies of Empowerment*, edited by Beth E. Schneider and Nancy Stoller. Philadelphia: Temple University Press.

Altman, Dennis. 1994. *Power and Community: Organizational and Cultural Responses to AIDS*. London: Taylor & Francis.

Andrews, K. T. 2001. "Social Movements and Policy Implementations: The Mississippi Civil Rights Movement and the War on Poverty, 1965–1971." *American Sociological Review* 66: 21–48.

Armstrong, Elizabeth A. 2002. *Forging Gay Identities: Organizing Sexuality in San Francisco, 1950–1994*. Chicago and London: University of Chicago Press.

Armstrong, Elizabeth, and Suzanna M. Crage. 2006. "Movements and Memory: The Making of the Stonewall Myth." *American Sociological Review* 71: 5, October, pp. 724–751.

Banaszak, Lee Ann. 2011. *The Women's Movement Inside and Outside the State*. New York: Cambridge University Press.

Beamish, T. D., and A. J. Luebbers. 2009. "Alliance Building across Social Movements: Bridging Difference in a Peace and Justice Coalition." *Social Problems* 56:4, pp. 647–676.

Blee, Katherine, and Verta Taylor. 2002. "Semi-structured Interviewing in Social Movement Research." Pp. 92–117 in *Methods of Social Movement Research*, edited by Klandermans, Bert and Suzanne Staggenborg. Minneapolis and London: University of Minnesota Press.

Bob, C., and S. E. Nepstad. 2007. "Kill a Leader, Murder a Movement? Leadership and Assassination in Social Movements." *American Behavioral Scientist* 50:10, pp. 1370–1394.

Brah, Avtar, and Ann Phoenix. 2004. "'Ain't I a Woman? Revisiting Intersectionality." *Journal of International Women's Studies* 5:3, pp. 75–86.

Brier, Jennifer. 2009. *Infectious Ideas: U.S. Political Responses to the AIDS Crisis*. Chapel Hill: The University of North Carolina Press.

Bullert, B. J. 1997. *Public Television: Politics & the Battle over Documentary Film*. New Brunswick, NJ: Rutgers University Press.

Burawoy, Michael. 1991a. Introduction. Pp. 1–7 in *Ethnography Unbound: Power and Resistance in the Modern Metropolis*, edited by Michael Burawoy, et al. Berkeley: University of California Press.

1991b. The extended case method. Pp. 271–287 in edited by Michael Burawoy, et al. Berkeley: University of California Press.

Carastathis, Anna. 2013. "Identity Categories as Potential Coalitions." *Signs* 38:4, pp. 941–965.

Carbado, Devon. 2013. "Colorblind Intersectionality." *Signs* 38:4, pp. 811–845.

Carroll, Tamar. 2015. *Mobilizing New York: AIDS, Antipoverity, and Feminist Activism.* Chapel Hill: University of North Carolina Press.

Chappel, Louise. 2006. "Comparing Political Institutions: Revealing the Gendered 'Logic of Appropriateness.'" *Politics and Gender* 22, pp. 223–235.

Cho, Sumi, Kimberlé Williams Crenshaw, and Leslie McCall. 2013. "Toward a Field of Intersectionality Studies: Theory, Applications, and Praxis." *Signs* 38:4, pp. 785–810.

Choo, Hae Yeon, and Myra Marx Ferree. 2010. "Practicing Intersectionality in Sociological Research: A Critical Analysis of Inclusions, Interactions, and Institutions in the Study of Inequalities. *Sociological Theory* 28:2, pp. 129–149.

Chun, Jennifer Jihye, George Lipsitz, and Young Shin. 2013. "Intersectionality as a Social Movement Strategy: Asian Immigrant Women Advocates." *Signs* 38:4, pp. 917–940.

Clemens, Elizabeth S. 1993. "Organizational Repertoires and Institutional Change: Women's Groups and the Transformation of U.S. Politics, 1890–1920." *The American Journal of Sociology* 98:4, January, pp. 755–798.

Cobble, Dorothy Sue. 2004. *The Other Women's Movement: Workplace Justice and Social Rights in Modern America.* Princeton, NJ: Princeton University Press.

Cohen, Peter F. 2013. *Love and Anger: Essays on AIDS, Activism and Politics.* New York and London: Routledge

Combahee River Collective. 1979. "Why Did They Die? A Document of Black Feminism." *Radical America* 13:6, November–December, pp. 40–47.

1981. A Black feminist statement. Pp. 210–218 in *This Bridge Called My Back: Writings by Radical Women of Color*, edited by Cherríe Moraga and Gloria Anzaldúa. Watertown, MA: Persephone Press.

Corea, Gina. 1992. *The Invisible Epidemic: The Story of Women and AIDS.* New York: HarperCollins.

Crenshaw, Kimberlé. 1989. "Demarginalizing the Intersection of Race and Sex: A Black Feminist Critique of Antidiscrimination Doctrine, Feminist Theory, and Antiracist Politics." *University of Chicago Legal Forum* 1989, pp. 139–167.

1991. "Mapping the Margins: Intersectionality, Identity Politics, and Violence against Women of Color." *Stanford Law Review* 436, pp. 1241–1279.

1995. "Mapping the margins: Intersectionality, identity politics and violence against women." Pp. 357–383 in *Critical Race Theory: The Key Writings that Formed the Movement*, edited by Kimberlé Crenshaw, Neil Gotanda, Gary Peller, and Kendall Thomas. New York: The New Press.

Davis, Kathy. 2008. "Intersectionality as Buzzword: A Sociology of Science. Perspective on What Makes a Feminist Theory Successful." *Feminist Theory* 9: 1, pp. 67–85.

Davis, Mike. 1990. *City of Quartz: Excavating the Future in Los Angeles.* London: Verso.

Diani, Mario. 2003 "Networks and Social Movements: A Research Programme." Pp. 299–319 in *Social Movements and Networks: Relational Approaches to Collective Action*, edited by Mario Diani and Doug McAdam. New York: Oxford University Press

Diani, M., and I. Bison. 2004. "Organizations, Coalitions, and Movements" *Theory and Society* 33, pp. 281–309.

Dixon, M., and A. W. Martin 2012. "We Can't Win This on Our Own: Unions, Firms, and Mobilization of External Allies in Labor Disputes." *American Sociological Review* 77:6, pp. 946–969.

Duggan, Lisa. 1992. "Making It Perfectly Queer." *Socialist Review* 22:1, January/March, pp. 11–31.

Epstein, Steven. 1996. *Impure Science: Aids, Activism, and the Politics of Knowledge.* Berkeley: University of California Press.

2009. *Inclusion: The Politics of Difference in Medical Research.* Chicago: University of Chicago Press.

Faderman, Lillian, and Stuart Timmons. 2009. *Gay LA: A History of Sexual Outlaws, Power Politics, and Lipstick Lesbians.* Berkeley: University of California Press.

Ferree, Myra Marx. 2009. Inequality, intersectionality and the politics of discourse: Framing feminist alliances." Pp. 86–104 in *The Discursive Politics of Gender Equality: Stretching, Bending and Policy-making*, edited by Emanuela Lombardo, Petra Meier, and Mieke Verloo. New York: Routledge.

Ferree, Myra Marx, and Silke Roth. 1998. "Gender, Class and the Interaction between Social Movements. A Strike of West Berlin Day Care Workers." *Gender & Society* 12:6, pp. 626–648.

Fraser, Michael R. 1996. "Identity and Representation as Challenges to Social Movement Theory: A Case Study of Queer Nation." Pp. 32–44 in *Mainstreams and Margins: Cultural Politics in the '90s*, edited by Michael Morgan and Susan Leggett. Westport, CT: Greenwood Publishing.

Freeman, Jo. 1972–1973. "The Tyranny of Structurelessness." *Berkeley Journal of Sociology* 17, pp. 151–165.

Gamson, Joshua. 1989. "Silence, Death, and the Invisible Enemy: AIDS Activism and Social Movement 'Newness.'" *Social Problems* 36:4, October, pp. 351–367.

1996. Must identity movements self-destruct? A queer dilemma. Pp. 399–420 in *Queer Theory/Sociology*, edited by Steven Seidman. Cambridge, MA: Blackwell Publishers.

Ghaziani, Amin. 2008. *The Dividends of Dissent: How Conflict and Culture Work in Lesbian and Gay Marches on Washington*. Chicago and London: University of Chicago Press.

Glaser, Barney G., and Anselm Strauss. 2012[1967]. *The Discovery of Grounded Theory: Strategies for Qualitative Research*. Chicago: Aldine Publishing Company.

Gould, Deborah B. 2009. *Moving Politics: Emotion and ACT UP's Fight Against AIDS*. Chicago and London: University of Chicago Press.

2002. "Life during Wartime: Emotions and the Development of ACT UP." *Mobilization: An International Journal* 7:2, pp. 177–200.

Guenther, Katja. 2010. *Making Their Place: Feminism After Socialism in Eastern Germany*. Stanford, CA: Stanford University Press.

2009. "The Politics of Names: Rethinking the Methodological and Ethical Significance of Naming People, Organizations, and Places." *Qualitative Research* 9:4, pp. 411–421.

Halcli, Abigail. 1999. "AIDS, Anger, and Activism: ACT UP as a Social Movement Organization." Pp. 135–150 in *Waves of Protest: Social Movements Since the Sixties*, edited by Jo Freeman and Victoria Johnson. Lanham, MD: Rowman & Littlefield Publishers.

Hartmann, Susan M. 1999. *The Other Feminists: Activists in the Liberal Establishment*. New Haven and London: Yale University Press.

Highleyman, Liz. 2002. "Radical queers or queer radicals? Queer activism and the global justice movement. Pp. 106–120 in *From ACT UP to the WTO: Urban Protest and Community Building in the Era of Globalization*, edited by Benjamin Shepard and Ronald Hayduke. London and New York: Verso Press.

Hill Collins, Patricia. 1998. *Fighting Words: Black Women and the Search for Justice*. Minneapolis and London: University of Minnesota Press.

Hollibaugh, A. 1994. Lesbian denial and lesbian leadership in the AIDS epidemic: bravery and fear in the construction of a lesbian geography of risk. Pp. in 219–230 in *Women Resisting AIDS: Feminist Strategies of Empowerment*, edited by Beth E. Schneider and Nancy E. Stoller. Philadelphia: Temple University Press.

Jasper, James, and Francesca Polletta. 2001. "Collective Identity and Social Movements." *Annual Review of Sociology* 27, pp. 283–305.

Jenkins, J. Craig. 1977. "Radical Transformation of Organizational Goals." *Administrative Science Quarterly* 22, December, pp. 568–586.

Jenson, J. 1987. Changing discourse, changing agendas: Political rights and reproductive policies in France." Pp. 64–88 in *The Women's Movements of the United States and Western Europe*, edited by Mary Fainsod

Katzenstein and Carol McClurg Mueller. Philadelphia: Temple University Press.

Jordan-Zachery, Julia S. 2007. "Am I a Black Woman or a Woman Who Is Black? A Few Thoughts on the Meaning of Intersectionality." *Politics and Gender* 3:2, pp. 254–263.

Juris, Jeffrey S. 2008a. "Spaces of Intentionality: Race, Class, and Horizontality at the United States Social Forum." *Mobilization* 13:4, December 2008.

2008b. *Networking Futures: The Movements against Corporate Globalization*. Durham, NC: Duke University Press.

Kane, Melinda. 2010. "You've Won, Now What? The Influence of Legal Change on Gay and Lesbian Mobilization, 1974–1999." *The Sociological Quarterly* 51, pp. 255–277.

Katzenstein, Mary F. 1990. "Feminism within American Institutions: Unobtrusive Mobilization in the 1980s." *Signs* 16, pp. 27–54.

1998a. Stepsisters: Feminist movement activism in different institutional spaces. Pp. 195–216 in *The Social Movement Society: Contentious Politics for a New Century*, edited by David S. Meyer and Sidney Tarrow. Lanham, MD: Rowman & Littlefield Publishers.

1998b. *Faithful and Fearless: Moving Feminist Protest inside the Church and Military*. Princeton, NJ: Princeton University Press.

Kauffman, L. A. 2002. A short history of radical renewal." Pp. 35–40 in *From ACT UP to the WTO: Urban Protest and Community Building in the Era of Globalization*, edited by Benjamin Shepard and Ronald Hayduk. London and New York: Verso Books.

Keck, Margaret, and Kathryn Sikkink. 1998. *Activists beyond Borders: Advocacy Networks in International Politics*. Ithaca, NY: Cornell University Press.

Kenney, Moira Rachel. 2001. *Mapping Gay LA: The Intersection of Place and Politics*. Philadelphia: Temple University Press.

King, Deborah H. 1988. "Multiple Jeopardy, Multiple Consciousness: The Context of a Black Feminist Ideology." *Signs* 14:1, Autumn, pp. 42–72.

Klawiter, Maren. 2008. *The Biopolitics of Breast Cancer: Changing Cultures of Disease and Activism*. Minneapolis: University of Minnesota Press.

Krinsky, Johna, and Ellen Reese. 2006. "Forging and Sustaining Labor-Community Coalitions: The Workfare Justice Movement in Three Cities." *Sociological Forum* 21:4, pp. 623–658.

Kosbie, Jeffrey. 2013. "Beyond Queer vs. LGBT: Discursive Community and Marriage Mobilization in Massachusetts." Pp. 103–132 in *The Marrying Kind? Debating Same-Sex Marriage within the Lesbian and Gay Movement*, edited by Mary Bernstein and Verta Taylor. Minneapolis: University of Minnesota Press.

Laurence, Leslie, and Beth Weinhouse. 1997. *Outrageous Practices: How Gender Bias Threatens Women's Health*. New Brunswick, NJ: Rutgers University Press. pp. 160–161.

Lewis, Gail. 2013. "Unsafe Travel: Experiencing Intersectionality and Feminist Displacements." *Signs* 38:4, pp. 869–892.

Loyd, Jenna M. 2014. *Health Rights Are Civil Rights: Peace and Justice Activism in Los Angeles, 1963–1978*. Minneapolis: University of Minnesota Press.

MacKinnon, Catherine A. 2013. "Intersectionality as Method: A Note." *Signs* 38:4, pp. 1019–1030.

Mayer, B., P. Brown, and R. Morello-Frosch. 2010. "Labor-Environmental Coalition Formation: Framing and the Right to Know." *Sociological Forum* 25:4, pp. 746–768.

McAdam, Doug. 1988. *Freedom Summer*. Oxford: Oxford University Press.
　1989. "The Biographical Consequences of Activism." *American Sociological Review* 54, pp. 744–60.

McAdam, Doug, and Ronnelle Paulsen. 1993. "Specifying the Relationship Between Social Ties and Activism." *American Journal of Sociology* 99, pp. 640–667.

McAdam, Doug, Sidney Tarrow, and Charles Tilly. 2001. *Dynamics of Contention*. New York: Cambridge University Press.

McCall, Leslie. 2005. "The Complexity of Intersectionality." *Signs: Journal of Women in Culture and Society* 30:3, pp. 1771–1800.

McCarthy, John D., and Mayer Zald. 1977. "Resource Mobilization and Social Movements: A Partial Theory." *American Journal of Sociology* 82, pp. 1212–1241.

McCorkel, Jill A., and Kristen Myers. 2003 "What Difference Does Difference Make? Position and Privilege in the Field." *Qualitative Sociology* 26:2, pp. 199–231.

Meyer, David, and Catherine Corrigall-Brown. 2005. "Coalitions and Political Context: US Movements against Wars in Iraq." *Mobilization: An International Quarterly* 10:3, pp. 327–344

Meyer, David S., and Sidney Tarrow, editors. 1998. *The Social Movement Society: Contentious Politics for a New Century*. Lanham, MD: Rowman & Littlefield Publishers.

Meyer, David S., and Nancy Whittier. 1994. "Social Movement Spillover." *Social Problems* 41:2, May, pp. 277–298.

Melucci, Alberto. 1989. *Nomads of the Present: Social Movements and Individual Needs in Contemporary Society*. London: Hutchinson Radius.

Michels, Roberto. 1959. *Political Parties: A Sociological Study of the Oligarchical Tendencies of Modern Democracy*. Translated by Eden Paul and Cedar Paul. 1915; reprint. New York: Dover.

Mitchell, Anne. 1992. "AIDS Activism: Women and AIDS in Victoria Australia." *Feminist Review* 41 Summer.

Mix, R. L., and S. Cable. 2006. "Condescension and Cross-Class Coalitions: Working Class Activists' Perspectives on the Role of Social Status." *Sociological Focus* 39:2, pp. 99–114.

Mohanty, Chandra Talpade. 2013. 'Transnational Feminist Crossings: On Neoliberalism and Radical Critique." *Signs* 38:4, pp. 967–991.

Molotch, H. 1979. Media and movements. Pp. 71–93 in *The Dynamics of Social Movements*, edited by Mayer N. Zald and John D. McCarthy. Cambridge, MA: Winthrop Publishers.

Moore, Mignon. 2011. *Invisible Families: Gay Identities, Relationships, and Motherhood among Black Women*. Berkeley: University of California Press.

Morgen, Sandra. 2002. *Into Our Own Hands: The Women's Health Movement in the United States, 1969–1990*. New Brunswick, NJ: Rutgers University Press.

Morris, Aldon D. 1984. *The Origins of the Civil Rights Movement: Black Communities Organizing for Change*. New York: Free Press.

Newman, J. 2012. *Working the Spaces of Power. Activism, Neoliberalism and Gendered Labour*. London: Bloomsbury Academic.

Nguyen, Vinh-Kim. 2010. *The Republic of Therapy: Triage and Sovereignty in West Africa's Time of AIDS*. Durham and London: Duke University Press.

Ostrander, Susan A. 1999. "Gender and Race in a Pro-Feminist, Progressive, Mixed-Gender, Mixed-Race Organization." *Gender & Society* 13:5, October, pp. 628–642.

Patil, Vrushali. 2013. "From Patriarchy to Intersectionality: A Transnational Feminist Assessment of How Far We've Really Come." *Signs* 38:4, pp. 847–867.

Phelan, Shane. 1989. *Identity Politics: Lesbian Feminism and the Limits of Community*. Philadelphia: Temple University Press.

Pulido, Laura. 2006. *Black, Brown, Yellow, and Left: Radical Activism in Los Angeles*. Berkeley: University of California Press.

Raeburn, Nicole C. 2004. *Changing Corporate America from Inside Out: Lesbian and Gay Workplace Rights*. Minneapolis: University of Minnesota Press.

Rapp, R. 1990. "Is the Legacy of Second-Wave Feminism Postfeminism?" Pp. 357–362 in *Women, Class, and the Feminist Imagination: A SocialistFeminist Reader*, edited by Karen V. Hansen and Ilene J. Philipson. Philadelphia: Temple University Press.

Ray, Raka. 1999. *Fields of Protest: Women's Movements in India*. Minneapolis and London: University of Minneapolis Press.

Roth, Benita. 1998. "Feminist Boundaries in the Feminist-Friendly Organization: The Women's Caucus of ACT UP/LA." *Gender & Society* 12:2, April. pp. 129–145.

　　2004. *Separate Roads to Feminism: Black, Chicana, and White Feminist Movements in America's Second Wave*. New York: Cambridge University Press.

　　2006. Gender inequality and feminist activism in institutions: Challenges of marginalization and feminist fading. Pp. 157–174, in *The Politics of*

Women's Interests: New Comparative Perspectives, edited by Louise Chappell and Lisa Hill. New York: Routledge.

2010. 'Organizing one's own' as good politics: Second wave feminists and the meaning of coalition. Pp. 99–128 in *Strategic Alliances: Coalition Building and Social Movements*, edited by Nella Van Dyke and Holly J. McCammon. Minneapolis: University of Minnesota Press.

Roth, Silke. 2008. Dealing with diversity: The coalition of labor union women. Pp. 213–231 in *Identity Work, Sameness and Difference in Social Movements*, edited by R. Einwohner, J. Reger, and D. Myers. Minneapolis: University of Minnesota Press.

2003. *Building Movement Bridges. The Coalition of Labour Union Women*. Greenwood, CT: Praeger.

Sacks, Karen. 1989. "Toward a Unified Theory of Class, Race and Gender." *American Ethnologist* 16:3, pp. 534–550.

Santoro, Wayne A., and Gail M. McGuire. 1997. "Social Movement Insiders: The Impact of Institutional Activists on Affirmative Action and Comparable Worth Policies." *Social Problems* 44:4, November, pp. 503–519.

Saunders, Clara. 2013. *Environmental Networks and Social Movement Theory*. London: Bloomsbury Academic.

2007. "Using Social Network Analysis to Explore Social Movements: A Relational Approach." *Social Movement Studies: Journal of Social, Cultural and Political Protest* 6:3, pp. 227–243.

Scharf, E., and Toole, S. 1992. "HIV and the Invisibility of Women: Is There a Need to Redefine AIDS?" *Feminist Review* 41, pp. 64–67.

Schneider, Beth E., and Nancy E. Stoller. 1994. Introduction: Feminist strategies of empowerment. Pp. 1–22 in *Women Resisting AIDS: Feminist Strategies of Empowerment*, edited by Beth E. Schneider and Nancy Stoller. Philadelphia: Temple University Press.

Schulman, Sarah. 1994. *My American History: Lesbian and Gay Life During the Reagan/Bush Years*. New York: Routledge.

Scott, Joan W. 1991. "The Evidence of Experience." *Critical Inquiry* 17, Summer, pp. 773–797.

Seidman, Steven. 2005. "From Outsider to Citizen." Pp. 225–243 in *Regulating Sex: The Politics of Intimacy and Identity*, edited by Elizabeth Bernstein and Laurie Schaffner. New York and London: Routledge.

Shepard, Benjamin, and Ronald Hayduk. 2002. Introduction. Pp. 1–10 in *From ACT UP to the WTO: Urban Protest and Community Building in the Era of Globalization*, edited by S. Benjamin and R. Hayduk. London and New York: Verso Press.

Simmons, L., and S. Harding. 2009. "Community-Labor Coalitions for Progressive Change." *Journal of Workplace Behavioral Health* 24, pp. 99–112.

Sitrin, Marina. 2006. *Horizontalism: Voices of Popular Power in Argentina.* Oakland, CA/Edinburgh, Scotland: AK Press.

Snow, D., and Benford, R. D. 1992. Master frames and cycles of protest. Pp. 133–155, in *Frontiers in Social Movement Theory*, edited by Aldon Morris and Carol Mueller. New Haven: Yale University Press.

Sontag, Susan. 1988. *Illness as Metaphor and AIDS and Its Metaphors.* New York: Anchor Books.

Spelman, Elizabeth V. 1982. "Theories of Race & Gender: The Erasure of Black Women." *Quest: A Feminist Quarterly* 5:4, pp. 36–62.

Stacey, J. 1990. Sexism by a subtler name? Postindustrial conditions and postfeminist consciousness in Silicon Valley. Pp. 338–356, in *Women, Class, and the Feminist Imagination: A Socialist-Feminist Reader*, edited by Karen V. Hansen and Ilene J. Philipson. Philadelphia: Temple University Press.

Staggenborg, Suzanne. 1988. "The Consequences of Professionalization and Formalization in the Pro-Choice Movement." *American Sociological Review* 53, pp. 585–606.

1986. "Coalition Work in the Pro-Choice Movement: Organizational and Environmental Opportunities and Obstacles." *Social Problems* 33:5, June, pp. 374–390.

Stein, Arlene. 1992. "Sisters and Queers: The Decentering of Lesbian Feminism." *Socialist Review* 1, pp. 33–55.

2013. What's the matter with Newark? Race, class, marriage politics, and the limits of queer liberalism. Pp. 39–66 in *The Marrying Kind? Debating Same-Sex Marriage with the Lesbian and Gay Movement*, edited by Mary Bernstein and Verta Taylor. Minneapolis: University of Minnesota Press.

Stockdill, Brett. 2003. *Activism against AIDS: At the Intersections of Sexuality, Race, Gender and Class.* Boulder, CO: Lynne Reinner.

Stride, H., and S. Lee. 2007. "No Logo? No Way. Branding in the Non-Profit Sector." *Journal of Marketing Management* 23:1–2, pp. 107–122.

Strub, Sean. 2014. *Body Counts: A Memoir of Politics, Sex, AIDS, and Survival.* New York: Scribner.

Taylor, Verta. 1989. "Social Movement Continuity: The Women's Movement in Abeyance." *American Sociological Review* 54, October, pp. 761–775.

Taylor, Verta, and Nicole C. Raeburn. 1995. "Identity Politics as High-Risk Activism: Career Consequences for Lesbian, Gay, and Bisexual Sociologists." *Social Problems* 42, May, pp. 252–273.

Taylor, V., and N. Whittier. 1992. Collective identity in social movement communities: Lesbian feminist mobilization. Pp. 104–129 in *Frontiers in Social Movement Theory*, edited by Aldon Morris and Carol Mueller. New Haven: Yale University Press.

Taylor, Verta, and Katrina Kimport Andersen. 2013. Mobilization through marriage: The San Francisco wedding protest. Pp. 219–262 in *The*

Marrying Kind? Debating Same-Sex Marriage within the Lesbian and Gay Movement, edited by Mary Bernstein and Verta Taylor. Minneapolis: University of Minnesota Press.

Thorne, B. 1975. "Women in the Draft Resistance Movement: A Case Study of Sex Roles and Social Movements." *Sex Roles* 1:2, pp. 179–195.

Thornton Dill, Bonnie. 1983. "Race, Class and Gender: Prospects for an All-inclusive Sisterhood." *Feminist Studies* 9:1 Spring: 131–150.

Touraine, Alain. 1981. *The Voice and the Eye: An Analysis of Social Movements*. Cambridge: Cambridge University Press.

Turner, Ralph. 1972. The theme of contemporary social movements. Pp. 586–599 in *Sociology, Students, and Society*, edited by Jerome Rabow. Pacific Palisades, CA: Goodyear Publishing.

Turner, Ralph H., and Lewis M. Killian. 1987. *Collective Behavior*. Englewood Cliffs, NJ: Prentice Hall.

Valentine, Gill. 2007. "Theorizing and Researching Intersectionality: A Challenge for Feminist Geography." *The Professional Geographer* 59:1, pp. 10–21.

Valocchi, Steve. 2001. "Individual Identities, Collective Identities, and Organizational Structure: The Relationship of the Political Left and Gay Liberation in the United States." *Sociological Perspectives* 44:4, pp. 445–467.

Van Dyke, Nella. 2003. "Crossing Movement Boundaries: Factors that Facilitate Coalition Protest by American College Students, 1930–1990." *Social Problems* 50:2, pp. 226–250.

Van Dyke, Nella, and Holly J. McCammon. 2010. Introduction: Social movement coalition formation. Pp. xi–xxviii in *Strategic Alliances: Coalition Building and Social Movements*, edited by Nella Van Dyke and Holly McCammon. Minneapolis: University of Minnesota Press.

Verloo, Mieke. 2013. "Intersectional and Cross-Movement Politics and Policies: Reflections on Current Practices and Debates." *Signs* 38:4, pp. 893–915.

Yuval-Davis, Nira. 2006. "Intersectionality and Feminist Politics." *European Journal of Women's Studies* 13:3, pp. 193–209.

Wachter, Robert M. 1991. *The Fragile Coalition: Scientists, Activists, and AIDS*. New York: St. Martin's Press.

Whalen, Jack, and Richard Flacks. 1989. *Beyond the Barricades: The Sixties Generation Grows Up*. Philadelphia: Temple University Press.

Whittier, Nancy. 1997. "Political Generations, Micro-Cohorts, and the Transformation of Social Movements." *American Sociological Review* 62, pp. 760–778.

2011. *The Politics of Child Sexual Abuse: Emotion, Social Movements, and the State*. New York: Oxford University Press, USA.

Winnow, J. 1992. "Lesbians Evolving Health Care: Cancer and AIDS." *Feminist Review* 41, pp. 68–76.

Wood, Lesley J., and Kelly Moore. 2002. Target practice: community activism in a global era. Pp. 21–34 in *From ACT UP to the WTO: Urban Protest and Community Building in the Era of Globalization*, edited by Benjamin Shepard and Ronald Hayduke. London and New York: Verso Press.

Zald, Mayer N., and Roberta Ash. 1966. "Social Movement Organizations: Growth, Decay and Change." *Social Forces* 44:3, March, pp. 327–341.

Index